Cardiac/Vascular Nursing Review and Resource Manual, 2nd Ed.

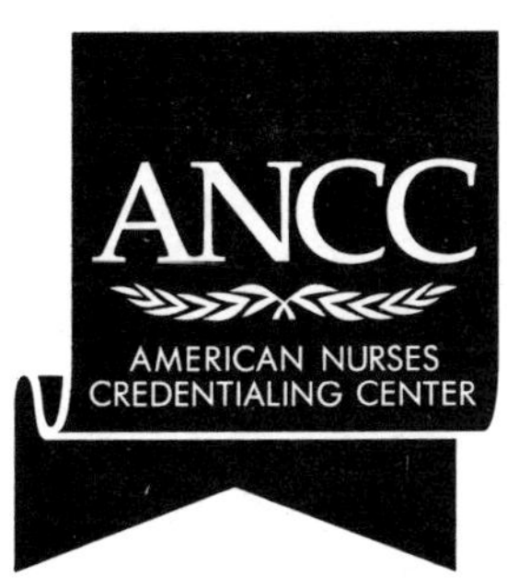

Library of Congress Cataloging-in-Publication Data

Cardiac/vascular nursing review and resource manual. -- 2nd ed.
p. ; cm.
Includes bibliographical references and index.
ISBN-13: 978-0-9768213-8-0
ISBN-10: 0-9768213-8-9
1. Cardiovascular system--Diseases--Nursing--Handbooks, manuals, etc. 2. Heart--Diseases--Handbooks, manuals, etc. 3. Heart--Nursing--Handbooks, manuals, etc. I. American Nurses Credentialing Center.
[DNLM: 1. Cardiovascular Diseases--nursing--Handbooks. 2. Cardiovascular Diseases--nursing--Outlines. WY 18.2 C2665 2006]
RC674.C3744 2006
616.1'0231--dc22

2006032072

ISBN 13: 978-0-9768213-8-0
ISBN 10: 0-9768213-8-9

Cardiac/Vascular Nursing Review and Resource Manual, 2nd Ed.

September 2006

Please direct your comments and/or queries to:
revmanuals@ana.org

The health care services delivery system is a volatile marketplace demanding superior knowledge, clinical skills, and competencies from all registered nurses. Nursing autonomy of practice, and nurse career marketability and mobility in the new century hinge on affirming the profession's formative philosophy which places a priority on a lifelong commitment to the principles of education and professional development. The knowledge base of nursing theory and practice is expanding, and while care has been taken to ensure the accuracy and timeliness of the information presented in the **Cardiac/Vascular Nursing Review Manual,** clinicians are advised to always verify the most current national treatment guidelines and recommendations and to practice in accordance with professional standards of care used with regard to the unique circumstances that apply in each practice situation. In addition, every effort has been made in this text to insure accuracy and, in particular to confirm that drug selections and dosages are in accordance with current recommendations and practice, including the ongoing research, changes to government regulations and the developments in product information provided by pharmaceutical manufacturers. However, it is the responsibility of each nurse practitioner to verify drug product information and to practice in accordance with professional standards of care. In addition, the editors wish to note that provision of information in this text does not imply an endorsement of any particular products, procedures or services. As a review text, this content is provided at a level that describes what a FNP should know upon entry into practice. NPs may object, for religious or other reasons, to the provisions of certain services. That decision, too, must be left to the individual NP.

Therefore, the authors, editors, American Nurses Association (ANA), American Nurses Association's Publishing (ANP), American

Nurses Credentialing Center (ANCC), and the Institute for Credentialing Innovation cannot accept responsibility for errors or omissions, or for any consequences or liability, injury and/or damages to persons or property from application of the information in this manual and make no warranty, express or implied, with respect to the contents of the **Cardiac/Vascular Nursing Review Manual.**

Published by: The Institute for Credentialing Innovation
8515 Georgia Avenue, Suite 400
Silver Spring, MD 20910-3402
www.nursecredentialing.org

The American Nurses Credentialing Center would like to acknowledge the editors, contributors and reviewers who assisted in development of the first edition of the Cardiac/Vascular Nursing Review and Resource Manual

Editors

Barbara S. Levine, PhD, CRNP, CS
Kathleen H. Miller, EdD, RN, ACNP

Contributors and Reviewers

Mary K. Alexander, EdD, RN, ANP
Marie Bosak, MS, RN, ACNP
Joanne Dalton, PhD, RN, CS
Doris Denison, MSN, NP, ACNP
Michelle Fey, MS, RN, ACNP
Pritesh J. Gandhi, Pharm D, BCPS
Polly Gardner, MN, ARNP, ACNP, CS
Susan D. Householder-Hughes, MSN, RN, CCRN, CS, FAHA
Annette Jakubisin Konicki, MS, RN, APRN, CCRN
Debra Laurent-Bopp, MN, ARNP, ACNP, CS
Patricia A. Kent, MS, RN, ACNP
Virginia F. Mason, PhD, RN, CS, CCRN
Theresa Mazzarelli, MS, RN, ACNP, CCRN
Sandra Oliver-McNeil, MSN, ACNP, CS
Pamela Vesta Meredith, MSN, RN, NP
Sandra Adams Motzer, PhD, RN
Janice Polletta, MS, RN, ACNP
Michael E. Rhodes, PhD
Sarah Shannon, PhD, RN
Patricia J. Simonowicz, MS, RN, ACNP, CCRN
Terri Simpson, PhD, RN
Maryellen Wrubleski, MS, RN, ACNP, CCRN

The American Nurses Credentialing Center would also like to acknowledge the Preventive Cardiovascular Nurses Association whose support guided the first edition of this manual.

Introduction to the Continuing Education (CE) Contact Hour Application Process for *Cardiac/Vascular Nursing Review and Resource Manual, 2nd Edition*

The Institute for Credentialing Innovation now offers the continuing education contact hours for this manual online at www.NursingWorld.org, the American Nurses Association's Web site. This process involves answering approximately 50 questions that test knowledge of the information contained within this manual. The continuing education contact hours can be completed at any time and a certificate can be printed from the Web site immediately upon successful completion of the test.

The ***Cardiac/Vascular Nursing Review and Resource Manual*** is designed to meet the following objectives:

1. Describe the key components, including risk assessment, health history, ethical issues, for care of the patient with cardiac/vascular disease.
2. Analyze the pharmacologic and invasive and noninvasive treatments for selected cardiac/vascular diseases.
3. Discuss the nurse's role in the care of acute and chronically ill patients with cardiac/vascular diseases.

Upon completion of this manual **and** the online CE test, a nurse can receive a total of 30 continuing education contact hours. **The entire process—online test and evaluation form—must be completed by December 31, 2008 in order to receive credit.** To begin the process, please e-mail revmanuals@ana.org or go to the ANCC website at www.nursecredentialing.org for specific instructions. Your patience with this new process is greatly appreciated.

Inquiries or Comments

If you have any questions about the CE contact hours, please e-mail The Institute at: revmanuals@ana.org. You mail also mail any comments to Barbara Burnham, RN, BSN, MA, Editor/Project Manager, at the address listed below.

Duplicate CE Certificates

Once you have successfully passed the CE test on NursingWorld, you may go back and re-print your certificate as often as you wish.

The Institute for Credentialing Innovation
American Nurses Credentialing Center
Attn: Editor/Project Manager
8515 Georgia Avenue, Suite 400
Silver Spring, MD 20910-3492
Fax: (301) 628-5342

The American Nurses Association is accredited as a provider of continuing nursing education by the American Nurses Credentialing Center's Commission on Accreditation. and approved by the California Board of Registered Nursing, Provider Number CEP6178.

Table of Contents

CHAPTER 1

Ethical and Legal Issues

Nurses are required to provide ethical and legal patient care that demonstrates respect for others. This chapter reviews the application of ethical theories and principles in clinical practice. The professional and legal regulation of practice is also discussed.

Ethics

1. Ethics is the systematic study of moral conduct and provides the framework for studying and examining moral dilemmas.
2. Bioethics, also called biomedical ethics or medical ethics, is the study of moral conduct within the context of health care.
3. Morality refers to norms about right and wrong human conduct that form a social consensus.
   a. Moral virtues are socially valued character traits.
   b. Five moral virtues for health professionals
      1) Compassion combines active regard for another's welfare with an emotional response of sympathy, tenderness, and discomfort at another's misfortune or suffering.
      2) Discernment involves the ability to make judgments and decisions without being unduly influenced by extraneous considerations (eg, fears, personal attachments).
      3) Trustworthiness involves ability and strength of character, dependability and reliability.
      4) Integrity involves firm adherence to moral and ethical principles.
      5) Conscientiousness involves careful, dependable, competent practice.

Ethical Principles

1. Beneficence means to do good.
   a. Promote the well-being of the patient
   b. Prevent harm
2. Nonmaleficence means to refrain from harm.
   a. Obligates the clinician to avoid inflicting harm directly or intentionally

   b. Balanced with beneficence — maximize benefits while minimizing harm
3. Autonomy refers to the human right to make one's own decisions. Clinicians show respect for autonomy when they engage in the following behaviors:
   a. Tell the truth
   b. Respect the privacy of others
   c. Protect confidential information
   d. Obtain consent for interventions with patients
   e. When asked, help others make important decisions
4. Justice is the principle of fairness
   a. To treat equals equally
   b. To refrain from discrimination

Code of Ethics for Nurses

Table 1–1 lists the 9 provisions of the Code. The full document includes interpretative statements related to each provision.

Selected Issues in Clinical Practice

Informed consent is based on respect for autonomy. There are 5 elements of informed consent.

1. **Decisional capacity** includes the ability to understand and make decisions.
   a. Decisional capacity is specific, not global. It depends on the match between the patient's abilities and the specific decision-making task.
   b. Decisional capacity may vary over time and be intermittent.
      1) Physiological (eg, illness, hypoxia) and situational factors (e.g., medically naive person admitted to the Emergency Department) may affect decision-making capacity.
      2) If the patient's decisional capacity can not be established initially, it is appropriate to assess his or her understanding, deliberative capacity, and coherence over time, and to consult with an expert when necessary.
      3) Surrogate decision-makers are authorized to make decisions for patients when decisional capacity is impaired.
         a) If possible, the surrogate decision maker is required to make the decision that the incompetent patient would have made if competent. This is the "substituted judgment" standard. Surrogates may have written evidence of an individual's wishes (eg, a Living Will or letter), verbal evidence (ie, conversations), or they may make inferences based on the individual's history of relevant choices.

b) If the surrogate has no way of knowing what choice a individual would have made, then the 'best interests' standard should be used. That is, the surrogate should choose the option that appears to be in the best interests of the patient. Hence, surrogates are held to a higher standard of decision making than competent individuals. Competent individuals may make health care choices that are eccentric, poorly reasoned, biased, etc. but, unless evidence exists to support such a choice, a surrogate is compelled ethically and legally to act in the patient's best interests.

TABLE 1–1.
Code of Ethics for Nurses

1. The nurse, in all professional relationships, practices with compassion and respect for the inherent dignity, worth, and uniqueness of every individual, unrestricted by considerations of social or economic status, personal attributes, or the nature of the health problem.
2. The nurse's primary commitment is to the patient, whether an individual, family, group, or community.
3. The nurse promotes, advocates for, and strives to protect the health, safety, and rights of the patient.
4. The nurse is responsible and accountable for individual nursing practice and determines the appropriate delegation of tasks consistent with the nurses obligation to provide optimum patient care.
5. The nurse owes the same duties to self as to others, including the responsibility to preserve integrity and safety, to maintain competence, and to continue personal and professional growth.
6. The nurse participates in establishing, maintaining, and improving health care environments and conditions of employment conducive to the provision of quality health care and consistent with the values of the profession through individual and collective action.
7. The nurse participated is the advancement of the profession through contributions to practice, education, administration, and knowledge development.
8. The nurse collaborates with other health professionals and the public in promoting community, national, and international efforts to meet health needs.
9. The profession of nursing, as represented by associations and their members, is responsible for articulating nursing values, for maintaining the integrity of the profession and its practice, and for shaping social policy.

Reprinted with permission from Code of Ethics for Nurses with Interpretive Statements. 2001, American Nurses Association: Washington, DC.

4) The order of surrogate authority varies slightly by state but generally specifies the following list in descending order of priority:
   a) Court-appointed guardian
   b) Durable Power of Attorney
   c) Spouse
   d) Adult children (usually requires unanimous consensus)
   e) Parents (usually requires unanimous consensus)
   f) Adult siblings (usually requires unanimous consensus)

2. **Disclosure** includes a core set of information about the treatment or research procedure including the following:
   a. Facts or descriptions that patients usually consider relevant when making a decision to refuse or consent.
   b. Information the clinician believes to be relevant (eg, alternate treatments).
   c. The clinician's recommendation
   d. The purpose of seeking consent
   e. The nature and limits of consent (eg, Research studies include the right to withdraw from study without penalty.)
   f. Patients have the right to refuse to be informed regarding their health care decisions however. In that situation, the clinician should document the refusal in the medical record.
3. **Understanding** is difficult to assess. Patients and research subjects should understand at least what the clinician or researcher believes the patient needs to understand to authorize the procedure.
4. **Voluntariness** implies that the patient agrees to the intervention without undue influence.
5. **Consent** is the acceptance or refusal of the treatment or research study after the patient is adequately informed.
   a. Consent can be withdrawn at any time
   b. A written form documenting that consent has occurred is required for some health care decisions such as sterilization, injection of a radioactive substance, surgery, etc. Which procedures and decisions require written evidence of consent is mandated occasionally by law and usually by institutional policies.
   c. Regardless of whether written consent is required, all health care should be delivered using the model of informed consent including nursing controlled activities such as ambulation following surgery, preoperative teaching, etc. Written evidence of consent for such non-invasive activities is not required.

Advance directives

An individual while competent, can complete a directive documenting his or her health care wishes or values or selecting a surrogate to make decisions during periods of incapacity.

1. Living wills are directives that specify preferred treatment during periods of incapacity. They represent written evidence of a patient's wishes.
2. Durable power of attorney for health care (DPAHC) is a legal document in which one individual assigns authority to another to act as his or her surrogate if he or she is unable to make health care decisions.
   a. In general, only the DPAHC includes health care decision making authority.
3. The Patient Self-Determination Act of 1990 requires health care facilities to develop programs to inform patients and staff about advance directives.

Access to Care

Access to care is a major ethical and political issue confronting the US and is based in the principle of justice.

1. Access is limited, in part, by economic considerations. Different insurance plans provide different reimbursement for and therefore different access to care.
   a. Approximately 18% of the non-older adult US population lack health insurance of any kind.
   b. Approximately 25% of the US population has publicly supported care (eg, Medicare, Medicaid) or insurance unconnected to employment.
   c. Approximately 60% of the US population has employer-based insurance.
2. Principle of justice — fair distribution of resources; equals are treated equally — implies a right to health care.
3. The dilemma confronting the US is how to fund and distribute health care fairly.

Nurse/health care team/patient relationships

1. **Veracity** obligates the nurse to be truthful with patients and members of the health care team. A current example is the increased emphasis on the need to disclose health care errors to colleagues, the institution, the patient, and in some cases to government agencies.

2. **Privacy** obligates the clinician to appropriately restrict access to the patient and to the health record. A current privacy issue is the need to restrict clinicians' access to the electronic medical record of any patients with whom they are not directly involved in care. This includes hospitalized colleagues, employees, public figures, and family or friends.
3. **Confidentiality** requires clinicians to share information about the patient only with the patient and those health professionals who are involved in caring for the patient.
4. **Fidelity** refers to faithfulness in keeping a promise. The nurse makes an implied promise to care for a patient based on the social contract the profession of nursing has established with the public. Fidelity requires that the nurse put the patient's interests above other interests, such as financial, personal, or other people involved in the patient's care or life.

Withholding and Withdrawing Treatment

Questions about withholding and withdrawing treatment derive from the principles of beneficence and nonmaleficence.

1. Medical futility is a controversial concept.
   a. Quantitative medical futility describes a situation where research and practice would suggest that there is less than a 1% chance that the treatment will have the intended effect, ie, CPR in a cachectic patient with metastasized cancer. Quantitatively futile treatments are not obligatory.
   b. Qualitative futility describes situations where the treatment will have the intended effect but will not achieve a desired benefit (ie, tube feeding a patient who has suffered a severe stroke will provide nutrition but will not restore neurological function.)
2. Ordinary versus extraordinary treatments
   a. The traditional rule is that extraordinary treatment can be withheld but ordinary treatment cannot.
   b. The distinction between ordinary and extraordinary treatments is not clear and of uncertain moral and ethical meaning.
3. Double-effect — A single act may have two effects, one beneficial and one harmful. For example, a patient requiring high doses of a narcotic analgesic for pain control (intended, beneficial effect) may be at risk for respiratory depression (unintended, harmful effect). Questions to consider:
   a. Is there an alternate treatment that provides the intended effect (pain control) without the unintended effect (respiratory depression)?

b. Is the treatment provided for its intended effect (pain control not respiratory depression)?
c. Does the intended effect (pain control) outweigh the unintended effect (respiratory depression)?

Ethical Reasoning

Application of a systematic way of thinking about an ethical dilemma will help to reach a conclusion. Steps in the reasoning process include:

1. Review facts and assumptions about the case or situation
   a. Clinical data and treatment options
   b. Relevant law
   c. Patient preferences and beliefs
   d. Goal of treatment
2. Define the ethical dilemma in specific terms
   a. An ethical dilemma requires a choice between courses of action that involves fundamental concepts of right and wrong.
   b. Ethical dilemmas usually involve concepts of rights, duties and responsibilities.
   c. An ethical dilemma is not a difference of opinion about treatment or different appraisals of clinical facts.
3. List possible courses of action
4. Choose a course of action, considering:
   a. Patient preferences
   b. Professional standards
   c. Relevant law
   d. Personal values and principles
5. Evaluate the choice
   a. Consistent with ethical principles?
   b. Consistent with decisions made in similar cases?
   c. Consistent with values and principles of those affected, i.e., culturally sensitive?
   d. Consequences of the decision?

Ethical Decision-making Resources

1. Ethics committees are multidisciplinary groups that are responsible to review ethical dilemmas and advise clinicians.
2. Ethics consultation services provide "on-call" assistance to patients, families and clinicians when confronted by ethical dilemmas.
3. Formal educational programs in ethics provide clinicians with an understanding and a framework for decision-making.
4. Policies related to ethical issues (eg, Do Not Attempt Resuscitation policy) guide institutional practice.

Patient's Rights

1. Patient's rights are derived from the ethical theory of Liberal Individualism
2. In 1990, the American Hospital Association codified the following in the Patient's Bill of Rights.
   a. Right to considerate and respectful care
   b. Right to information about diagnosis, treatment and prognosis
   c. Right to make decisions about the plan of care
   d. Right to have advance directives
   e. Right to privacy
   f. Right to confidentiality
   g. Right to review clinical records
   h. Right to responsible care and services including the right to transfer
   i. Right to information about business relationships among the hospital, educational institutions, and payers that might influence care and treatment.
   j. Right to reasonable continuity of care
   k. Right to be informed of hospital policies and procedures that regulate patient care, treatment and responsibilities. Includes the right to grievance and dispute resolution.

Regulation of Nursing Practice

Professional Regulation

1. Professional practice standards are authoritative statements by which the nursing profession describes the responsibilities of nurses.
   a. **Standards of care** describe a competent level of nursing care as demonstrated by the nursing process. (Includes assessment, diagnosis, outcome identification, planning, implementation and evaluation.)
   b. **Standards of professional performance** describe a competent level of behavior in the professional role. (Includes activities related to quality of care, performance appraisal, education, collegiality, ethics, collaboration, research and resource utilization.)
2. Nursing's social policy statement describes the discipline of nursing, its scope and the profession's responsibility to society.
   a. The 1980 Social Policy Statement defined nursing as "the diagnosis and treatment of human responses to actual or potential health problems."
   b. Since that time definitions of nursing acknowledge 4 essential features:

        1) Attention to the full range of human experiences and responses to health and illness (ie, not limited to actual or potential health problems)
        2) Integration of objective data with understanding of the patient's subjective experience
        3) Use of scientific knowledge in the process of diagnosis and treatment
        4) Provision of a caring relationship that facilitates healing
    c. Scope of basic nursing practice involves promoting, supporting, and restoring health; preventing illness; and assisting with activities that contribute to a peaceful death.
        1) Nurses in basic practice coordinate care, prepare patients for tests and procedures, and monitor the patient's response to various treatments.
        2) Nurses in basic practice provide care in a variety of settings including hospitals, homes, schools, places of employment, correctional facilities, nursing homes, and community-based healthcare facilities.

Professional Certification

1. Private (not governmental) agencies sponsor programs to certify that individuals meet certain criteria and are prepared to practice in that discipline or clinical area.
2. Certification recognizes specialized knowledge and skills beyond that which is required for safe, basic practice.

Legal Regulation of Nursing Practice

1. Protects the public health, safety, and welfare
    a. All states require licensure for nursing practice (eg, registered nurse, licensed practical nurse).
    b. Most states have additional requirements for advanced clinical nursing practice (ie, nurse practitioner, clinical nurse specialist, nurse anesthetist, and nurse midwife).
2. Nurse practice acts are state laws that grant the right to practice nursing to individuals who meet predetermined standards (eg, education).
    a. Regulatory boards (eg, Board of Nursing [BON]) are created under the nurse practice act and govern nursing practice in the state.
    b. The BON is responsible for:
        1) Determining eligibility for licensing and relicensing
        2) Approving and supervising educational programs

3) Enforcing the statute (ie, the nurse practice act and the BON regulations)
4) Writing rules and regulations governing the practice of nursing

c. Basic grounds for disciplinary action:
   1) Fraud in obtaining a license
   2) Unprofessional, illegal, dishonorable, or immoral conduct
   3) Performance of specific actions prohibited by the act
   4) Conviction of a felony or crime of moral turpitude
   5) Drug or alcohol addiction rendering the individual incapable of performing duties

d. Possible sanctions if found guilty of the above include:
   1) Revocation of license
   2) Suspension of license for a specified period of time
   3) Suspension of license for an unspecified period of time with the opportunity to reapply after a specified program of study or treatment
   4) Prohibition of work in specified settings

Legal Aspects

Individual Accountability

1. The individual is personally responsible for his or her own actions.
2. The person who actually causes the harm has the primary responsibility.
3. Duty to communicate may be most important duty of the nurse.
   a. Communicate change in the patient's condition to the physician
   b. Communicate concern about impaired practice to the nurse manager or supervisor
   c. Communicate concerns about short staffing to the appropriate person every time the situation occurs

Employer and Supervisor Accountability

1. An employer is liable for the actions of its employees within their scope of employment.
   a. The employer may not be responsible if the employee is acting beyond his or her scope of employment.
   b. Employer and supervisor responsibility does not eliminate individual responsibility.

2. A supervisor may be liable for harm caused by an incompetent nurse, if the supervisor failed to assess the nurse's ability, if the employee has a known problem that can affect performance (eg, alcoholism), or if the supervisor failed to provide adequate supervision.
3. A health care facility is obligated to carefully monitor the credentials and competence of employees and independent contractors.

Independent Contractor Accountability

1. The independent contractor is responsible for his or her own actions.
2. The health care facility or organization may be liable also if it has reason to know that the independent contractor was incompetent and failed to act.

Torts

1. A tort is a civil action for financial damages for injury to a person, property or reputation.
2. Negligence, an unintentional tort, is the most common cause of cases involving nurses.
   a. Failure to adhere to the standard of nursing care (negligent practice) results in harm to the patient
   b. Four elements must be proved to establish a claim of negligence
      1) Duty
         a) It must be proved that the nurse had a duty (responsibility) to care for the patient.
         b) The scope or limits of that duty must be proved. Published standards of care and the actions of a "reasonably prudent nurse" (expert witness) are used to establish scope of duty.
      2) Breach of duty — it must be proved that the nurse deviated in some manner from the standard of care.
      3) Injury or harm to the patient must result. Harm may be physical, emotional or financial.
      4) Causation — the breach of duty must be proved to be the proximate cause of injury.
   c. Protect yourself against negligent practice:
      1) Know your practice area and remain current
      2) Know your abilities and limitations
      3) Know and follow the standards of care in your area
      4) Know and follow your facility's policies and procedures

5) Know your patients and their families — build good relationships

d. Statute of limitations specifies the time limit within which a suit must be filed.
   1) Established under state law
   2) Varies by nature of the complaint. In most states, a complaint of negligence must be entered within 2 years of the time the patient (or patient's representative) becomes aware of the injury.

3. Torts generally result in financial settlements. The BON may take action regarding licensure in addition to the financial settlements resulting from a successful civil tort (malpractice) claim. Crimes carry the possibility of jail sentences.
4. In some states, Good Samaritan Laws extend a degree of immunity to individuals providing care gratuitously in an emergency situation.
5. Intentional torts contain purposeful action and the intent to do an act — the intent does not have to be hostile or malicious. There must be an understanding that the harmful outcome is highly likely or that the act was done with reckless disregard for the interest of the patient.
   a. Assault and battery
      1) An assault is a credible threat that causes another to become apprehensive of being touched in a manner that is offensive, insulting, provoking, or physically injurious.
      2) If the threat (assault) is carried out, the act is battery.
   b. Defamation is the wrongful injury to the reputation of another person
      1) Oral defamation is libel.
      2) Written defamation is slander.
      3) Statement must be made to a third person; statements made directly to the person are not defamatory.
      4) Best protection against defamation: truth and privilege.
         a) True statements are not basis for legal action.
         b) A privileged statement is one that could be considered defamatory in other situations, but is not because of a legally recognized higher duty that the person making the communication must honor.
   c. Invasion of privacy occurs when an unauthorized person has access to confidential information.
      1) Information about a patient is confidential and should not be released without permission of the patient.
      2) Mandatory reporting of communicable diseases, suspicion of child or elder abuse, and other matters required by law

to the appropriate officials is not invasion of privacy.

a) Disclosure to the general public, media, or other interested parties is invasion of privacy.

b) Clinicians who access information about patients for whom they do not have direct responsibility are invading the privacy of those patients and may be subject to institutional or civil penalty.

d. Fraud and misrepresentation are false or misleading statements that the patient relies on to his or her detriment.

e. False imprisonment is the unlawful restriction of the freedom of a person, including physical restraint.

CHAPTER 2
Theory

This chapter reviews theories from nursing and other disciplines that apply directly to the practice of cardiac and vascular nursing. A brief discussion of theory, in general, is followed by theories of human behavior, individual behavior change, and organizational change. The chapter ends with theories about individuals' and families' response to illness. The use of theory in clinical nursing increases the probability of good outcomes and provides support for implementing changes in practice.

Nursing and Health

Nursing Theory

Theory is to nursing practice as a road map is to a cross-country car trip. Theory, like a road map, provides direction to facilitate successful outcomes.

1. Theory is a set of concepts, definitions, and propositions that projects a systematic view of phenomena by defining specific interrelationships among the concepts for purposes of describing, explaining, and predicting phenomena.
2. A concept is a word or phrase that describes an abstract idea or mental image of a phenomenon. Concepts are the building blocks of theory. For example, concepts with special relevance to nursing are "health" and "cardiovascular fitness."
3. A proposition is a statement about a concept or the relationship between two or more concepts. For example, a descriptive proposition related to health is "health is more than the absence of disease." A relational proposition is "cardiovascular fitness is a component of health."
4. The purpose of theory is to describe, explain, or predict phenomena. Theory serves the discipline of nursing in several ways:
    a. As an organized reservoir for knowledge and research findings.
    b. To explain observations and predict outcomes.
    c. To stimulate new directions in practice and research.
    d. To develop research questions for testing.

5. Theory improves nursing practice by increasing understanding of phenomena; understanding influences behavior. Learning to think differently about phenomena enables one to try different approaches.

Health and Illness

Health and illness are key concepts in nursing theory, research, and practice. In 1974 the World Health Organization (WHO) defined health as follows. "Health is a state of complete physical, mental, and social well-being and not merely the absence of disease and infirmity."

1. This definition changed the conceptualization of health from an illness model to a competence model. Health became a positive condition to be attained.
2. Four general conceptualizations of health are found in the nursing literature.
   a. Clinical: Health is the absence of disease or injury.
   b. Role: Health is the ability to perform role functions.
   c. Adaptive: Health is adaptation or adjustment to life's demands.
   d. Eudaimonistic: Health is the expression of the maximum potential of the individual. The WHO definition is an example of eudaimonistic definition.
3. Holistic theorists define health as a state or process in which the individual experiences a sense of well-being and the integration of body, mind, and spirit interacting harmoniously with the environment.
4. Illness and disease are different concepts. Illness is the subjective experience of the symptoms and suffering to which the individual assigns meaning. Disease is a discrete entity causing specific symptoms.
   a. Some scholars conceptualize health and illness as existing on a single continuum, from optimum health to terminal illness.
   b. Others conceptualize health and illness on two distinct, but interacting, continua. One continuum is anchored by no illness and terminal illness; the other by optimum health and poor health.

Human Behavior

Theories of human behavior have been used to describe, explain or predict health-related behavior. Theories and models that focus on individuals describe, explain or predict the choices that individuals make about health-related behavior.

Maslow's Hierarchy of Needs

Maslow's hierarchy depicts human need as a pyramid with survival needs at the base and the most sophisticated needs at the apex of the pyramid. As needs are met at each level, the next higher level provides motivation for behavior. Layers of the pyramid, from most basic to most sophisticated are:

1. Physiological survival needs — food, air, sleep, and shelter;
2. Safety needs — freedom from fear of threat to survival;
3. Belonging needs — affiliation and love; and
4. Self-actualization needs — maximizing one's potential and achieving personal fulfillment.

Social Cognitive Theory

Social Cognitive Theory (SCT) examines the mental processes through which thoughts, beliefs and attitudes are converted into behavior. Perceived self-efficacy is a significant determinant of behavior.

1. Perceived self-efficacy is an individual's assessment of his or her ability to perform the actions necessary to achieve a desired outcome.
2. Perceived self-efficacy is a thought or belief that is unrelated to actual skill-level.
3. Perceived self-efficacy is behavior specific — an individual's perceived self-efficacy for engaging in exercise may differ from his perceived self-efficacy for dietary change.
4. Efficacy information is obtained from four sources.
    a. Mastery experience is the most powerful source and comes from engaging in the behavior and evaluating personal performance.
    b. Vicarious experience comes from watching others perform a task and hearing their self-evaluation and feedback.
    c. Physiological cues provide information to the individual through his level of autonomic arousal. Individuals use physiological cues related to anxiety, fear, and tranquility to judge their competence.
    d. Verbal or social persuasion is information presented by others to convince the individual that he or she possesses the capacity to carry out a specific course of action. Verbal or social persuasion is the least powerful source of efficacy information.
5. SCT and perceived self-efficacy have been used in several studies of the resumption of activity after an acute cardiac event. In general, perceived self-efficacy for a specific behavior is moderately-to-highly correlated with achievement of the behavior.

Health Belief Model

The Health Belief Model (HBM) explains why healthy people use health-protecting and disease-preventing services. The HBM has been refined and extended to explain individual responses to preventive services and illness treatment.

1. In the HBM, three sets of variables interact and determine individual response.
   a. Individual perceptions
      1) Perceived vulnerability of the individual
      2) Perceived seriousness of the disease
      3) Perceived benefits of preventive action
      4) Perceived barriers to preventive action
   b. Modifying factors
      1) Demographics: Age, gender, and ethnicity
      2) Psychosocial characteristics: Personality, social class, and peer group pressure
      3) Structural characteristics: Knowledge about the disease and prior contact with disease
   c. Cues to action
      1) Media campaigns
      2) Advice from others
      3) Postcard reminders
2. The interaction of individual perceptions, modifying factors, and cues to action determines whether or not a person engages in a health-promoting behavior.
3. The HBM has been used to explain health-related behavior and to guide program development to increase the likelihood of success.
4. Across studies, perceived barriers to preventive action have been most consistently associated with health-promoting behaviors. When perceived barriers are high, the likelihood of adopting the preventive behavior is low.
5. The HBM has been criticized for several reasons:
   a. It places responsibility for action exclusively on the individual;
   b. It focuses on avoiding negative behavior, as opposed to embracing positive health behaviors; and
   c. The motivation for behavior change comes from perceived threat or fear related to illness.

Health Promotion Model

The Health Promotion Model (HPM) focuses on health-seeking rather than disease-preventing behaviors.

1. In the HPM, two sets of variables interact and determine individual commitment to action:
   a. Individual characteristics and experiences (including expectations); and
   b. Behavior-specific thoughts and feelings
      1) Perceived benefits of action
      2) Perceived barriers to action
      3) Perceived self-efficacy
      4) Activity-related affect.
2. The commitment to action may be modified or broken by competing demands and preferences.
3. In general, studies that used the HPM produced evidence that supports the relationships between perceived self-efficacy, benefits of and barriers to action, and health-related behavior.

Transtheoretical Model

The Transtheoretical Model (TTM) describes a 6-stage process of behavior change. The motivation to change and effective interventions to promote change differ by stage. Progression through the stages is not linear. The average person recycles through the stages several times before behavior change is achieved.

1. In the **precontemplation** stage, the client has no intention of changing.
   a. The client may deny that change is needed, blame others for the problem, or feel overwhelmed and demoralized.
   b. Clinicians are most effective if they are empathetic and patient while offering hope for change.
2. In the **contemplation** stage, the client acknowledges the need to change but is ambivalent and anxious about the change.
   a. Clinicians can provide information, acknowledge ambivalence, help clarify goals, and eliminate barriers to change.
3. In the **preparation** stage, the client begins to explore different options or ways to change the behavior. He or she is actively planing to change within the next month.
   a. Clinicians can assist the client to make realistic plans about how to handle relapse while focusing on the future and the benefits of change.
4. In the **action** stage, the client changes the behavior.
   a. Clinicians assist the client to substitute alternate behaviors. Affirmation and support are helpful at this stage.
5. In the **maintenance** stage, the client continues the change. If a lapse occurs it may result in fear and decreased self-efficacy.

   a. Clinicians assist the client to view a lapse as a learning opportunity without imposing guilt. A lapse is not a defeat.
6. In the **termination** stage, the client revises his self-image and the former behavior is no longer a threat.
   a. Clinicians remain alert to risks for old behavior and continue to promote the client's self-efficacy for the behavior.
7. The TTM developed through studying the process of smoke cessation with adults. Subsequent studies have shown its applicability to exercise and other behavior changes.

Community-level Behavior Change

Social Ecology Theory

Social Ecology Theory (SET) examines the way people influence and are influenced by their environment and pays particular attention to the interface between person and environment.

1. Responsibility for health is shared between individuals and community systems.
2. Health promoting strategies are developed through community action and public policy. Programs based on SET focus on creating healthier communities to produce healthier people.
   a. The role of the clinician is consultant and supporter of the change process.
   b. The Minnesota Heart Health Program is an example of a community-based behavior change program. Strategies employed included community-level health education programs related to smoking cessation, exercise, and nutrition.

Organizational Change

Lewin's Planned Change

Lewin's process of planned change is the classic theory of organizational change.

1. Successful change involves unfreezing existing structures, introducing the change and moving to a new level, and re-freezing the structures to incorporate the change.
2. Successful change requires identifying forces driving the change and those restraining the change. Change is accomplished by strengthening driving forces and reducing restraining forces.

Strategies for Organizational Change

Strategies for organizational change reflect individual change theories.

1. Empirical–rational strategies for organizational change reflect the Theory of Reasoned Action
   a. The logic is as follows: Organizations are comprised of people. People are rational. To create change, provide education and disseminate knowledge. Once the people see the benefit they will adopt the change.
2. Normative–reeducative strategies of organizational change reflect social cognitive theory.
3. Power–coercive strategies of organizational change reflect motivational theories. The impetus for change is authority or organizational power. Change occurs because it reduces pain or harm as opposed to increasing pleasure or benefit.

Barriers to Organizational Change

Forces restraining acceptance of organizational change include the following:

1. Threat to self-interest — the change will be harmful in some way.
2. Inaccurate perceptions of the effect the change will have.
3. Disagreement about the value of the change.
4. Low tolerance for change and uncertainty, which may be related to lack of self-confidence.
5. Time — a system that has been stable for a long time is resistant to change.

Drivers for Organizational change

Forces facilitating acceptance of organizational change include the following:

1. People believe that the change is their idea or agrees with their ideas.
2. People are part of the change process.
3. Other people who are important to the individual support the change.
4. The change reduces burden or work.
5. The change is introduced as a pilot with evaluation.
6. The change is implemented using skillful, enthusiastic leadership that emphasizes communication and participation.

Family Dynamics

1. Families are important in nursing practice. Families are conceptualized as the context within which the individual exists and as the client for therapeutic intervention.
2. Family may be defined as a small group of intimates related biologically, legally or emotionally — a family is as it defines itself.
3. Cardiovascular and other health risk factors cluster within families. The Framingham Heart Study found a higher than expected concordance between spouses for blood pressure, cholesterol, triglyceride, blood sugar, smoking, and pulmonary function.

Family Systems Theory

1. Members of the family interact as a functional whole. Change in one element of the family system affects the whole system.
   a. The family as a whole is greater than (and different from) the sum of its parts.
   b. Individuals are best understood within the family context.
2. The family system is in contact with the environment with input and output across its boundaries.
   a. Families function to transmit culture.
   b. Family members occupy a variety of roles and functions that may assume varying importance at different familial developmental stages.
   c. Family members, especially the spouse, are the most important source of social support.
      1) Social support has a direct effect on health.
      2) The quality of family relationships has an indirect effect on health by buffering stress.
3. Problems and symptoms occurring within family members reflect the family's adaptation to its total structure and environment at a given point in time.
4. Adaptive efforts of family members effect the biological, interpersonal, and intrapsychic connections with the family (nuclear and extended) and the society.
   a. Concurrent events in different parts of the family are connected in some way.
5. There are normative expectations related to timing of major transitions within the family, such as leaving home, marriage, and childbirth.
   a. "On time" events create less strain within the family than "off time" events.

Family Life Cycle

1. As with individuals, family development follows a predictable course.
   a. Unattached young adult
   b. Newly married couple
   c. Family with young children
   d. Family with adolescent children
   e. Family launching children and moving on
   f. Later life family
2. Families oscillate between periods of closeness (centripetal) and periods of distance (centrifugal). These periods reflect the needs of the family within its developmental stage. For example, a family with young children requires high cohesion (centripetal) while a family that is launching children requires more distance (centrifugal).

Family Response to Serious Illness

Family response to serious illness depends on when the illness occurs within the family life cycle, which family member falls ill and the family's usual coping style. For example, a myocardial infarction may have different meaning to a family with young children versus a later life family. Family stress related to role change may differ by whether it is the husband or the wife who becomes ill.

Crisis Theory

Crisis is a response to hazardous events and is experienced as a painful state. A situation becomes a crisis because the individual perceives it as threatening in a highly significant way. Clinicians describe crisis as a clinical syndrome involving emotional upset, increased tension, unpleasant affect, ineffective coping strategies, and impaired functioning.

1. Life events associated with loss and threat can precipitate situational crisis.
   a. Examples include death, divorce, major illness, job loss, rape, and trauma.
   b. Positive events such as marriage and childbirth create conflicts that can lead to crisis. For example, differences in values related to family or religion. The arrival of the first child creates major change in the couple's relationship, which can cause conflict and stress related to loss.

2. Developmental crises occur at predictable points at which new behavior must be learned in order for the individual to move to the next level. Erickson identified three developmental tasks with potential for crisis that occur in adulthood:
   a. Intimacy versus isolation in young adults,
   b. Generativity versus self-absorption in middle-aged adults, and
   c. Integrity versus despair in older adults.
3. Crisis occurs when the usual coping strategies are unable to control effectively or resolve the tension generated by the situation. Each individual usually functions within a specific range of effectiveness and personal satisfaction. In a crisis, there is overwhelming emotional distress that interferes with effective problem solving.
   a. A crisis is self-limited and some resolution occurs in 4 to 10 weeks.
   b. All of the individual's energy and resources focus on resolution of the crisis and reduction of the pain.
4. The individual in crisis is generally more open to accepting help. Minimal help may produce meaningful results.

Crisis Intervention

1. Crisis intervention consists of short-term psychotherapy with specific goals:
   a. To keep the individual safe — prevent harm to self or others.
   b. To return the individual to the pre-crisis level of functioning or higher.
   c. To enhance the coping repertoire and self-esteem.
2. Crisis intervention techniques include reassurance, suggestion, support, environmental manipulation, and psychotropic medications.

CHAPTER 3
Leadership

This chapter focuses on the leadership roles and responsibilities of cardiac and vascular nurses. Methods to improve the quality of care of patients with cardiac and vascular ilnesses are discussed.

Leadership

Leadership is the personal characteristics or qualities that the leader uses to influence others to achieve an identified goal. Key attributes of a leader that promote the achievement of the identified goal are:

1. The leader works effectively with members of the group or team.
2. The leader facilitates communication among members of the group or team.
3. The leader motivates the members of the group or team.

Leadership Styles

1. **Autocratic leadership** uses power to influence group members. The leader makes the decision and gives minimal consideration to the ideas or suggestions of members.
2. **Participative leadership** uses the democratic process for decision-making with group members. The leader encourages the participation of members and provides consistent feedback.
3. **Laissez-faire leadership** uses minimal guidance and provides little feedback to group members. The leader is unwilling to make decisions and consequently does not initiate change.
4. **Transactional leadership** focuses on daily activities and is comfortable with the status quo. The leader rewards group members for work completed and deals with problems after they have occurred.
5. **Transformational leadership** articulates a vision and commitment to the organization's goals. The leader empowers members to achieve the goals and vision.

Leadership in Cardiovascular Care

Cardiovascular (CV) nurses assume a leadership role as they coordinate care. The complexity of cardiac and vascular care is increasing and there is a great need for interdisciplinary collaboration to meet patient care needs. Participative and transformational leadership styles facilitate group or team processes to achieve desired outcomes in patient care.

Team Building

Team building involves many factors that promote good working relationships among team members. Teams collaborate to promote the efficiency of the organization and to optimize patient outcomes. Teams develop the highest potential of its members so that they contribute in significant ways, accept more responsibility, and share a commitment to the organizational goals and structure.

Team

1. A team is a group of people committed to an identified, shared purpose, with common goals, complementary or shared skills, and a similar approach to completing the work. Each member is accountable to the team for the completion of assigned tasks.
2. Attributes of a successful team include the ability to self-regulate, awareness of team member roles including strengths and weaknesses, adaptability to changing events, accountability for evaluating actions, and responsibility for revising the plan as necessary.

Team Building Models

1. The Traditional Model of Team Effectiveness views the team as a series of components that include team building, team processes, and team effectiveness. This model examines the symptoms of team effectiveness but does not look at the actual reasons such as motivation or cognitive processes, that drive the team towards attainment of its goals.
   a. Assumptions are that the team is passive, stable, and a behavioral entity.
   b. Team building is geared towards redesigning behavioral processes by examining the signs of team effectiveness rather than the causes.
   c. Team processes include communication, social integration, role clarification, and goal setting.
   d. Process, attitudinal, and perceptual indicators measure team effectiveness.
2. Cognitive Motivational Model of Team Effectiveness (CoMMTE) is based on the premise that each of the variables (ie, assumptions, team causes, team processes, team effectiveness, and team building)

are interdependent and can be used to evaluate and redesign team developed interventions.

a. CoMMTE assumes that the team is an active, dynamic, fluid, and cognitive-motivational entity.
b. Team causes or purposes include shared goals and actions, the ability to evaluate its actions, and to redesign its interventions.
c. Team processes are self-regulated and have diagnostic perogative.
d. Team effectiveness is measured by the achievement of results.
e. Team building focuses on redesigning cognitive functioning by analyzing team effectiveness.

Benefits of Team Building in Health Care

1. Nursing, medicine, and other health care professionals must provide integrated care that supports optimal use of health care resources to improve patient outcomes.
2. Collaboration among nurses provides continuity of care by focusing on a plan that promotes teamwork to enhance positive patient outcomes and to coordinate care delivery.
3. Interdisciplinary collaboration involves the joint contributions of professionals from other disciplines such as nursing and medicine working towards the common goals of improving quality of care and outcomes for patients.
4. Teams can streamline health care services for patients while avoiding duplication or gaps in their care.

Team Building and Teamwork

1. Clear expectations about the roles, skills, and goals of the team and its members enhance teamwork, reduce conflict, and promote success.
2. Participative learning experiences foster collaboration among the members of the team.
3. Effective communication among team members promotes team effectiveness.
4. Support, encouragement, respect, and commitment among members facilitate teamwork.
5. Recognition of one member of the team as the leader by other members enhances group processes.

Barriers to Team Building and Team Work

1. Health care professionals have not been taught about teamwork or team building.

2. Sex role stereotyping and gender hierarchy have a negative effect on interdisciplinary groups.
3. Role status of team members has the potential to impede communication within the group.
4. Team members with traditional views of organizational roles may have difficulty with teamwork.
5. Situations that promote lack of communication, support, and respect for team members impair teamwork.

Team Building for CV Care

1. The formation of teams and subsequent team building are beneficial for the management of acute and chronically ill patients with cardiac and vascular health problems.
2. Decreased length of stay for cardiac surgical patients mandates that health care services are coordinated within the hospital among nursing, cardiology, cardiac surgery, anesthesia, physical therapy, dietary, and respiratory therapy. The development of fast track protocols for early extubation and discharge of these patients require interdisciplinary collaboration.
3. The formation of teams to address the needs of hospitalized CV "outliers" has also been effective. Nurses used primary nursing to manage the nursing care needs while interdisciplinary teams developed clinical pathways. For example, the development of ventilator weaning and extubation protocols has decreased the duration of mechanical ventilation and hospitalization for patients after cardiac surgery.
4. Teamwork has also been effective in coordinating the care of patients with chronic CV diseases (such as heart failure). Intra- and interdisciplinary team efforts provide continuity in the transition from hospital to home.

Case Management

Definitions

Nursing uses case management to coordinate the care of patients. Case management is defined differently by different professional organizations.

1. The Case Management Society of America states that case management is "a collective process which assesses, plans, implements, coordinates, monitors and evaluates the options and services required to meet an individual's health needs using communica-

tions and available resources to promote quality, cost-effective outcomes." This definition, while broad enough to encompass the different disciplines involved in case management, does not address nursing's unique role.

2. The American Nurses Credentialing Center defines nursing case management as "a dynamic and systematic collaborative approach to providing and coordinating health care services to a defined population. It is a participative process to identify and facilitate options and services for meeting individuals' health needs, while decreasing fragmentation and duplication of care and enhancing quality, cost-effective clinical outcomes.

Case Management Models

1. Nursing case management models evolved from primary nursing and were traditionally used in acute care settings.
   a. Nurse case managers coordinate each patient's care throughout hospitalization as the patient moves to different locations throughout the institution.
   b. Nursing case management plans use DRG length of stay, critical pathway reports, and variance analysis, along with interdisciplinary collaborative group practice arrangements, to provide health care services to these patients.
2. Community-based case management models use case managers to coordinate the care of patients from the hospital to the community and to long-term care settings, if indicated. These patients have chronic health conditions and need long-term health care services. Community-based models provide care and resources to high-risk patients across the continuum of care.
3. Case management models have been modified to accomodate the needs of patients in a variety of community settings.
   a. **Long-term health care models** are used for prior authorization screening or direct service.
   b. **Rehabilitation case management** targets chronic medical or psychosocial health problems that have a longer recovery or treatment time than acute health problems.
   c. **Occupational health care models** focus on employee health with return to work and wellness as the major goals.
   d. **Private case management** involves subcontracting with individuals or groups for the coordination of services, advocacy, and counseling.
   e. **Insurance case management** emphasizes the linkage of resources for patient care but is not involved with direct care.

f. **Managed care** and **HMO case management models** monitor access to services and advocate cost effective alternatives to services. In some cases, permission for costly services is required but not necessarily granted.

Role of Case Managers

1. Establish a professional case management relationship with the patient and family.
2. Assist the patient and family in adapting to the health problem.
3. Advocate for the patient and family.
4. Ensure that patient and family education needs associated with the health problems are met.
5. Manage, coordinate, and facilitate the health care services that the patient and family need.
6. Make sure that health care services are appropriate, delivered within the required time frames, and coordinated across the continuum of care.
7. Evaluate the quality and cost-effectiveness of health care services delivered to patients and their family.

Case Management for CV Care

Driving forces that will reshape case management delivery systems in the future for CV patients include managed care, rising health care costs, and efforts to improve the quality of health care services and outcomes. The emphasis on acute and episodic care will shift to include the long-term management of chronic illnesses such as heart failure, hypertension and stroke. Health promotion and strategies for risk identification and reduction will be emphasized. Information systems and telehealth will influence the redesign of case management models. Nurses will use computer software for risk identification and remote transmitters for monitoring. Other factors that will affect the future of case management include:

1. The **aging of the population** will have major effects on the health care system. It has been projected that the number of people age 65 years and older in the US will more than double to 70 million by the year 2030 while the number of centenarians will increase from 65,000 to 381,000 people. The incidence of many diseases such as coronary heart disease and peripheral vascular disease increase with aging. More people will need health care services for cardiac and vascular health problems.
2. The **shortage of nurses** will have a profound effect on the way that health and nursing care are delivered. Hospitals are already experiencing decreasing numbers of nurses particularly in the

areas of acute and critical care. The nursing shortage will also have an effect on other settings such as home care agencies and long-term care facilities.

3. **Decreasing numbers of allied health care personnel** is affecting the current delivery of health care services. Many health care systems are experiencing shortages or limited numbers of applicants for technical positions in radiology, respiratory therapy, and surgery.
4. The **growth of managed care companies** will generate greater demand for nursing case managers.
5. **New technology** used in the home setting, such as monitoring of patients weights, blood sugars, and cardiac rhythms, will affect the future of case management.
6. **Reduced reimbursement** for health care services due to government efforts at cost containment.
7. **Increased use of information systems.** Computer networks can be used to provide 24-hour support, monitoring, information, and reminders about medications and appointments.

Total Quality Management

1. Total quality management (TQM) is a way to run complex organizations to achieve the aims or mission of the organization.
2. TQM emphasizes empowerment of employees
   a. An underlying principle is that most people are trying quite hard to do their best work, further the mission of the organization, and meet the needs of the customers.
3. TQM recognizes that an organization or department has multiple customers who may have competing needs.
   a. A customer is anyone who depends on a department to provide a service. Customers of nursing service include patients and families (external), but also physicians and other clinicians (internal).
   b. TQM focuses on meeting the needs of both internal and external customers.
4. Quality problems occur when good people get caught in broken processes or systems that don't work.
   a. The people doing the work have the most information about how the work gets done
   b. Quality is cost effective. Fewer resources are required to do the job right the first time, than are required to do it multiple times until it is right.
5. A key strategy of TQM is to involve the worker in improving the work processes through continuous quality improvement.

Continuous Quality Improvement

1. Continuous quality improvement (CQI) is an approach to improve quality that focuses on how the work gets done (process) rather than on who is doing the work (people).
2. A process is a sequence of actions leading to an outcome that is important to customers (eg, patients) who depend on the process.
3. It often happens with complex processes that no one individual or department understands the whole process. Therefore, CQI requires an interdepartmental team.
   a. Suppose, for example, that it took too long for a patient who was experiencing a stroke to get from the Emergency Department (ED) to the angiography suite where a thrombolytic agent could be administered. A CQI team formed to address this quality problem might require representation from the ED, business office (patient registration), nursing (triage), medicine, transportation, and radiology.
4. CQI empowers health care workers to reduce the cost and improve the quality of their work.

Shewart Cycle

1. Shewart Cycle (also known as the Deming Cycle) is the planning and improvement process in widest use in US health care organizations today. The cycle has four steps: plan, do, check, act (PDCA).
2. The CQI team plans change by studying the process, deciding what could improve it, and identifying data to be used in monitoring the process.
3. The team tests the proposed change by doing a small-scale trial or data simulation exercise. The team checks the effects of the trial by studying the results and modifies the planned change if necessary.
4. The team acts to improve the process by implementing the change.
5. The cycle repeats continuously. Small changes are implemented and evaluated until the process is as efficient as can be achieved. In the time from ED to angiography suite example:
   a. **Plan:** The team measured the average time from ED check-in to throbolytic injection. They studied the process and determined that time waiting for transport was a critical factor.
   b. **Do:** The team assigned a transporter to the ED for one month and continued to monitor time to thrombolytic injection.
   c. **Check:** Pre- and post-intervention data were analyzed and the team found that time to throbolytic injection was reduced by 25 minutes. The team consensus was that further reduction was possible.

d. **Act:** The one-month trial of the transporter was extended another month and preprinted physician orders were implemented also. Time-to-thrombolytic-injection data were gathered continually.
e. **Repeat:** The data showed further reduction in time; the team continued to examine the process to identify further potential improvement.

CQI Relies on Data

1. Quality issues are identified from data.
2. Local and national data are used to establish benchmarks for quality care.
3. Data are collected and analyzed to determine the effect of the change on the process of care.

Barriers to Implementing CQI Programs

1. Organizational barriers include:
   a. Resistance to change.
   b. Culture is so deeply engrained that the behavioral change is in conflict with the organization's philosophy.
   c. There is limited time for the change to take place.
   d. Lack of organizational support for CQI.
2. Management barriers include:
   a. Management not accepting of role change associated with CQI.
   b. Organization's goals not clearly communicated to management.
   c. Lack of managerial support.
3. Process barriers include:
   a. Data are not available.
   b. National or local benchmarks have not been defined.
4. CQI team barriers include:
   a. Inadequate team building.
   b. Key departments not represented.
   c. Lack of understanding by team members of the CQI process.
   d. Personal agendas.

CQI in CV Care

CQI programs have improved the care of CV patients. Quality improvement models will continue to evolve to address the complex resources needed by CV patients and their families. The acuity of patients receiving CV invasive procedures has increased because of the success of most of these interventions. Health care providers need to continually evaluate care to ensure the quality that is being delivered to patients and to redesign this care, if necessary.

Outcome Evaluation

Outcome evaluation is important for patients, health care providers, and the health care system. It can be used to evaluate the effect of care on the patient's recovery from cardiac and vascular procedures. This process can also be used to enhance the knowledge of health care providers, establish the criteria for clinical decision-making, evaluate the effectiveness of interventions, and to identify areas for improvement.

An outcome is a change in status between two points in time. The change may be positive or negative.

1. Frequently used patient outcomes include:
   a. Morbidity or incidence of complications
   b. Mortality
   c. Hemodynamic parameters (eg, pulmonary artery pressures, central venous pressures)
   d. Laboratory values (eg, blood sugar, prothrombin time, INR)
   e. Symptoms (nausea, vomiting, pain, fatigue, angina, anxiety, depression)
   f. Functional status (eg, activities of daily living, sexuality, family function, employment)
2. Frequently used health care provider outcomes include:
   a. Change in knowledge or skill-level
   b. Compliance with practice standards
3. Frequently used system outcomes include:
   a. Service utilization
   b. Length of hospital stay or duration of services
   c. Cost of care or services

Outcome Evaluation in CV Care

1. Outcome evaluation was used to identify factors associated with more complications after cardiac surgery. Practice changes were implemented, such as tighter glycemic control for diabetic patients, and the number of complications was reduced.
2. Interdisciplinary models need to be evaluated to determine the positive and negative patient outcomes based on collaboration of health care providers to deliver coordinated services for health promotion and disease management.

3. System or organization outcomes need to be evaluated to determine untoward effects such as medication errors, infection rates, and treatment failure along with indicators of quality of care and cost-effectiveness. This process should involve intra- and interdisciplinary collaboration along with the use or development of benchmarks for the care of cardiovascular patients by national organizations.

CHAPTER 4

Research

The primary function of nursing research is to develop the scientific knowledge base for nursing practice. Baccalaureate-prepared nurses are readers and users of nursing research. This chapter reviews the steps of the research process, qualitative and quantitative research methods, and evidence-based practice.

Problem Identification

Sources of Ideas for Research Problems

1. Clinical practice
   a. The idea emerges: For example, how can the nurse relieve patient and family anxiety about early hospital discharge?
   b. Brainstorm with colleagues: Do others perceive anxiety about early discharge to be a problem? Why is it a problem? Does it have bad outcomes?
   c. Review the literature: Has the question been answered? Is the answer definitive? Are observable variables suggested or supported by the literature?
   d. Identify variables: What concepts contained in the questions have the ability to vary?
      1) Possible patient-related variables: Age, gender, procedure, and pre-hospitalization anxiety.
      2) Possible nurse-related variables: Age, gender, education, and experience.
      3) Possible system-related variables: Discharge planning procedure, length of hospital stay, and referral to home care.
2. Continuous quality improvement trends
3. Theory
   a. Some scholars believe that the purpose of nursing research is to generate and test theory, and research that is unrelated to theory is trivial.
4. Literature
5. Priorities set by professional organizations and funding agencies
6. Conferences and colleagues

Problem Evaluation

1. Does the problem occur frequently? or Does it occur infrequently but have a significant effect on outcome?
2. Can the problem or question be answered by collecting observable data?
3. Will answering the question result in better care?
4. Are the resources necessary to answer the question available? Is it feasible, practical?
5. Is the question ethical? Will some good come to the participant or society? Are the risks outweighed by the benefits of participation?
6. Is the nurse's level of interest in the question sufficient to sustain the effort?

Stating the Question or Problem

1. A research question is a concise statement, worded in the present tense, that includes one or more variables (or concepts).
2. Kinds of research questions
   a. Descriptive: For example, "How is anxiety related to early discharge manifested in patients and families?"
   b. Exploratory or relational: For example, "What is the relationship between predischarge anxiety and postdischarge behavior?"
   c. Predictive: For example, "Does self-efficacy, predischarge anxiety, or family structure, best predict postdischarge behavior?"
   d. Experimental or quasi-experimental: If one can predict the outcome, the next step would be to modify the outcome. If one knew, for example, that self-efficacy predicted postdischarge behavior, then one could prescribe a self-efficacy enhancement intervention to influence postdischarge behavior.

Research Method

The research question and the existing knowledge about the phenomena of interest determine the research method used.

1. Qualitative methods are inductive; quantitative methods are deductive.
2. Qualitative methods are used in the following situations.
   a. When the question is broad and little is known about the subject. For example, "How do mid-life women decide to use natural as opposed to pharmaceutical estrogen replacement?"
   b. To achieve a deep, rich understanding of the phenomena — discovery, exploration, and description of the phenomena. For

example, "What factors contribute to women's delay in seeking emergency care when experiencing symptoms of myocardial infarction?"
   c. In combination with quantitative methods — for triangulation or as a complement.
   d. For instrument development.
   e. To generate hypotheses about relationships for subsequent testing.
3. Quantitative methods are used to:
   a. Explain and predict phenomena.
   b. Generate evidence of cause and effect.
   c. Test theory or instruments.
   d. Evaluate the effectiveness of interventions.

Qualitative Methods

General Characteristics

1. Qualitative methods allow the researcher to gain insight through discovering meaning.
2. Qualitative methods are a way to explore the richness and complexity of phenomenon.
3. Qualitative data are expressed in words rather than numbers.
4. Data collection and analysis occur concurrently.
5. Theoretical or purposive sampling is used. Using insights from the data, the researcher selects informants with particular characteristics to increase theoretical understanding of the phenomenon.
6. Researchers are concerned with the trustworthiness of qualitative studies

Assuring Trustworthiness

1. Credibility is the truth-value of the study. It has been compared to the internal validity of a study using quantitative methods. When assessing the credibility of the study, the reviewer considers the period of engagement with the study, the use of multiple data sources (triangulation), and if the researcher checked with the informants and included their response before publishing the study.
2. Transferability of a study has been compared to the external validity of a study using quantitative methods. In general, the result of a qualitative study is deep, rich description of a phenomenon or process. Results are not directly transferable to other settings or populations. The understanding gained may be used to inform other studies or practices.

3. Dependability of a study has been compared to the reliability of a quantitative study. The researcher maintains scrupulous records about methods and decisions that can be reviewed and verified in a process audit.
4. Confirmability of a study has been compared to the objectivity of a quantitative study. The issue here is the extent to which the meanings assigned to the data are grounded in the events and the culture rather than in the researcher's experience. "Would another analyst find similar meaning in the data?"

Phenomenological Research

Phenomenological research is used to describe experiences as they are lived from the perspective of the study participant.

1. Phenomenology is not just a research method but also a philosophy that guides the research process.
2. The first step in conducting a phenomenological study is to identify the phenomena of interest.
3. The research question asks "What is the human experience and meaning of this phenomena?"
4. Sampling requires locating and identifying people living with the phenomena who are willing to share their thoughts, feelings, and experiences with the researcher.
5. Data are generated and collected through observation, interview, videotape, and descriptions written by participants.
6. Analysis consists of attaching meaning to statements and the outcome is a theoretical statement responding to the research question.
   a. Excerpts from the data are used to support the theoretical statement.
   b. Many nurses are familiar with Benner's phenomenological study of nursing knowledge acquisition, *From Novice to Expert.*

Grounded Theory

Grounded theory is a research method used to understand basic social processes. It has its roots in sociology.

1. The first step is to identify the social process of interest.
2. Data are generated and collected through participant-observation and intensive interviewing.
3. Data are coded and categorized.
   a. Constant comparative analysis compares each piece of data with every other piece.

b. The categories are found within the data — not preconceived.
c. Data are collected until all of the characteristics of the category are revealed.
4. The outcome is a theory explaining the social process of interest that is grounded in the data from which it was derived.

Ethnography

Ethnography is a research method used to understand a culture (or subculture) from its own perspective. Ethnography has its roots in anthropology.

1. The first step with ethnography is to identify the culture to be studied.
2. Literature review provides a background for the study.
   a. The researcher seeks a general understanding of the phenomena to be examined specifically within the culture.
   b. Studies of health-behavior and experiences of homeless people may use ethnographic methods, for example.
3. Data generation and collection require access to the culture and key informants.
   a. Key informants are members of the culture who are willing to share their knowledge of the culture and the phenomena.
   b. The researcher becomes immersed in the culture through active participation.
4. Data are collected through observation and interview.
5. Analysis involves identifying meaning attached to the data and events by the informants. Members of the culture validate meaning before the results are final.
6. The outcome is detailed description of the phenomena as experienced within the culture.

Historiography

Historiography examines past events.

1. The first step is to select the topic and questions to be examined.
2. Next the researcher must identify sources of data and obtain access to these sources.
   a. Data may include letters, memos, and mementos.
3. Analysis involves synthesis of the data collected.
4. The outcome is a cogent retelling of historical events and their meaning.
   a. Examples of historical studies include *We Band of Angels* and *Critical Care Nursing*.

Content Analysis

Content analysis is a method used to classify words in text by their theoretical importance.

1. Content analysis differs from other qualitative methods as it uses numbers to represent frequency, order, or intensity of words, phrases or sentences.
2. Content analysis is sometimes used in historical research.
3. Theoretically significant categories are identified. Data are classified into categories and the number of data bits assigned to the category is determined.
4. Descriptive statistics may be used to count and summarize data.

Quantitative Methods

General Concerns and Issues

1. Variables
   a. An **independent variable** is the stimulus or activity that is manipulated by the researcher to create an effect on the dependent variable.
      1) Control is very important in experimental and quasi-experimental designs.
      2) The greater the amount of control the researcher has, the stronger the evidence from the study.
   b. A **dependent variable** is the response, behavior, or outcome that the researcher wants to predict or explain.
   c. **Extraneous variables** are all of the other factors that can vary and may influence the dependent variable.
      1) The researcher uses research design amd statistical methods to reduce the effect of extraneous variables.
   d. **Demographic variables** are characteristics of the subjects that are collected for descriptive purposes.
2. Causality — support for causal relationships.
   a. Correlation or association alone does not prove causality.
   b. Three conditions must be met to establish causality:
      1) Strong correlation between the proposed cause and effect.
      2) Proposed cause must precede the effect in time.
      3) Proposed cause must be present every time the effect occurs.
   c. Multicausality — multiple factors contribute to the effect or outcome.
   d. Probability addresses relative, rather than absolute, causality. It describes the likelihood that one factor caused another.

3. Validity of a study is a measure of the truth or accuracy of the study. There are multiple aspects of validity that contribute to strength of the evidence provided by a study.
   a. Statistical conclusion validity is concerned with whether the conclusions made through statistical analyses accurately reflect the real world.
      1) **Type I error** occurs when the researcher concludes that there is a difference between two groups when in reality there is no difference.
         a) The risk of Type I error increases when the researcher conducts multiple statistical analyses of relationships or differences.
         b) Some relationships or differences may be found by chance within the sample that do not reflect true population relationships or differences.
      2) **Type II error** occurs when the researcher concludes that there is no difference between two samples when there is a true difference.
         a) Low statistical power is the most common cause of Type II error.
   b. Internal validity is the extent to which the effect detected in a study results from the relationship between the independent and dependent variable and not from some extraneous factor.
   c. Construct validity is the goodness of the fit between the definition of a concept of interest and its method of measurement.
   d. External validity describes the extent to which study findings can be generalized beyond the sample used in the study.

Quantitative Designs

1. Descriptive designs are used when the purpose is to delineate characteristics of a sample or setting. The purpose is not to generalize to a larger population.
2. Correlational designs study a population by systematically examining a representative sample. Findings may be generalized to the population represented by the sample.
   a. Cross-sectional designs collect data at one point in time.
   b. Longitudinal designs collect data at more than one point in time.
   c. Correlational designs may be used also to describe relationships between or among factors when the intent is not to make inferences about a larger population.

3. Quasi-experimental and experimental designs are used to test hypotheses about causal relationships.
   a. Control is a basic characteristic of experimental and quasi-experimental designs. Control is the ability of the researcher to manipulate the independent variable and to eliminate, hold constant, or measure the effect of extraneous variables.
   b. Elements of a true experimental design include:
      1) At least two groups — experimental and control.
      2) Random assignment of the sample to the experimental and control groups.
      3) Pre-tests before the manipulation of the independent variable.
      4) Post-tests following manipulation of the independent variable.
   c. When all 4 elements cannot be met, the design is quasi-experimental.

Sampling

Sampling involves selecting a group of people or elements to participate in a study.

1. Population refers to the entire set of people or elements that meet the sampling criteria. Accessible population refers to the set of people or elements that meet the sampling criteria to which the researcher can gain access.
2. Sampling criteria are the characteristics essential for inclusion in the target population.
   a. Inclusion criteria are characteristics that must be present for a subject to be included in the population.
   b. Exclusion criteria are characteristics that when present cause a subject to be excluded from the population.
3. Representativeness is the extent to which the sample is like the population
4. Adequate sample size for a study is determined by the anticipated effect size, power of the statistical tests, and significance level.
   a. Effect size is the amount of an impact or the strength of the relationship between the independent and dependent variables.
   b. Power is the capacity of the statistical test to detect significant differences or relationships that exist between groups in the sample. The minimal acceptable power for a study is .80, meaning there is an 80% probability of correctly discerning a difference between two groups.
   c. The significance level is set by the researcher and determines the probability of making a Type I error (concluding that there

is a difference between two groups when in reality there is no difference). In general, researchers use a probability of 0.05 or less when analyzing data. When a test of difference is significant at the 0.05 level, the researcher may conclude that there is a 95% probability that the two groups are different.

Sampling Error

Parameters describe population characteristics or attributes; statistics describe sample characteristics.

1. Sampling error is the difference between a sample statistic and a population parameter.
   a. If the sample does not reflect the population, sampling error will be large.
   b. Random variation is the expected difference that occurs when one measures a variable in different subjects from the same sample.
   c. Systematic variation occurs when subjects vary in some specific way from the population as a whole.
2. Random sampling is a way to assure that every individual in the population has an equal chance to be selected into the sample.
   a. Random sampling assures that the sample represents the population and minimizes systematic variation.
   b. Random samples include simple random samples, stratified random samples, and cluster samples.
3. In non-probability sampling, every individual in the population does not have an equal chance to be selected.
   a. Non-probability sampling reduces the likelihood that the sample represents the population. There is an increased risk of systematic variation.
   b. Non-probability samples include convenience and quota samples.
      1) Random assignment to group is used in an attempt to control systematic bias within convenience samples.

Measurement

Measurement is the process of assigning numbers to objects, events or situations according to a rule.

1. Levels of measurement
   a. Nominal scale is the lowest level of measurement. Numbers function as labels or categories and cannot be used for calculation. For example, the numbers on baseball players' shirts are labels only. And when the variable gender is measured

using 1 for female and 2 for male the numbers represent categories only.
   1) The categories are mutually exclusive.
   2) All of the data fit in one of the categories (exhaustive).
b. Ordinal scale represents sequence or order — members of a set are ordered from most to least with respect to some characteristic. For example, a graduating student may be first or tenth in a class. The number is significant in terms of relative position.
   1) Categories are mutually exclusive and exhaustive.
   2) Categories can be ordered, but intervals are not equal.
c. Interval scale has order and equal numerical distance between intervals. For example, temperature is measured on an interval scale. The difference between 70 degrees and 80 degrees is the same as the difference between 50 degrees and 60 degrees. A temperature of 0 degrees does not indicate the absence of temperature, however.
   1) Categories are mutually exclusive and exhaustive.
   2) Categories can be ordered.
   3) Intervals are equal, but the scale does not contain absolute zero.
d. Ratio scale is the highest form of measurement and exists on a continuum. Weight, length and volume are examples of ratio-level measurements. Zero represents the absence of weight, length, or volume. Because absolute zero is contained in the scale, one can say that 10 lb is twice as heavy as 5 lb.
   1) Categories are mutually exclusive and exhaustive.
   2) Categories can be ordered.
   3) Intervals are equal.
   4) Scale contains absolute zero.

Measurement Issues

It is not possible to measure a concept perfectly. Measurement error is the difference between the concept in reality and as measured by an instrument.

There are 3 components to a measured score: the true score, the observed score, and the error score. The observed score equals the true score plus the error score.

There are 2 components to the error score — **random error** and **systematic error**.

1. **Random error** causes the observed score to vary around the true score.
   a. According to measurement theory, the sum of random errors is zero. Some observed scores will be higher than the true scores

and some will be lower, but taken together the errors will add up to zero.

b. Random error is not correlated with the true score. Random error will not cause the mean score to be higher or lower than the true mean but will increase the amount of unexplained variance around the true mean. Random error cannot be eliminated.

2. Systematic error causes the observed score to vary from the true score in a consistent (systematic) way. For example, a scale that consistently weighs subjects as 2 lb heavier than their true weight adds systematic error. Systematic error effects mean scores.
   a. The goal in measurement is to reduce systematic error as much as possible.
3. Reliability of a measure reflects the consistency or reproducibility of scores obtained with the measure.
   a. Reliability testing provides an indication of the amount of random error inherent in the measurement of the concept within the sample.
   b. Reliability of a measure is expressed as a correlation coefficient with 1.00 representing perfect reliability and 0.00 representing no reliability.
   c. Estimates of reliability are specific to the sample being tested.
      1) Reliability testing is performed on each instrument used in a study before other statistical analyses are done.
      2) A reliability coefficient of 0.80 is the minimal acceptable level for established instruments. For newly developed instruments, a reliability coefficient of 0.70 may be accepted.
4. Validity of a measure reflects the extent to which an instrument represents the concept being measured within the specific situation. Validity of a measure determines the appropriateness, meaningfulness, and usefulness of inferences made from scores on the measure.
   a. Systematic error reduces the validity of measures.
   b. Evidence for the validity of an instrument develops through repeated use over time in a variety of situations. Traditionally, the various means of accumulating evidence have been grouped into categories. The use of category labels does not indicate different kinds of validity, but different types of evidence.
      1) Content-related evidence examines the extent to which the method of measurement includes representative elements from a domain of content.
         a) Content-related evidence often relies on expert judgment to identify appropriate elements for inclusion.

b) Factor analysis is a statistical method that examines clusters of relationships among items. Once the clusters are identified mathematically, the analyst explains theoretically why the items grouped as they did.

2) Criterion-related evidence examines the performance of an instrument in comparison with other measures, preferably a "gold standard."

3) Evidence of validity accrues from differential prediction of future or concurrent events.

a) The ability to predict future performance.

b) The ability to differentiate between groups known to be high and low in the concept of interest.

5. Sensitivity is the ability of a measure to detect relevant change in the concept.

Data Collection Strategies

1. Observation
   a. Answers questions about overt human behavior — actions, facial expressions, body language, etc.
   b. Allows phenomena to be studied in their natural environment.
2. Self-report — interviews, questionnaires, and surveys.
   a. Answers questions about facts, beliefs, feelings, and attitudes.
   b. Individuals may be unwilling or unable to answer the questions. Questions may not be answered truthfully.
3. Existing data — public records, medical records, national data bases.
   a. Existing data may be used to answer a new question. For example, an investigator might use census data to explore a health-related question.
   b. Personal health (medical) records are often used in case series. Health records may contain biases of the health care clinician.
4. Physiological measures — blood pressure, heart rate, blood tests, etc.

Protection of Human Rights

1. Informed consent
2. Anonymity and confidentiality
3. Risks and benefits

Data Analysis

1. The research question, methods used to obtain data, and characteristics of the data determine the appropriate statistical tests to be used.

2. Descriptive statistics provide precise, standard ways to summarize and communicate complex information about a sample.
   a. Measures of central tendency
      1) The mode is the numerical value or score that occurs with the highest frequency.
      2) The median is the score at the exact center of the distribution. Exactly 50% of scores is above the median and 50% of the scores is below the median.
      3) The mean is the sum of scores divided by the number of scores included in the sum.
   b. Shape of the distribution
      1) Symmetry — left side of the curve is a mirror image of the right side of the curve. When a curve is symmetrical all three measures of central tendency are equal. When a curve is not symmetrical it is skewed.
         a) Positive skew — the largest portion of data falls below the mean; the curve has a tail extending to the right.
         b) Negative skew — the largest portion of data falls above the mean; the curve has an initiating tail.
      2) Modality — a curve may be unimodal, bimodal or multimodal. Symmetric curves are usually unimodal.
      3) Kurtosis — describes the peakedness of the curve, which is related to the spread or variability of the scores.
   c. Measures of dispersion
      1) The range is the mathematical difference between the highest and lowest scores.
      2) The standard deviation is the average amount by which scores vary around the mean.
      3) The variance is the average of the squared standard deviations. It is frequently used in statistics but is difficult to interpret as a measure of dispersion.
   d. Measures of association
      1) Contingency tables or cross tabulations allow visual comparison of summary data related to two variables within the sample.
         a) Contingency tables are used to examine nominal or ordinal level data.
         b) Chi-square is a statistic designed to test for differences between cells in contingency tables.
      2) Correlation coefficients provide information about the direction, strength, and shape of relationships. Values range from –1.00 (a perfect and inverse correlation) to +1.00 (a perfect and positive correlation.)

3. Inferential statistics allow the investigator to go beyond description of the sample and make probabilistic inferences about the population.
   a. Parametric statistics require assumptions about the distribution of data — normality and homogeneity of variance, for example.
   b. Non-parametric statistics make no assumptions about the shape of the distribution.
      1) Non-parametric statistics are particularly relevant when the distribution is not normal or the sample size is small.
      2) Non-parametric statistics are commonly used to analyze nominal and ordinallevel data.
   c. Hypothesis testing of differences and association between variables.
      1) Tests of difference
         a) Parametric: t-test, ANOVA
         b) Non-parametric: Mann Whitney U test, sign test
      2) Tests of association
         a) Parametric: Pearson correlation coefficients
         b) Non-parametric: Spearman and Kendall correlation coefficients

Evidence-based Practice

Evidence-based practice is the synthesis and use of scientific information to direct practice.

Sources and Kinds of Evidence

1. National guidelines may be research based, represent the consensus of experts, or more commonly both.
   a. The Agency for Healthcare Policy and Research, now the Agency for Healthcare Research and Quality, published practice guidelines that summarized evidence related to specific topics. Some guidelines are now outdated and archived, but can be viewed online from the websites (www.ahrq.gov or www.guideline.gov). Evidence-based guidelines:
      1) Contain comprehensive review and summary of existing research.
      2) Rate the quality of the evidence; place highest value on evidence from randomized clinical trials (RCT).
         a) Strongest evidence rating A — results of two or more RCTs.
         b) Rating B — results of two or more controlled clinical trials.

c) Rating C — results of one controlled trial, two case series or descriptive studies, or expert opinion.
3) Expert panel makes practice recommendations based on evaluation of the evidence.

2. Professional organizations publish research-based protocols. For example, Nurses Improving Care for Health System Elders (NICHE) sponsored by the Hartford Foundation at NYU.
3. Research utilization: Before using research in practice a comprehensive analysis should be performed.
   a. Locate relevant clinical nursing research.
   b. Critique the research to determine transferablity, feasibility and readiness for use in practice.
      1) Assess quality of the research — the strength of the evidence and applicability to clinical practice.
      2) Studies that have been replicated generate more confidence in outcomes.
4. Local data — Continuous Quality Improvement (CQI)
   a. Revise systems and processes on the basis of data about the process itself.
   b. CQI measures the current status, locates comparative data and establishes bench marks.
   c. Change in practice is initiated; data continue to be gathered and analyzed; additional change is implemented as indicated.
   d. The improvement process is continuous and cyclical.

Outcomes Evaluation

The growing expense of health care led to focus on outcomes — how to maximize the benefit associated with the resources used in health care.

An outcome is a change in patient health status between two or more points in time.

1. Health status encompasses physiologic, functional, cognitive, emotional and behavioral health.
2. Outcomes can be positive, negative or neutral changes in health status.

Outcome is a function of baseline condition of the individual and treatment factors.

Frequently used outcome measures

1. Patient satisfaction measures
2. Functional health status
3. Mortality rates

CHAPTER 5
Education and Counseling

The purpose of patient education and counseling is to provide the patient with knowledge needed for self-care. Today's major health problems are the result of chronic and acute conditions that can be influenced positively by individual and community behaviors. While avoiding blaming the individual for his or her disease, the clinician must provide information and support to facilitate behavior change. This chapter will address principles of adult learning, the processes of patient education and counseling, and information needed for self-management of health. Discharge planning is used as an example of the teaching/learning process in clinical practice.

Adult Learning

Adult learning is a persistent change in behavior based on experience.

Characteristics of Adult Learners

1. Adult learners come with problems to solve and learn best when content is related to the immediate need, problem, or deficit.
   a. Adult learners are self-directed.
   b. Adult learners are motivated and have a need to know.
2. Adult learners have life experience that can hinder or facilitate learning.
   a. Learning is enhanced when new content builds on past experience and is related to something the learner knows.

Domains of Learning

1. Cognitive learning deals with the intellectual or knowledge area and involves acquiring facts, reaching conclusions, or making decisions.
2. Affective learning consists of changing the attitudes, feelings, and interests the individual has toward an object or idea.
3. Psychomotor learning involves mastering physical skills or motor activities.

Conditions for Learning

1. Learning depends on three conditions: motivation to learn, ability to learn, and the learning environment.
2. Motivation describes the effect of internal and external forces on the individual that initiate, direct and maintain behavior.
   a. Motivation to learn is based on previous knowledge, attitudes, and sociocultural factors.
   b. Motivation is the willingness of the individual to learn.
   c. Six theories of motivation offer insight about why people may learn or change.
      1) A desired behavior is reinforced or rewarded.
      2) A behavior change satisfies a need for food, shelter, love, or self-esteem.
      3) Changing the behavior relieves cognitive dissonance.
         a) Cognitive dissonance is the tension felt when a deeply held belief is challenged by an inconsistent behavior.
      4) The causal explanations or attributions an individual makes about the situation affect his or her motivation to change.
         a) For example, patients who attribute their heart attack to a high-fat diet may be more likely to change their diet than those who attribute their heart attack to bad luck or genetics.
         b) Locus of control is a key concept in attribution theory.
            1. People with an internal locus of control attribute success or failure to their own efforts.
            2. People with an external locus of control attribute success or failure to external factors, such as luck, fate, or difficulty of the task.
      5) Individual differences in personality may influence motivation to learn or change.
         a) Optimism is a personality trait that has been positively associated with information seeking and changing behavior.
         b) Learned helplessness causes a person to believe he or she will fail no matter what is tried, thus making the person less likely to learn or change.
         c) Coping style may be a part of personality structure, although coping style may also be learned.
      6) The individual's perceived ability to achieve the goal affects motivation.
         a) Self-efficacy is correlated positively with activity level after a heart attack.

3. Ability to learn reflects the learner's developmental level, physical wellness, and intellectual thought processes.
   a. Developmental level refers to the stage of life of the individual. Each stage is accompanied by developmental tasks and concerns. For example, a young adult is concerned with establishing intimacy and close personal relationships. An older adult understands his or her purpose in life and seeks to share accumulated wisdom.
      1) Literacy level involves reading, comprehension, problem solving, math calculation, and the application of these abilities.
         a) Illiteracy is found among all ethnic groups and at all socioeconomic levels.
         b) Health literacy is the level of literacy required to function in the health environment. Health literacy cannot be predicted from educational level.
         c) Cues to low health literacy include:
            1. Withdrawing or avoiding learning situations.
            2. Excuses when asked to review printed material — too tired, forgot my glasses, gave it to my partner to take home, for example.
            3. Listening and observing very carefully to memorize how things work.
      2) Language. Does the learner speak and understand English? If not, are the interpreter's skills sufficient to explain?
   b. Physical wellness includes the required level of strength, coordination, and sensory acuity for learning.
      1) Physical size and strength must match the task to be performed or the equipment to be used.
      2) Coordination is the dexterity required for complex motor skills. Consider, for example, the dexterity required to prepare and administer insulin injections. If dexterity is inadequate an alternate method of administration must be found.
      3) The sensory acuity level needed to receive information and respond appropriately to teaching includes vision, hearing, touch, taste,and smell.
         a) Instructor awareness can compensate for some reduced or impaired sensory acuity. (See Table 5–1.)
   c. Multiple intellectual processes are necessary for learning to occur. For example, the ability to pay attention, to understand language, to manipulate symbols, to retrieve information from memory, and to transfer learning to novel situations.

1) Intellectual ability can be affected by health status (eg, person with receptive aphasia due to a stroke), developmental stage (eg, child versus adult), and genetic factors (eg, person with Down syndrome).

4. The environment can have a significant impact on the ability to learn. Many factors may need to be addressed to facilitate learning and minimize barriers to learning.
   a. Teacher/learner ratio
      1) Some individuals may learn better in a group but a group may be too distracting for others.
      2) Some may learn better in small, interactive groups while others learn better in large groups where there is more anonymity.

TABLE 5–1
Sensory impairments with implications for patient teaching

Sensory impairment	Implications for teaching
Reduced hearing acuity	• Get the individual's attention before beginning to speak. • Use simple sentences. • Face the patient and stand not more than 6 feet away. • Refrain from standing in front of a window or bright light, which may cast a shadow across your face or glare in patient's eyes. • Request feedback frequently to assure the patient heard and understood what was said. • If the patient has hearing aid(s), be certain they are functioning, adjusted properly, and in use.
Reduced visual acuity	• Vision enhancing devices: clean glasses, adequate light, or magnifying glasses. • Adequate contrast: black ink on white paper. • Adequate font size for written materials (14 point). • Avoid blue, blue-green, and violet hues in printed materials and posters. • Consider using audio tapes to enhance auditory learning.

3) Groups provide the opportunity for adult learners to learn from one another's experiences and understanding of the material presented.
4) Much patient education is presented in a 1:1 — nurse to patient — session. One-to-one teaching is sometimes called counseling. It tends to be more responsive to individual concerns and approaches.

b. Privacy and the assurance of confidentiality are necessary when addressing sensitive issues (eg, HIV status, genetic counseling).

c. Comfortable physical environment
   1) Moderate temperature
   2) Sufficient lighting that minimizes glare
   3) Minimal extraneous noise
   4) Adequate ventilation
   5) Appropriate and comfortable furniture

Patient Education Process

The patient education process parallels the nursing process

Assessment

Assessment data are used to define learning needs and develop a teaching plan to meet the needs of the individual.

1. Assessment of need to learn
   a. What does the patient know, feel, and believe about his or her health condition?
   b. What does he or she need to know?
2. Assessment of motivation to learn
   a. What motivates this individual to learn or change?
      1) The learner with an **internal locus of control** may be eager to change his or her health behavior because the change will enhance feelings of control.
      2) The learner with an **external locus of control** may be difficult to involve in learning and behavior change. He or she does not believe that individual behavior affects health status.
      3) The learner who believes someone else controls his or her health, (eg, the nurse or a family member), may expect "someone else" to correct the condition.
   b. Are there health-related cultural beliefs that may affect learning? Who should be included in the teaching and decision-making processes?

3. Assessment of readiness to learn
   a. Are there attitudes or beliefs that may hinder the ability to learn?
      1) Some individuals do not believe or deny that health behaviors effect health status, (eg, individuals who continue to smoke with peripheral vascular disease.) Others believe that it does not matter what they do; illness is going to happen.
      2) Perceived benefits of changing behaviors differ among learners. Some individuals may not want to devote the time and energy to change a behavior that they do not believe will improve their quality of life. Others may feel that any effort to change is good.
      3) Teaching strategies and techniques used for affective learning (changing attitudes and beliefs) differ from those used for cognitive learning (attaining facts and information).
   b. Does the learner have the necessary energy and endurance or will fatigue hinder learning?
      1) Patient fatigue often limits the amount of information that can be presented in one session.
   c. Is the learner comfortable?
      1) Is pain controlled and the patient mentally alert?
      2) Does the patient feels safe with the instructor and in the setting?
         a) Privacy and confidentiality assured.
         b) Patient perceives the instructor as knowledgeable.
   d. Are there sensory impairments for which the instructor must compensate?
   e. Does the patient have the physical maturity and coordination needed to learn psychomotor skills?

Diagnostic Statement and Objectives

1. Nursing diagnoses provide broad diagnostic statements. The following NANDA diagnoses may require educational intervention.
   a. Deficient knowledge (specify)
   b. Ineffective coping
   c. Ineffective health maintenance
   d. Noncompliance
2. Learning objectives are developed in the cognitive (facts and information), affective (attitudes and beliefs) and psychomotor (skills) domains.
3. Learning objectives are developed in behavioral terms that specify performance, conditions, and outcome.

a. Performance: Action verbs describe what the learner will do. For example, make a list or solve a problem.
b. Conditions: Identify specific circumstances that will be included in the action. For example, place, time of day or equipment and tools to be used.
c. Criteria: Indicate how achievement of the objective will be evaluated or measured. For example, test score, accuracy, or frequency.

4. Although objectives are developed and written by the instructor, they must be relevant to the learner. Mutual objective setting helps to assure relevance.

Intervention: Teaching-learning

1. The role of the instructor is to facilitate learning. The role of the student is to learn.
2. Structured teaching has been shown to be more effective than unstructured teaching.
3. The instructor selects teaching strategies that help the learner to achieve his or her objectives.
4. Teaching strategies may be more or less effective depending upon the learning domain, learner characteristics, the learning environment, and the skill of the instructor.
   a. Lecture is commonly used when teaching groups.
      1) Lecture is an effective method for presenting facts (cognitive learning), but is less effective for affective or psychomotor learning.
      2) Lecture combined with discussion is more effective than lecture alone.
         a) Discussion allows the learner to express personal feelings and concerns, to ask questions, and to clarify misunderstandings.
   b. Question and answer (Q & A) sessions focus the discussion on specific learner needs.
      1) Q & A sessions can facilitate both cognitive and affective learning.
      2) Q & A sessions are effective in teaching groups and in 1:1 teaching.
         a) In groups, individuals may learn from others' questions.
      3) Q & A sessions require active learner participation.
      4) Q & A sessions are not effective unless the learner has prior knowledge about the subject. The learner must know enough to recognize and ask questions.

c. Demonstration with return demonstration is an effective strategy for teaching psychomotor skills.
   1) Explanation while slowly demonstrating the skill evolves into offering cues to the learner while he or she practices the skill.
   2) Repeated practice with praise reinforces the behavior and helps the learner to move toward independent functioning.
   3) Supervised return demonstration assists with evaluation of learning.
   4) Demonstration/return demonstration is effective with small groups and in 1:1 teaching.

d. Role-playing is an effective strategy for teaching in the affective domain.
   1) The learner responds to a stimulus based on his or her experience while the teacher offers guidance and feedback.
   2) The role-playing may need to be repeated several times before the learner is able to internalize the behavior.
   3) In role-modeling, the instructor may take the role of the patient and demonstrate an appropriate response.

e. Oral or written tests may be used for evaluation of cognitive and psychomotor learning.
   1) Tests can be used as a part of assessment (pretests) and as an evaluation method to check progress.
   2) Oral may be better than written tests when literacy is a concern.
   3) Some learners are intimidated by written tests.

f. Simulation or case study method can be used to teach and evaluate the application of material to different situations.
   1) Simulation may be computer-based or may use actors to create the scenario.
   2) The scenario is presented and the learner interacts with the computer or actor.
   3) Solutions and recommendations offered by the learner in response to the scenarios allow instructors to evaluate the effectiveness of their teaching.

g. Teaching tools include books, pamphlets, pictures, films, slides, audio and video tapes, models, programmed instruction, and computer-assisted learning modules.
   1) Selection of effective teaching tools depends on the planned instructional method, learning needs assessed, and the learning ability of the student.
   2) The instructor must evaluate tools for content, format, reading level, and appropriateness of illustrations before use.

a) Content must match the patient's reading level and present the subject material clearly and logically.
   1. Avoid technical language.
   2. Standardized assessment formulas can be used to establish readability, (eg, SMOG).
b) Content must be relevant to the situation and contain accurate, current information.
c) Format of the materials affects learning. In general, materials should:
   1. Be organized with important general points presented first.
   2. Progress to specific information based on general points.
   3. Be logical and "user friendly" (eg, Q & A format.)
d) Illustrations enhance learning by emphasizing and reinforcing the written message. They increase motivation by attracting attention, adding variety, and providing breaks in the text.
   1. Illustrations should focus on the crucial aspects of the content.
   2. Effective illustrations:
      a. Are simple, uncluttered, and labeled legibly.
      b. Graphic symbols may help if there are language barriers
      c. Colors should be accurate and portray a realistic image.
   3. Learner interpretation of illustrations may be influenced by literacy level, cultural beliefs, and prior experience.
e) Layout and design of printed material can greatly influence its effectiveness.
   1. Font should be clear and easy to read.
   2. Type size should be 12–14 point, especially for the older adult learner.
   3. Maintain case contrast, avoid all capitals. Use bold or underline for emphasis.
   4. Ink color should offer sufficient contrast with the paper color.
   5. Glossy paper may produce glare and make reading difficult.
   6. Adequate spacing of text, illustrations, and "white space" makes the materials easier to read.

Evaluation and Reteaching

1. Evaluation is used to measure learning and health-related outcomes, monitor performance, and determine competence. Information gathered during evaluation is used to redirect teaching with the goal of improving responses and outcomes.
2. Direct and indirect measurement are used for evaluation.
   a. **Direct measurement** involves observing the learner and recording behaviors. The observer may use tools to guide the observations and rate behavior, such as:
      1) Rating scales (eg, Likert, numerical [1–10, 0–5, 1–100] or visual analog scales).
      2) Checklists of required behaviors.
      3) Anecdotal notes (ie, written observations of behavior.)
   b. **Indirect measurement** makes the assumption that learning has occurred when learners have achieved at a predetermined level. Indirect measurement does not measure behavior directly.
      1) Oral questioning is a flexible form of indirect measurement.
         a) Oral questioning allows immediate feedback to the learner and the correction of areas of weakness by the instructor.
         b) Oral questioning may be difficult for the learner if oral expression or language is a problem.
      2) Written tests are an indirect measure of cognitive learning. The most effective tests are well written, based on identified learning objectives, and involve increasing levels of difficulty.

Documentation

1. Document in the clinical record the content presented, written materials provided, and the patient's understanding of the information.

Patient Education and Counseling

1. Knowledge is necessary, but not sufficient, to change health behavior.
2. Patient education and counseling often occur in busy practice settings.

Strategies

1. Several patient education/counseling strategies have been described that can be implemented in brief periods of time during routine health visits.
   a. Frame the teaching to match the patient's perceptions.
   b. Fully inform patients of the purposes and expected effects of interventions and when to expect these effects. For example, when a smoker quits smoking risk for cardiac and vascular mortality drops significantly in the first year and then more gradually through ensuing years.
   c. Suggest small changes rather than large ones. Loss of 3–4 pounds in 4 weeks is better than recommending loss of 25 pounds in 6 months.
   d. Be specific. If a patient is walking a mile 3 days a week, recommend increasing frequency to 5 days a week.
   e. It is sometimes easier to add new behaviors than to eliminate established behaviors. It may be easier to add moderate exercise than to reduce caloric intake.
   f. Link new behaviors to established behaviors. For example, linking riding an exercise bicycle for 30 minutes to watching the evening news.
   g. Use the power of the profession. Direct, explicit, simple measures are powerful. For example, the message "You have smoked your last cigarette" may be effective if given by a trusted health professional.
   h. Get explicit commitments from the patient.
   i. Use a combination of strategies. Educational efforts that incorporate individual counseling, group classes, and written materials are more likely to be effective than single strategies.
   j. Involve office staff. Patient education and counseling is a shared responsibility of physicians, nurses, health educators, dietitians, and allied health professionals. The provision of educational materials in the waiting area may stimulate interest and discussion of health-related topics.
   k. Refer — an increasing number of educational programs are available through community agencies, national voluntary organizations, and health facilities.
   l. Monitor progress through follow-up contact. Inquire at each visit about progress and challenges. Telephone calls initiated by the professional to the patient to assess progress may provide external motivation for change.

Health Self-management

Health self-management issues include health maintenance, disease prevention, and health promotion.

Health Maintenance

Health maintenance activities are behaviors that maintain or improve health over time. Health maintenance depends on three characteristics: perception of health, motivation to change when needed, and adherence to prescribed interventions.

1. Perception of health involves an individual's understanding of current health status and having the knowledge to manage positive health behaviors.
   a. Health perceptions include the importance of health, the ability to control health, and the benefits of and barriers to healthy behavior.
   b. Factors affecting health perception include age and developmental stage, personality characteristics and physical wellness.
2. Motivation to change is determined by the responsibility that the learner assumes for health.
3. Adherence to (or compliance with) prescribed intervention requires making the decision to change or comply, setting goals, and making the actual therapeutic lifestyle changes.
   a. Making a decision and commitment to change may be difficult to achieve but is an essential first step
   b. Goals need to be set that are realistic and achievable. Failure occurs when the goals are unrealistic and too difficult to achieve.
   c. Making and maintaining lifestyle changes over time is often difficult.
      1) Negative life events (eg, the death of a spouse, family member, or close friend) can weaken the patient's resolve and old behaviors may resurface.
      2) The professional helps the patient to view the reoccurrence of old behavior as a temporary lapse rather than as a failure.
   d. A positive social support system helps the patient focus on the treatment goals.

Disease Prevention

Disease prevention is the organized effort to limit the development and progression of lifestyle-related illness. Three areas of disease prevention are primary, secondary, and tertiary.

1. **Primary prevention** precedes the occurrence of disease and is used with healthy populations.
   a. Primary prevention aims to decrease the probability of disease.
   b. Primary prevention includes immunizations, health education programs, and fitness activities such as eating a healthy diet, avoiding alcohol and tobacco products, and exercising regularly.
2. **Secondary prevention** involves screening to detect and treat disease in its earliest stages, ie, before symptoms are present.
   a. Early detection and treatment are associated with improved health outcomes and reduced morbidity and mortality.
   b. Secondary prevention includes screening programs such as, cholesterol screening, vision/hearing screening, and blood pressure screening.
3. **Tertiary prevention** attempts to reduce complications and disability from established disease thereby improving quality of life.
   a. In rehabilitation the goal is to minimize residual dysfunction and to maximize functional level.

Health Promotion

Health promotion refers to risk reduction strategies applied at the population level (macro level). Nurses have major roles as educators for the prevention of disease and enhancement of quality of life and as citizens to influence health policy.

1. Passive health promotion requires no action by the individual. For example:
   a. Fluoridation of municipal drinking water.
   b. Fortification of milk with vitamin D.
   c. Addition of iodine to table salt.
2. Active health promotion is the adoption of and participation in health programs by the individual (micro level). For example:
   a. Achieving and maintaining an ideal weight.
   b. Eating a healthy diet.
   c. Not smoking or using tobacco.
   d. Exercising regularly.
   e. Reducing stress.

Discharge Planning

Discharge planning facilitates the patient's transition between settings along the continuum of care. Discharge planning usually begins with admission to an institutional setting (hospital or nursing home) and continues until full recovery occurs, or the patient's condition is stabilized at the highest possible functional level.

Key Elements

Key elements addressed in discharge planning include changes in the patient's condition, coordination and facilitation of care, and negotiation of roles and responsibilities.

1. Transitions involve changes in patient condition. These changes may require adjustment by patients and their families.
   a. Mobility may be altered due to disease, surgery, or trauma. For example, an independent older adult patient may require a walker after surgery for an injured hip.
   b. Self-concept may change and need to be addressed. For example, an individual may feel 'damaged' and less confident after MI or heart surgery.
   c. Role-performance may be altered permanently or temporarily after a stroke or aneurysm repair. The individual may be unable to return to his or her former occupation and roles within the family and community may need to be renegotiated.
   d. Similarly, self-care deficits may be present for the stroke patient either short- or long-term.
2. Coordination of care is the identification, implementation, and direction of treatment prior to discharge.
   a. In the acute care setting, coordination of care is facilitated by the use of multidisciplinary care paths or critical pathways.
      1) Care paths or critical pathways sequence interventions to achieve expected outcomes over a projected length of stay for specific case types.
      2) If care is provided according to these guidelines and variance from the guideline is addressed promptly, the patient will be discharged in a timely manner and in as healthy a condition as possible.
   b. Home care and long-term care agencies use similar case-specific, clinical guidelines for care coordination.
3. Facilitation of care and discharge requires the anticipation of discharge needs upon admission.
   a. Initial assessment of potential discharge needs is done when the patient is admitted to the facility or service.
   b. Initial assessment of family resources and caregiving ability must occur also.
4. Negotiation is the process by which discharge goals and roles and responsibilities are determined or assigned.
   a. Negotiation may be formal or informal.
   b. Negotiation may be necessary when:

1) The patient who is unable to manage at home may need supportive care, eg, a visiting nurse, temporary nursing home placement, or outpatient rehabilitation.
2) The patient's health problems may require more family involvement, eg, 24-hour supervision. The family may select a responsible person or multiple family members may agree to be present for specified times.

Levels of Discharge Planning

Levels of discharge planning vary based on patient needs, family support, and financial resources. There are three levels of discharge planning currently used in hospitals: basic, simple, and complex.

1. Basic discharge planning may require only patient teaching.
   a. The clinical nurse may do the teaching, (eg, wound care or medication actions).
   b. Specialists, (eg, dietitians, enterostomal nurses, lactation nurses, diabetic educators), may be involved with the teaching.
2. Simple discharge planning involves referring the patient to community resources. This usually involves giving the necessary information to the patient or family, such as:
   a. Sources for durable medical equipment.
   b. Private-pay, in-home service agencies.
   c. Sources for outpatient therapies (eg, speech, physical or occupational therapy).
3. Complex discharge planning involves interdisciplinary collaboration, coordination, and negotiation. The discharge planner, the patient (when possible), and the family work together with community based, sub-acute, or long-term care services to formulate the most appropriate discharge plan.
   a. Community based care may be needed when the patient remains in the home environment but requires supervision or therapy on an intermittent basis. For example:
      1) Day care programs for the cognitively impaired adults
      2) Home care services may include nurses, aides, therapists, and durable medical equipment companies.
   b. Sub-acute care is designed for patients who are too ill to be discharged from the hospital to a traditional extended care facility or home. There are four types of sub-acute care facilities.
      1) Transitional units are an alternative to continued hospital stays for patients with complex nursing or medical care needs, (eg, deep wound management, complicated vascular or cardiac surgery).

2) General units are for stable patients who require a moderate level of care, (eg, long-term intravenous therapy).
3) Chronic units are for patients with little or no hope of recovery, (eg, ventilator-dependent patients).
4) Long-term transitional units are for patients with medically complex conditions when recovery is expected, (eg, acute ventilator support with difficulty weaning).

c. Nursing homes offer care to patients experiencing debilitating acute or chronic illnesses, (eg, multiple sclerosis, muscular dystrophy, surgery, or trauma).
   1) Skilled nursing facilities provide care that requires licensed health care professionals such as nurses or therapists, (eg, tube feedings, care of stage 3 and 4 wounds).
   2) Nursing facilities care for patients who cannot independently perform activities of daily living.
   3) Residential facilities such as assisted-living centers and group homes offer supervision of patients who are fairly independent and able to perform most or all self-care activities.

CHAPTER 6
Community Health

Community health practice is concerned with promoting health and preventing disease and disability for individuals, families, groups, and communities. This chapter reviews the components of community health practice and the roles in which community health nurses participate in that practice. Private and governmental (US) initiatives influencing cardiac and vascular health are discussed.

Community Health Practice

- Community health practice provides the organizational structure, health care resources, and interdisciplinary collaboration to promote healthy people and communities.

- Community health providers focus on individuals, families, populations, and the community using public health science.

- Community health practice involves the identification of needs and improvement of health for people in communities.

- Community health principles promote the positive connections between populations, their environment, and health of the community.

Community Health Clients

1. Individuals
2. Families
3. Populations are composed of people who occupy or live in a certain area but can also include those with similar attributes or characteristics. The homeless and frail older adults are examples of vulnerable populations.
4. Aggregates are groupings of individuals who are loosely associated with one another by characteristics such as by age, gender, race, risk factors, or health problems. Women with heart disease and people who smoke cigarettes are examples of aggregates.

Types of Communities

1. Geographic communities are defined by the boundaries of towns, cities, or neighborhoods.
2. Common interest communities are collections of people with similar interests or goals that are usually health related, such as smoking cessation or 911 emergency care for acute coronary syndromes.
3. Community of solution is a group of people who come together to solve a problem such as the lack of health care for indigent populations.

Building a Healthy Community

- People work together in a group to identify the needs of the community.
- The group identifies and agrees on goals.
- The group reaches consensus on the strategies to achieve the goals.
- The group collaborates on the actions to attain the desired outcomes.

Levels of Prevention

1. **Primary prevention** includes actions used to keep an illness from occurring.
   a. Altering the susceptibility of people to illness.
   b. Decreasing exposure to substances that may cause disease
   c. Examples are public education on risk factors for coronary heart disease (CHD) or strategies for smoking cessation.
2. **Secondary prevention** includes those actions that are used in the early detection and treatment of health problems. These actions may include hypertension or cholesterol screening, for example.
3. **Tertiary prevention** includes actions to decrease the severity of health problems that have occurred.
   a. The goals are to minimize disability and to preserve or restore function.
   b. These actions may include treatment and rehabilitation for those people who are recovering from a stroke.

Components of Community Health Practice

Health Promotion

1. Health promotion involves efforts to promote optimal health in individuals, families, populations, and communities to:
   a. Increase the period of healthy living for people of all age groups.
   b. Decrease health disparities in groups of people especially for those at high risk for health problems such as cardiovascular diseases.
      1) For example, black women have higher risk for stroke than white women. A program directed specifically to black women might be used to reduce this disparity.
   c. Increase access to clinical preventive services for all people to decrease the incidence or increase early detection of health problems.

Disease Management (DM)

This component of community health practice focuses on disease and illness.

1. Treatment of usually chronic diseases according to clinical guidelines that have been shown to be effective for a majority of the people with the disease.
2. Goal of DM is to prevent medical crises through education, monitoring, and early intervention.
3. DM has demonstrated benefit in populations with diabetes, hypertension, CHD, and heart failure.
4. DM may be accomplished in several ways.
   a. Nursing and other health care services may be provided to individuals with the disease such as home visits from a health care agency, clinics at a homeless shelter or mobile van, or screening, education, counseling, and referrals offered at neighborhood health centers.
   b. Individuals may be offered assistance to obtain treatment such as nutritional counseling for those affected by elevated cholesterol or appointments with cardiologists for problems such as hypertension.

Rehabilitation

This component focuses on reducing disability and restoring function for individuals, families, populations, and communities.

1. Interventions include cognitive and functional assessment, realistic goal setting, counseling and intensive education, physical occupational and speech therapy, environmental modification, and outcome evaluation.
2. Health care organizations involved in rehabilitation include subacute hospitals, long-term care facilities, and home care agencies.
3. For some individuals and their families, participation in groups such as "The Mended Hearts" provides needed support and guidance as they recover from cardiovascular procedures.

Program Development

1. Community health providers develop programs for individuals, families, populations, and communities. Programs may also be aimed at the individuals involved with building healthy communities such as the lay public, interdisciplinary health care providers, and administrators of health care agencies.
2. These programs may focus on screening individuals for health problems, educating people about risk factors or diseases that may impact their health, and teaching community health providers about changes in care delivery or community issues. For example, a community education program that highlights the symptoms of myocardial infarction and emergency care may be developed to increase the public's awareness of this health problem and to improve survival by prompt treatment.

Practice Evaluation

1. Practice evaluation involves the analysis of community health practice and, if indicated, the identification of need for change.
2. There are several types of evaluation that may be used for this process.
   a. Outcome evaluation involves analysis of the impact of community health practice on patient/family knowledge, incidence of disease, recovery from illness, health care visits, and complications. This process can be used to evaluate the quality of care based on the numbers of positive and negative outcomes.
   b. Structure and process evaluation involves the formation and operation of a treatment plan with established performance standards.

1) Structures include the resources to meet the identified needs of the community or goals of the plan. Structures include provider qualifications, licensing, certification, and program funding.
2) Process is the way in which services are delivered.

Community Health Nursing

1. Community health nursing synthesizes theories from public health science, nursing science, and community health practice to address the needs of communities and vulnerable populations.
2. Community health nurses use the nursing process to identify client, family, and group needs, set goals, plan and provide services, and evaluate the impact of their care.
   a. They formulate health promotion strategies for clients, families, and groups.
   b. Community health nurses encourage client and family self-care and independence.
   c. They use aggregate data and analysis to guide and evaluate their work with groups and populations.
3. Community health nurses work collaboratively with health care providers from other disciplines to manage the care of clients.

Roles of Community Health Nurses

1. The **clinician role** includes the care that is provided to individuals, families, groups, and populations. Health care services are focused on holistic practices that integrate principles of health promotion, disease management, and rehabilitation.
2. The **educator role** includes the instruction and counseling of individuals, families, groups, and populations. Community health nurses incorporate principles of adult learning into the educator role. They evaluate the effect of their teaching through program evaluation.
3. The **collaborator role** includes working with health care providers from other disciplines and with different groups of people to meet the needs of individuals, families, groups, and populations.
4. The **researcher role** involves examining community health problems by collecting and analyzing data. Data collection and analysis may be for continuous quality improvement or to answer a research question.
5. The **leadership role** focuses on initiating healthful change with different groups within the community. Community health nurses facilitate the achievement of goals by guiding the work of the

group. Additionally, community health nurses have a leadership role beyond the community by influencing health policies at the state and federal levels.

Practice Settings

1. Homes
2. Ambulatory care sites such as outpatient departments of hospitals, clinics, neighborhood health centers, day care centers, senior centers, health departments, migrant camps, and homeless shelters.
3. Public and private schools (eg, preschool, elementary, middle, secondary vocational, technical, specialized schools, and colleges).
4. Occupational health sites such as clinics in industry.
5. Residential settings including hospice, halfway houses, camps, assisted living, and long-term care facilities.
6. Parishes.

Emerging Needs of Aggregates

1. Aging of the population will have a major impact on community health nursing.
   a. The number of people age 65 years and older in the US will more than double to 70 million by the year 2030 while the numbers of centenarians will increase from 65,000 to 381,000 people.
   b. Many older adults have at least one chronic health problem that requires monitoring by health care providers.
   c. The increased acuity of illness in older adults together with the shortened length of hospital stays will continue to impact community health practice.
2. Increasing cultural diversity of the population is having a significant influence on community health nursing.
   a. The US is becoming more racially and ethnically diverse. The number of minorities living in the US has been projected to increase to 22% by 2020.
   b. Community health nurses and other clinicians need to be culturally competent to meet the needs of the growing African-American, Hispanic, Asian, and other populations.
3. The community mental health movement will continue to affect the responsibilities of community health nurses.
   a. There will be increasing numbers of people needing mental health and substance abuse services in diverse community health settings such as clinics, halfway houses, and residential facilities.

4. Communicable diseases will have a substantial effect on the practice of community health nurses as treatment changes occur. Additionally, there exists the possibility of the emergence of new diseases and the increased virulence of existing health conditions that will affect community health practice.
5. Bioterrorism is a renewed area of concern for the US.
   a. The exact risks associated with the use of biochemical weapons are not known.
   b. Bioterrorism could result in epidemics with the potential to infect large segments of the population because of the delayed onset of symptoms for certain diseases and the increased mobility of individual.

Healthy People 2010

This document identifies goals and objectives that target changes specific to age, gender, and race to improve the health of the US over the next decade. *Healthy People 2010* incorporates previous initiatives such as the 1979 Surgeon General's Report, *Healthy People* and *Healthy People 2000: National Health Promotion and Disease Prevention Objectives. Healthy People 2010* is available on-line at www.health.gov/healthypeople.

Goals

To increase quality and years of healthy life
To eliminate health disparities

Focus Areas

- Approximately 467 objectives were formulated within 28 focus areas. The objectives include interventions intended to achieve the goals by the year 2010.

- Focus areas are listed in Table 6–1.

Leading Health Indicators

1. Reflect the major health concerns in the US at the beginning of the 21st century.
2. Will be used to measure the health of the US over the next decade.
3. The leading health indicators are:
   a. Physical activity
   b. Overweight and obesity
   c. Tobacco use

d. Substance abuse
e. Responsible sexual behavior
f. Mental health
g. Injury and violence
h. Environmental quality
i. Immunization
j. Access to health care

TABLE 6–1.
***Healthy People 2010* Focus Areas**

Access to quality health care
Arthritis, osteoporosis, and chronic back conditions
Cancer
Chronic kidney disease
Diabetes
Disability and secondary conditions
Educational and community-based programs
Environmental health
Family planning
Food safety
Health communication
Heart disease and stroke
HIV
Immunization and infectious disease
Injury and violence prevention
Maternal, infant, and child health
Medical product safety
Mental health and mental disorders
Nutrition and overweight
Occupational safety and health
Oral health
Physical activity and fitness
Public health infrastructure
Respiratory diseases
Sexually transmitted diseases
Substance abuse
Tobacco use
Vision and hearing

Individuals, communities, professional organizations, and federal agencies are involved with *Healthy People 2010* and with measuring the improvement in the health of the people of the US.

Community Initiatives

National Organizations

1. The American Heart Association (AHA), a national voluntary organization, has sponsored several national campaigns to reduce the risk of cardiovascular disease (CVD) for individuals and communities.
   a. "My Heart Watch" is a community education program for preventing heart attack and stroke that includes risk assessment tools, cardiovascular health information, and chat rooms.
   b. "Take Wellness to Heart" is an initiative that is focused on increasing the awareness of women about their risk for heart disease and stroke.
   c. "Operation Heartbeat" is a community education program designed to increase community knowledge and support for emergency care related to cardiac arrest.
2. The National Heart, Lung, and Blood Institute sponsors several national initiatives that are focused on the goals of Healthy People 2010 and community education.
   a. "Act in Time to Heart Attack Signs" is a public education campaign to increase awareness about emergency care of heart attack victims.
   b. "National High Blood Pressure Education Program" is to increase public awareness of hypertension and its treatment.
   c. "Detection, Evaluation, and Treatment of High Blood Cholesterol in Adults (Adult Treatment Panel III)" is a national cholesterol education program to decrease the morbidity and mortality associated with CHD by lowering blood cholesterol.
   d. "Obesity Education Initiative" is to decrease the incidence of obesity and physical inactivity thus reducing the risk for CVD and diabetes.
   e. "Developing a Woman's Heart Health Education Action Plan" is a new cardiovascular education program for women, especially those at high risk.

State and Local Initiatives

State and local chapters of voluntary organizations such as the AHA promote cardiovascular initiatives through public and professional involvement in community education programs.

Other organizations, such as schools and health care agencies, are involved with community education programs to reduce the risk of cardiovascular diseases by increasing the public's awareness and by implementing screening initiatives.

Many state governments are using *Healthy People 2010* as a framework for building healthy communities. They are using the leading health indicators and objectives to promote healthy living for the people in their respective states and to reduce disparities in health. Another focus of the *Healthy People 2010* initiative is to make the community a healthier place to live.

CHAPTER 7
Cardiac and Vascular Risk

Coronary Heart Disease (CHD)

Risk Identification

1. The term "cardiac risk factor" describes the characteristics found in healthy individuals that are independently related to the subsequent development of CHD. These characteristics are termed modifiable and non-modifiable.
2. Modifiable cardiac risk factors include: hypertension, hypercholesterolemia, low highdensity lipoprotein cholesterol (HDL-C) level, diabetes mellitus, tobacco use, and obesity.
3. Non-modifiable cardiac risk factors include: age, gender, and a family history of premature CHD in a first degree relative (males <55 years, females <65 years).
4. Patients having experienced a CHD event have the highest risk of experiencing another event. This risk is greater than 20% over 10 years.
5. Patients with a CHD risk equivalent have the same level of CHD risk (>20% in 10 years), but have not yet experienced a CHD event.
6. There are 3 CHD risk equivalent groups:
    a. Patients with 2 or more cardiac risk factors.
    b. Patients with other forms of atherosclerotic vascular disease: peripheral vascular disease, abdominal aortic aneurysm, and symptomatic carotid artery disease.
    c. Patients with type 2 diabetes.
7. Patients with a 10 year risk of a coronary event 20% or greater should be treated as aggressively as people who already have CHD regardless of symptom profile.

Core Risk Factors

1. Modifiable
    a. Hypertension
        1) There is a 27% increase in risk for every 7 mmHg increase in diastolic blood pressure (BP).
        2) Isolated systolic hypertension (SBP >160 mmHg) markedly increases the risk for nonfatal myocardial infarction (MI) and

cardiovascular death among general population samples and low-risk groups.

3) Pulse pressure, a potential surrogate for vascular wall stiffness, predicts first and recurrent MI.
4) With effective antihypertensive therapy, CHD risk is reduced but not to baseline.
5) BP goal should be lower in people with diabetes and those with renal disease (eg, <130/85).

b. Dyslipidemia
1) Estimates suggest that half of American adults have cholesterol levels greater than 200 mg/dl and that 20% of American adults have cholesterol levels of 240 mg/dl or greater.
2) A 10% increase in serum cholesterol is associated with a 20–30% increase in risk for CHD.
3) The lower the concentration of HDL-C, the greater the risk of CHD.
   a) HDL-C below 40 mg/dl is classified as low.
   b) HDL-C above 60 mg/dl is classified as high and is associated with lower CHD risk.
4) Evidence supports elevated triglyceride (TG) level as an independent predictor of CHD risk.
   a) TG levels in the borderline high and high range (150 mg/dl to 500 mg/dl) are associated with increased CHD risk.
5) Saturated fatty acids increase low-density lipoprotein cholesterol (LDL-C) levels. Monounsaturated fatty acids lower LDL-C and do not affect HDL-C.

c. Diabetes Mellitus
1) Type 2 diabetes accounts for about 90% of all diabetes cases. Underlying causes of type 2 diabetes are obesity, physical inactivity, and genetics.
2) Diabetes is associated with an accelerated atheromatous process resulting in increased risk for atherosclerotic disease. This risk qualifies diabetes as a CHD risk equivalent (10 year risk of CHD event >20%).
3) Age-adjusted rates for CHD are 2–3 times higher among men with diabetes and 3–7 times higher among women with diabetes than among their counterparts without diabetes.
4) Three fourths of all deaths among individuals with diabetes result from CHD. By age 40, CHD is the leading cause of death in both men and women with diabetes.
   a) There is a 2-fold increase in mortality in those who have diabetes at the time of MI, as well as increased risk for heart failure.

5) Metabolic syndrome represents a constellation of lipid and nonlipid risk factors of metabolic origin. Metabolic syndrome is closely linked to a generalized disorder termed insulin resistance, implicating impaired insulin action.
   a) Excess body fat (particularly abdominal obesity) and physical inactivity promote the development of insulin resistance.
   b) The diagnosis of metabolic syndrome is made when 3 or more of the risk determinants are present:
      1. Waist circumference (at the iliac crest) >40 inches for men or ≥35 inches for women.
      2. Triglyceride ≥150 mg/dl.
      3. HDL-C <40 mg/dl for men and <50 mg/dl for women.
      4. BP ≥135 mm Hg systolic or ≥85 mm Hg diastolic.
      5. Fasting blood glucose ≥110 mg/dl.

2. Non-modifiable
   a. Age
      1) 85% of people who die of CHD are age 65 years and older.
      2) About 80% of CHD mortality in people below age 65 occurs during the first MI.
      3) Lifetime risk of developing CHD after age 40 is 49% for men and 32% for women.
      4) In general, men (ages 35–65) have a higher risk for CHD than women. In women, the onset of CHD is generally delayed by 10–15 years (ages 45–75).
   b. Gender
      1) The incidence of CHD in women lags behind men 10 years for total CHD and by 20 years for more serious clinical events such as MI and sudden death.
      2) In men, the 3 major presentations of CHD (angina, sudden death, and MI) are equally distributed. Women with CHD more frequently present with angina symptoms.
      3) CHD kills more women than all cancers combined.
      4) In 50% of men and 63% of women who died suddenly of CHD, there were no previous symptoms of this disease.
      5) 25% of men and 38% of women will die within 1 year after having an initial recognized MI.
      6) Within 6 years after a recognized heart attack 18% of men and 35% of women will have another heart attack.
      7) Women in the US are more likely to die of CHD than any other cause.
         a) CHD rates in women after menopause are 2–3 times those of women before menopause.

b) Women taking oral contraceptives who also smoke have an increased risk of CHD.

c. Ehnicity
   1) Blacks and Hispanics are the two largest minority groups in the US. In 1993, CHD death rates (per 100,000 population) were:
      a) 133.0 for white males and 139.3 for black males (4.7% higher in black than white males).
      b) 63.8 for white females and 85.7 for black females (34.3% higher in black than white females).
      c) For age 35–74 years, the death rate from MI for black women is more than 38% higher than that for white women.
   2) Among American Indians, ages 65–74, the rates (per 1,000 population) of new and recurrent heart attacks are 25.1 for men and 9.1 for women.
d. Family history
   1) Family history is considered positive when CHD events are confirmed in first-degree male relatives before age 55 years or first-degree female relatives before 65 years.
   2) Typically, the presence of premature CHD in the family history is accompanied by a family history of other cardiac risk factors.
e. Socioeconomic
   1) In developed countries, CHD is a disease concentrated in the lower socioeconomic, less educated sector of the population.
   2) In developing countries, CHD is a disease of urban middle and upper classes and is virtually unknown in the traditional country villages.
   3) Among the cardiovascular diseases, CHD is the leading cause of death in urban areas in rapidly industrializing countries (eg, China).

Life Habit Risk Factors (Modifiable)

1. Smoking
   a. Smoking is the most important modifiable risk factor for CHD accounting for 400,000 deaths annually.
   b. Compared to non-smokers, those who consume >20 cigarettes per day have a 2- to 3-fold increase in CHD risk.
   c. Smoking acts synergistically with oral contraceptives to increase CHD risk.
   d. Smoking may enhance oxidation of LDL-C, as well as decrease HDL-C, impair coronary vasodilation, increase C-reactive pro-

tein and fibrinogen, and enhance monocyte adhesion to endothelial cells.

e. Smoking increases risk for coronary spasm and for ventricular ectopic activity.
f. Smoking cessation decreases the risk of first MI by 65%.

2. Obesity
   a. Obesity adversely influences other vascular risk factors, causing hypertension, dyslipidemia, glucose intolerance, and insulin resistance.
   b. Obesity is independently associated with left ventricular hypertrophy (LVH), while weight loss can reduce left ventricular mass.
   c. Waist-hip ratio, a surrogate for abdominal obesity, is an independent marker of vascular risk for women and older men.
   d. Waist circumference measurements which indicate increased risk are >40" in men and >35" in women.
3. Physical Inactivity
   a. Mortality data suggests that >200,000 deaths result from inactivity annually.
   b. Physical inactivity is associated with other CHD risk factors including decreased HDL-C, insulin resistance, and hypertension.
   c. Physically fit but overweight people have a CHD risk similar to that of people without CHD risk factors.
4. Diet and Nutrition
   a. The effect of diet on risk is mediated through lipids, BP, and obesity.
   b. There is growing interest in the Mediterranean diet which is rich in monounsaturated fats as well as fruits and vegetables.
5. Alcohol Abuse
   a. The relative risk of death from CVD in moderate drinkers compared to non-drinkers was 0.7 in men and 0.6 in women.
   b. The protective effect of moderate alcohol intake on CVD may be mediated through increased HDL-C, decreased platelet aggregation, and fibrinolysis.
   c. Alcohol abuse leads to hypertension, hemorrhagic stroke, and sudden cardiac death.
6. Mental Stress
   a. Mental stress can cause coronary vasoconstriction, particularly in atherosclerotic arteries, reducing myocardial oxygen supply.
   b. Catecholamines promote alterations in thrombosis and coagulation, favoring clot formation.
   c. There have been documented increases in coronary deaths during missile attacks and earthquakes.

Emerging Risk Factors

1. Hyperhomocysteinemia
   a. Elevated homocysteine levels are independently associated with CVD.
   b. Mechanisms include endothelial toxicity, accelerated oxidation of LDL-C, impaired endothelial-derived relaxation factor, and decreased flow-mediated arterial vasodilation.
   c. Deficiencies in folate, Vitamin B–12 and B–6 lead to elevated serum levels of homocysteine while supplementation decreases levels.
2. Hypercoagulability
   a. Fibrinogen is positively associated with age, obesity, smoking, diabetes, and LDL-C, and inversely associated with HDL-C, alcohol abuse, physical activity, and exercise level.
   b. The relative risk of CV events is 1.8 times higher for individuals in the top as compared with the bottom third of base line fibrinogen concentration.
   c. Factor VII levels, plasminogen activator inhibition, and platelet aggregation have been associated with CVD risk.
3. Estrogen Status
   a. In premenopausal women, the age-adjusted incidence and mortality for CHD is lower than in men, however the rates converge after menopause.
   b. Aside from lipid benefits (deceased LDL-C with increased HDL-C, apo A1, and triglycerides), estrogen decreases LDL oxidation, promotes endothelial vasodilation, decreases fibrinolytic capacity, and enhances glucose metabolism.
   c. Post-menopausal hormone replacement therapy reduces CV risk by 35–45%.
   d. The HERS (Heart and Estrogen/Progestin Replacement Study) trial of women with preexisting coronary disease found no difference in risk for nonfatal MI or CV death between women assigned to HRT or placebo.
4. Lipoprotein (a) [Lp(a)]
   a. Studies suggest a positive association between Lp(a) and vascular risk, although levels are elevated after acute ischemia, making measurement unreliable.
   b. Limitations on the utility of Lp(a) screening include lack of testing standardization, variability of levels among racial groups, and unclear predictive value.
   c. LDL reduction markedly reduces any adverse hazard associated with Lp(a).

5. Triglyceride (TG)
   a. Elevated levels of TG are related to decreased HDL-C, elevated levels of small dense LDL particles, and procoagulant state.
   b. Lower triglyceride result in a significant reduction in CVD events.
6. Oxidative Stress
   a. Vitamin E, beta carotene, and other natural antioxidants have failed to show a beneficial effect on CHD risk or disease progression.
   b. American Heart Association discourages the use of antioxidant vitamin supplements, and recommends dietary modifications.
7. Left Ventricular Hypertrophy (LVH)
   a. The incidence of LVH increases with age, BP, and obesity.
   b. LVH is independently associated with increased incidence of CVD.
   c. There are no conclusive data to support the theory that a reduction in LV mass can improve CV outcome independent of a decrease in BP.
8. Inflammatory Processes
   a. Evidence linking inflammation to atherosclerosis stems from studies focusing on acute and chronic phases of CHD.
   b. Acute phase reactants such as high-sensitivity C-reactive protein (hs-CRP), ICAM–1 (adhesion molecules), and IL–6 and tumor necrosis factor (cytokines) are inflammatory markers measured in the plasma.
   c. hs-CRP and serum amyloid A have been shown in several studies to be markers of risk.
      1) Individuals with elevated hs-CRP levels had a relative risk of future vascular events 3–4 times higher than individuals with lower levels, effects that were independent of other risk factors.
   d. Numerous infectious agents are being considered as possible causes of vascular injury and inflammation (eg, cytomegalovirus, *Chlamydia pneumoniae, Helicobactor pylori,* herpes simplex virus).
   e. Extravascular foci of chronic infection might include gingiva, the bronchi, the urinary tract (including the prostate), or diverticular disease.

Risk Stratification

The Framingham Heart Study has developed and updated mathematical health risk appraisal models that relate risk factors to the probability of developing CHD.

1. The new sex-specific models incorporate primary and secondary, or subsequent, risk appraisal.
2. Primary models assess CHD risk in persons free of CV disease, including MI, coronary insufficiency, angina pectoris, stroke, TIA, heart failure, and intermittent claudication.
   a. Risk factors included in the Framingham model are triglyceride level, alcohol use, and menopausal status.
3. Subsequent CHD models are applicable for individuals with a history of CHD or ischemic stroke who have survived the acute period after the event.
   a. Risk factors include age, blood lipid levels (total cholesterol and HDL-C), diabetes, SBP, and smoking.
4. The probability of developing CHD within a 10-year period is calculated by assigning points to each risk factor. Points are summed and probability of CHD read from a Framingham Risk Table.
5. The risk tables are included in the appendix of the ATP-III Guidelines.

Example of a 55 year-old, male smoker with elevated cholesterol and high blood pressure.

Age	6 points
Total cholesterol/triglyceride	10 points
Non-diabetic	0 points
Smoker	4 points
SBP 140 mmHg on medication	4 points

Total points = 24 which indicates a 9% probability of a CHD event within 10 years.

Stroke

Risk Identification

1. Stroke is the third leading cause of death in the US.
2. There are 700,000 incident strokes annually.
3. 4.4 millions people are stroke survivors.
4. The most common variety of complete strokes is atherothrombotic brain infarcts (61% excluding TIAs) followed by cerebral embolus (24%).
   a. 83% were ischemic
   b. 10% were intracerebral hemorrhage
   c. 7% were subarachnoid hemorrhage
   d. 7.6% of ischemic strokes and 37.5% of hemorrhagic strokes result in death within 30 days.

Core Risk Factors

1. Nonmodifiable
   a. Age
      1) The risk of stroke doubles in each successive decade after 55 years of age.
      2) 28% of stroke victims are <65 years of age.
   b. Gender
      1) Stroke prevalence is higher in men than women with the exception of those 35 to 44 years old and those >85 years in whom women have slightly greater age-specific incidence than men.
      2) Fatality rates are higher in women than men; one in six women will die of stroke.
   c. Race/ethnicity
      1) Blacks and some Hispanic Americans have an almost 2-fold increased incidence of stroke in comparison with whites.
      2) The increased incidence of stroke in blacks is due to higher prevalence of HTN, obesity (in women), diabetes, increased LP(a) levels, smoking (in men), and low socioeconomic levels.
      3) Black men and women were more likely to die of stroke than white men and women.
      4) Chinese and Japanese men and women have a high incidence of stroke.
   d. Family History
      1) Paternal and maternal history of stroke may be associated with increased stroke risk.
      2) Mechanisms include genetic heritability of stroke risk factors, inheritance of susceptibility to effects of risk factors, and familial sharing of cultural, environmental and lifestyle factors.
      3) There is a 5-fold increase in stroke prevalence among monozygotic (identical) twins in comparison with dizygotic (fraternal) twins.
   e. Socioeconomic Factors
      1) In one study, women living in deprived areas had an increased risk of stroke.
2. Modifiable
   a. HTN
      1) Major risk factor for both cerebral infarct and intracerebral hemorrhage.
      2) The incidence of stroke increases in proportion to both systolic and diastolic BP.

3) Two-thirds of people who experience a first stroke have BP >160/95.
4) Isolated systolic hypertension (ISH) is an important risk factor for older adults.
5) ISH is defined by JNC VII as systolic BP >160 mmHg and diastolic BP <90 mmHg.
6) The SHEP (Systolic Hypertension in the Elderly Program) trial showed a 36% reduction in incidence of stroke with antihypertensive therapy.

b. Diabetes, Hyperinsulinemia, and Insulin Resistance
1) Individuals with insulin-dependent diabetes have an increased susceptibility to atherosclerosis and risk factors (eg, HTN, obesity, abnormal blood lipids).
2) Metabolic risk factors have been identified in some individuals with Type 2 diabetes known as the Metabolic Syndrome, which includes hyperinsulinemia and insulin resistance, and results in hyperglycemia, increased VLDL, decreased HDL, and HTN.
3) The relative risk of ischemic stroke in individuals with diabetes ranges from 1.8 to 8.0.
4) Individuals with glucose intolerance have double the risk of brain infarction compared to those with normal gluocose tolerance.
5) Tight control of HTN in individuals with diabetes significantly reduces stroke incidence.

c. Asymptomatic Carotid Stenosis
1) Cerebral ischemic events occurred more frequently among patients with severe (>75%) carotid artery stenosis, progressing carotid artery stenosis, or heart disease, and in men.
2) The annual risk of stroke was 3.2% over 5 years with 60–99% carotid artery stenosis.
3) Some studies suggest that the rate of stroke may be higher for patients with progressing stenosis and those with more severe stenosis, than in those with stable disease.
4) As with asymptomatic carotid bruit, an asymptomatic carotid artery stenosis is an important indicator of concomitant ischemic cardiac disease.

e. Atrial Fibrillation (A fib)
1) The annual risk of stroke for patients with nonvalvular A fib is 3–5% with the condition being responsible for 50% of thromboembolic strokes.
2) Two-thirds of strokes in A fib patients are cardioembolic.

3) Framingham Heart Study showed a dramatic increase in stroke risk with A fib in advancing age: in 50–59 year olds, the increase risk was 1.5% and in 80–89 year olds, the risk increased to 23.5%.
4) Predictors of high risk for stroke were advanced age, prior TIA or stroke, systolic HTN, history of HTN, impaired LV function, diabetes, and women >75 years of age.

f. Other Cardiac Diseases
   1) 20% of ischemic strokes are due to cardiogenic embolism from other cardiac diseases (eg, ischemic cardiomyopathy, valvular heart disease, and intracardiac congenital defects).
   2) MI
      a) 80% of men and 11% of women will have a stroke within 6 years after MI.
      b) Post-MI development of A fib is a common source of cardiogenic emboli.
      c) Overall occurrence of stroke in acute MI is 0.8%, with 0.6% being ischemic.
      d) Risk factors for stroke post-MI demonstrated preexisting factors such as previous stroke, A fib, old age, heart failure, and heart rate >100 bpm were more important than treatment with thrombolysis which was a borderline significant risk factor.

g. Cardiac Surgical Procedures
   1) Perioperative stroke occurs in 1–7% of patients having coronary artery bypass grafting.
   2) History of prior neurologic events, advanced age, female gender, diabetes, and A fib (only if accompanied by low cardiac output syndrome) were identified as risk factors for early and delayed stroke.
   3) Other factors include the duration of cardiopulmonary bypass and the presence of aortic atherosclerosis and macroemboli.
   4) Hospital mortality for stroke was 24.8% compared to 2% for the rest of the patient population.

h. Hyperlipidemia
   1) One study showed a continuous and progressive increase in thromboembolic stroke rates with rising levels of cholesterol.
   2) An inverse relationship exists between HDL-C level and stroke risk. (High HDL-C is associated with lower stroke risk.)

3) In the 4S trial (Simvastatin Survival Study), the simvastatin-treated group experienced a 51% reduction in ischemic nonembolic stroke.

i. Sleep Apnea
   1) Sleep-related breathing disorder appears to contribute as a risk factor for stroke.
   2) Pathogenic mechanisms are decreased cerebral perfusion, increased coagulability, and diurnal HTN.

j. Sickle Cell Disease (SCD)
   1) The prevalence of stroke by age 20 in patients with SCD is at least 11%.

Life Habit Risk Factors

1. Smoking
   a. Effects of smoking are multifactorial, affecting both systemic vasculature and blood rheology.
   b. Some effects include increased arterial wall stiffness, increased fibrinogen levels, increased platelet aggregation, decreased HDL, and increased hematocrit.
   c. Smokers have two times the relative risk of cerebral infarct in comparison with non-smokers.
   d. The relative risk of stroke among former smokers was 1.34 in the Nurses' Health Study and 1.26 in the Physician's Health Study.
   e. Stroke risk declined to the level of non-smokers at five years from cessation.
   f. Exposure to environmental tobacco smoke increased the risk of coronary events from 20–70%.
2. Obesity
   a. Obesity increases the risk of stroke due to the association with HTN, hyperglycemia, and abnormal blood lipids.
   b. Abdominal obesity in men is an indepedent risk factor for stroke.
   c. Weight gain in women is an independent risk factor for stroke.
3. Physical Inactivity
   a. Several studies have demonstrated an inverse association between levels of physical activity and stroke incidence.
   b. Protective effects of physical activity may be mediated through its role in controlling HTN, cardiovascular disease, diabetes, and body weight. Other mechanisms include decreasing fibrinogen and platelet activity, and increasing tissue plasminogen activator activity and HDL concentration.

4. Diet and Nutrition
   a. Data regarding the effects of general nutritional status on stroke are limited.
   b. An increment of one serving of fruit and vegetables per day was associated with a 6% decreased risk of stroke.
5. Alcohol Abuse
   a. There is a protective effect against stroke with 2 drinks per day (one drink = 12 oz beer, 4 oz wine, 1.5 oz 80-proof spirits, or 1 oz 100-proof spirits).
   b. Risk for stroke increases for those drinking >5 drinks per day compared to nondrinkers.
   c. There is a direct dose-dependent effect of alcohol consumption on hemorrhagic stroke.
6. Drug Abuse
   a. Studies examining the effects of illicit drug abuse on stroke risk have been neutral.
   b. Pathogenesis of stroke in this subset of patients is likely multifactorial; eg, sudden increases in BP, vasculitis, etc.

Emerging Risk Factors

1. Hyperhomocysteinemia
   a. Homocysteine concentrations increase with age, with men having higher levels than women, especially at younger ages.
   b. Case-controlled studies have shown an association between hyperhomocysteinemeia and stroke. However no randomized trials have been done to determine whether lowering levels decreases the risk of stroke.
2. Hypercoagulability
   a. Limited data exists on the association between antiphospholipid antibodies and cerebrovascular arterial thrombosis.
   b. In one study, elevated anticardiolipin antibody was demonstrated to be an independent stroke risk factor across three ethnic groups, conferring a 4-fold increased risk of ischemic stroke.
   c. Studies examining other coagulation abnormalities (factor V Leiden, protein C deficiency, protein S deficiency, antithrombin III deficiency) have been poorly adjusted for other stroke risks.
3. Hormone Replacement Therapy (HRT)
   a. The impact of postmenopausal HRT on stroke risk appears to be neutral with the exception of the Framingham Heart Study that found a 2.6-fold increase in the relative risk of atherothrombotic stroke among women receiving HRT compared to non-users.

4. Oral Contraceptive Use
   a. The risk of ischemic stroke is increased in oral contraceptive users, but the absolute increase in risk is small due to the low stroke incidence in this population.
5. Lipoprotein (a) [Lp(a)]
   a. Lp(a) is an independent risk factor for ischemic stroke especially in young adults. However, other studies have not supported this finding.
   b. The ratio of apolipoprotein b to apolipoprotein a–1 was associated with carotid atheroma.
6. Inflammatory Processes
   a. Atherosclerosis, the most common cause of stroke, is now believed to be a disease of chronic inflammation.
   b. *Chlamydia pneumoniae* has been identified in atherosclerotic carotid plaques and localizes to regions of altered plaque morphology.
      1) The relationship between serum anti-body titers to *C. pneumoniae* and stroke is likely due to its role in plaque progression and destabilizaton.
      2) The benefit of antibiotic therapy for *C. pneumoniae* is unclear.
   c. High-sensitivity C-reactive protein (hs-CRP) and serum amyloid A, markers of acute infection, may be associated with stroke.
      1) Levels are elevated in smokers and in healthy men with vascular risk factors.
      2) There is a significant and positive association between plasma hs-CRP levels and risk for stroke.

Risk Stratification

Framingham Heart Study has developed a health risk appraisal for the purpose of predicting the risk of stroke.

1. Risk factors measured include age, systolic BP, use of antihypertensive therapy, diabetes, smoking prior CVD (coronary heart disease, cardiac failure, intermittent claudication), atrial fibrillation, and LVH measured by electrocardiogram.
2. The 10-year probability of stroke is determined according to a point system. Points associated with each risk factor are summed. Risk associated with number of points is determined from a Framingham Stroke Risk Profile.

Example of a 70 year-old male, smoker with hypertension and diabetes.

70 y.o. male	5 points
SBP 180 mm Hg	7 points
On HTN therapy	2 points
Diabetic	2 points
Smoker	3 points
Total = 19 points = 32.9% probability	

This patient has a 32.9% 10-year probability of stroke equating to a stroke risk 2.4 time higher than average.

Peripheral Vascular Disease

Risk Identification

Peripheral vascular disease (PVD) is a manifestation of the atherosclerotic process that affects 12% to14% of the general population.

1. Approximately one half of the 8.4 million Americans with PVD are symptomatic.
   a. An estimated 840,000 present with critical leg ischemia.
   b. Approximately 3.4 million present with symptoms of intermittent claudication (IC).
2. The prevalence of symptoms of IC increases with age.
   a. 5% of men and 2.5% of women over age 60 years experience symptoms of IC.
   b. Three times as many have an abnormal ankle brachial index.
3. Symptoms of IC are usually stable over a 5 to 10 year period.
   a. 73% have no significant change in symptoms.
   b. 16% experience deterioration in symptoms.
   c. 7% require peripheral vascular bypass surgery.
   d. 4% have a major amputation.

Core Risk Factors

1. Diabetes
   a. Individuals with diabetes are 3 to 4 times more likely to develop PVD than those without diabetes.
   b. The atheromatous process in individuals with diabetes particularly affects smaller more distal vessels, making options for revascularization more difficult.

2. HTN
   a. Those with HTN are 1.5 to 2.5 times more likely to develop PVD than those without.
   b. HTN is a significant risk factor for atherosclerosis when it coexists with other risk factors such as smoking and diabetes.
3. Hyperlipidemia
   a. Relative risk for developing PVD is 1.1 per 10 mg/dL increase in total cholesterol.
4. Age
   a. The prevalence of PVD in Americans increases with age:18
      1) 3% ages 40–59 (about 2.1 million people).
      2) 8% ages 60–69 (about 1.6 million people).
      3) 19% age 70 and older (4.7 million people).
   b. In men, half of new cases of PVD present in the fifth decade. In general disease presentation is later in women. By the seventh decade, prevalence is similar.
5. Ethnicity
   a. Risks of developing PVD seem to be race neutral and are similar in white, African-American and Japanese-American people.

Life Habit Risk Factor

1. Tobacco use
   a. Cigarette smoking is the most prominent high risk behavior in developing PVD.
   b. Smokers are 2.5 to 3 times more likely to have PVD than non-smokers.

Emerging Risk Factor

1. Hyperhomocysteinemia
   a. Genetic and nutritional factors, such as deficiencies in folate, vitamin B12 and vitamin B6, are associated with increased levels of homocysteine (>15 mmol/l). It is suggested that hyperhomocysteinemia is an independent risk factor associated with PVD.
   b. The relative risk of developing PVD in those with hyperhomocysteinemia is 1.7–2.6.

Risk Stratification

1. PVD is an independent predictor of increased risk of cardiac death.
   a. Half of patients presenting with PVD have symptoms of CHD or electrocardiograghic abnormality.
   b. 90% of those with PVD have abnormalities on coronary angiography.
   c. 40% have duplex evidence of carotid artery disease.
2. All-cause mortality rates are 2–3 times higher for those with PVD than those without PVD.
3. Over 30% of cardiovascular patients have peripheral arterial occlusive disease.
4. Symptomatic PVD carries at least a 30% risk of death within 5 years and almost 50% within 10 years due primarily to MI (60%) or stroke (12%).
   a. Asymptomatic patients (ankle brachial index <0.9) have a 2 to 5-fold increased risk of fatal or nonfatal cardiovascular events.

CHAPTER 8

Risk Reduction

The presence of CVD is associated with characteristic modifiable and non-modifiable risk factors. There is general agreement, although not consensus, that modifying risk factors can reduce the likelihood of developing or slow the progression of CVD. This chapter provides guidelines for primary, secondary and tertiary prevention strategies for risk reduction.

Levels of Prevention

Levels of prevention comprise a 3-tiered model of intervention that promotes optimum health by promoting health, preventing disability or reducing disease progression, reducing morbidity and mortality, and preserving function and quality of life. The presence or absence of clinical disease defines the level of prevention and ***not*** the nature of the intervention.

Primary Prevention

1. Primary prevention is concerned with promoting health and delaying or preventing disease in the general population. Primary preventive interventions occur before there is a clinical indication of disease.
2. Primary prevention of CVD involves helping children make healthy lifestyle choices and avoid choices that increase risk (eg, tobacco use, physical inactivity, excessive body weight, and high-fat diet).
3. Primary prevention strategies include education, public law and policy (eg, no tobacco for people <18 years of age), the reduction of environmental hazards (eg, secondhand smoke), and chemoprophylaxsis (eg, aspirin use among individuals without known CVD).

Secondary Prevention

1. Secondary prevention is concerned with the early detection of disease or health problems and intensive treatment while the outcome can be favorably altered.
2. Secondary prevention of CVD involves detecting and treating risk factors such as HTN and dyslipidemia before a cardiac or vascular

event (eg, MI, stroke, or arterial occlusion) occurs. Secondary prevention includes intensive management of risk after an acute event for purposes of preventing subsequent events and death.

3. The goal of secondary prevention is to control risk factors and to achieve therapeutic protection of arteries from plaque rupture.

Tertiary Prevention

1. Tertiary prevention is concerned with the treatment of the disease or health problem to avoid negative sequelae and to return the individual to the highest possible functional level.
2. Tertiary prevention of CVD includes post-stroke rehabilitation programs and programs that modify work responsibilities to enable people to return to work after an acute cardiac event. (Cardiac rehabilitation programs use both secondary and tertiary prevention strategies. The emphasis on adopting a healthy lifestyle to prevent future events is an example of secondary prevention. The emphasis on resuming role responsibilities after an acute cardiac event is an example of tertiary prevention.)
3. The goals of tertiary prevention are to minimize disability and to preserve or restore function and quality of life.

CVD Prevention

1. Preventing CVD requires individual, community, and societal effort.
2. Data support the benefits of preventing and treating CVD.
3. CVD is present in almost fifty million Americans and is the leading cause of death for both men and women in the US.
4. CVD is a large source of the chronic disability and health costs encountered in the world making prevention a cost-effective goal with far reaching consequences.
5. Lifestyle modifications can reduce the risk of developing CVD by approximately 50%.
6. Mortality from CVD in all races has been reduced by about 50% from the 1960s. It is believed that this reduction represents the effect of multidisciplinary prevention and management strategies including changes in dietary and smoking habits, physical activity, and lipid and HTN management.
7. Future research should be multidisciplinary, aimed at prevention across the lifespan, and examine disease progression and precipitants of acute events among various ethnic, racial, and socioeconomic groups.

Risk Factor Modification

1. Many of the risk factors of CVD are modifiable: physical inactivity, tobacco use, obesity, HTN, diabetes, and lipid management.
2. Successfully applied preventive interventions can reduce mortality and morbidity, acute coronary event rate, and re-hospitalization for disease progression — thereby reducing health care costs.
3. An organized system to reduce risk through a variety of preventive strategies is more likely to be effective than single strategies applied unsystematically.
   a. Health needs assessment can identify populations at risk and prioritize individual and environmental interventions.
4. Health care professionals need to assess patient need for information, ability to comply, and barriers to successful change before selecting strategies to promote change in lifestyles.
5. Educating individuals about the benefits that can be obtained from risk factor reduction may motivate individuals to trial and then to adhere to lifestyle changes.

Relative Risk

Relative risk is the ratio of the likelihood of CHD developing with and without a given risk factor. Absolute risk is the probability of developing CHD in a specified finite period, meaning a high relative risk early in life may correspond to a high absolute risk later in life.

Exercise and Activity

Physical activity can be cost-effective, flexibly scheduled, and need not require special equipment or location.

Activity Guidelines

1. Physical activity is recommended for primary and secondary prevention of CVD.
   a. An active lifestyle from childhood is key to primary prevention of atherosclerosis.
   b. School programs should include aerobic activities (such as running, swimming, walking, and dancing) and resistance exercises with freeweights or exercise machines.
   c. Physical inactivity is associated with at least a 2-fold increase in risk for cardiac events.
2. Exercise and activity reduce CVD risk through lowering blood pressure, reducing platelet aggregation, raising HDL-C and improving glucose metabolism.

a. Physical activity also helps psychologically to improve mood (reduces feelings of depression and anxiety).
b. Personal satisfaction is an important consideration in selecting an activity that will become an almost everyday choice.
c. Intensity, duration, and frequency of exercise as well as mode and progression need to be included in exercise prescriptions.

3. Primary prevention
   a. All children and adults should accumulate at least 30 minutes of moderate physical activity on most, if not all, days of the week.
      1) Activities of moderate intensity include brisk walking, cycling, swimming, and yard work.
      2) Chilren (and adults) who already meet this standard of activity will receive additional benefits from increased duration or intensity of activity.
   b. The American Heart Association (AHA) recommends vigorous activity for at least 30–60 minutes, 3–4 days per week at 50–75% of maximum heart rate for most healthy individuals.
   c. Intensity may be measured by the onset of breathlessness or fatigue. The Borg scale rates perceived exertion (scaled from 6 to 20) and is used in outpatient cardiac rehabilitation programs.
   d. Individuals with acute illnesses such as influenza or upper respiratory infections should decrease or stop physical activity for up to 2 to 3 weeks, while recovery occurs.
   e. Exercise testing (measurement of functional capacity) is not required for primary prevention
   f. Physical activity can be accumulated in intervals of 10–15 minutes throughout the day to total 30 to 60 minutes.
   g. For those unable to maintain or increase intensity level, frequency and duration should be increased to compensate.
4. Secondary prevention

   Secondary prevention is physical activity occurring after a heart attack or stroke has occurred or for those at great risk of developing CVD. The goal is to prevent further cardiac and vascular events or disability from disease.
   a. Walking has been shown to increase survival, decrease recurrent events, and may slow the progression of CVD.
   b. Additional benefits of walking include improved quality of life, decreased incidence of hospitalization, and reduced need for repeat invasive procedures, such as angioplasty, stenting, or laser therapies.
   c. Walking for patients with intermittent claudication should be 60 minutes a day with stops for rest if pain develops.

d. Regular light or moderate physical activity started in middle age or older age has been shown to reduce mortality from CVD.

5. Tertiary prevention

   Tertiary prevention minimizes disability, improves function, and improves quality of life.

   a. Exercise testing is recommended before starting an exercise program after an acute cardiac event.

Safety Considerations

1. Risk should be assessed, preferably with an exercise test, prior to the initiation of an exercise prescription following a cardiac event.
2. In the early recovery period following a cardiac event, (eg, during the second week), the goal is to walk 5 to 10 minutes and perform nonresistive range of motion.
3. Later in recovery, activity is guided by the results of a symptom-limited exercise test and includes:
   a. Warm-up and cool-down periods before and after exercise involving large muscle groups performed for a total of 20 to 30 minutes at least 3 to 4 times per week.
   b. Low risk patients are characterized by the absence of ischemia and significant dysrhythmia.
      1) The majority of patients requiring secondary prevention is classified as low risk and can implement an exercise prescription at home or in the community.
      2) In low risk patients, primary prevention guidelines apply.
      3) Follow-up exercise testing is recommended on an annual basis.
   c. Activities progress as tolerated up to a moderate level of intensity.
   d. During early recovery from an acute event and in the initial stages of an exercise program, an increase of 20 beats per minute above resting heart rate may be used as a guideline for the progression of activity.
   e. Once a steady state of activity is tolerated without symptoms, dysrhythmia, or excessive tachycardia, the duration of exercise may be increased in 5-minute increments each week, while intensity can be increased at a frequency of 3–6 times weekly.
4. High-risk patients are encouraged to attend medically supervised exercise sessions.
   a. Moderate-to-high risk patients have ischemia and/or significant dysrhythmia on symptom-limited exercise testing.

1) Significant dysrhythmia includes ventricular tachycardia, symptom-producing dysrhythmia, and hemodynamic instability.
2) Signs of ischemia include the presence of chest pain, 2 mm ST-segment depression or elevation, or a decrease in systolic blood pressure ≥20 mm Hg from base line.

b. Exercise prescriptions for moderate-to-high risk patients require medical supervision, such as cardiac rehabilitation.
c. Exercise for older individuals may best be done under initial supervised conditions for a brief period of time.

Nutrition

Skills

Required skills for patients to engage successfully in dietary modification include reading food labels before purchasing groceries, selecting appropriate foods from restaurant menus, using appropriate cooking styles, and taking medications, if indicated.

Lipid Management

Normalizing blood lipids may reduce the rates of coronary events and death from CVD.

1. Diet, exercise, and drug therapy have been shown to be effective strategies in achieving optimum cholesterol levels.
   a. LDL-C 100 mg/dL
   b. HDL-C >40 mg/dL
   c. Triglyceride <200 mg/dL
2. Low fat, low cholesterol choices for a healthy diet include:
   a. 5 servings of a variety of fruits and vegetables daily.
   b. 6 or more serving of grain daily.
   c. Include fat-free or low-fat items.
   d. Balance daily caloric intake by calorie expenditure
      1) Multiply weight in pounds by 15 (if active) or by 13 (if sedentary).
3. Individuals without CVD, diabetes, or high LDL-C should consume
   <30% of their total calories as fat; <10% as saturated fat, and <300 mg of cholesterol per day.
4. Individuals with CVD, diabetes, or high LDL-C should consume <30% of total calories as fat, <7% as saturated fat, and <200 mg of cholesterol per day.

Weight Management

1. Body mass index (BMI) is used to define overweight and obesity.
   a. BMI = weight in kilograms divided by height in meters squared **or**
   b. Estimated BMI = (weight in pounds divided by height in inches squared) multiplied by 704.5
2. The healthy range for BMI is 18.5 to 24.9.
   a. Overweight is defined as a BMI of 25–29.9
   b. Obesity is defined as a BMI ≥30
3. Treatment goals for cardiovascular health are:
   a. BMI <25 throughout adult life. (BMI of 25 corresponds to 110% of ideal body weight).
   b. If BMI is 25–30, diet and exercise management is recommended.
      1) A caloric deficit of 400 calories per day should result in weight loss of 0.45kg (1 lb) per week. The recommended weight loss rate is 1 lb per week.
      2) Pharmacologic agents may be indicated for BMI >30.
4. A threshold level of BMI is not entirely appropriate, because the distribution of adipose tissue to the abdomen effects the risk of CHD more than distribution in the pelvic area.
   a. BMI does not take into account distribution of body fat.
   b. Research shows that increased waist circumference and waist-to-hip ratio predict comorbidities and mortality from obesity.
      1) Desirable waist circumference is <35 inches (88 cm) for women and <40 inches (102 cm) for men.
      2) Waist-to-hip ratio is the waist measurement divided by the hip measurement. Desirable waist-to-hip ratio is <0.8 for women and ≤1.0 for men.
5. BMI or obesity independently predicts coronary atherosclerosis in whites. The relationship between obesity and CVD morbidity and mortality is less clear for non-whites.
   a. Weight loss is associated with improved lipid levels, less insulin resistance, and lower BP.
   b. Cardiac rehabilitation may aim for a reduction of 5 to 10% of body weight to improve risk factors.
6. Prevention of obesity by diet and regular physical activity is a high priority to reduce CVD risk.
7. Obesity is associated with a number of comorbidities, which include heart disease.
8. Heredity may explain 30% to 70% of obesity, but environmental factors must be considered as contributors to the increasing prevalence of obesity.

9. Weight loss is particularly important for patients with HTN, elevated triglycerides, or elevated blood glucose levels.

Metabolic Syndrome

1. Metabolic syndrome is a clustering of several metabolic risk factors in one patient, which predisposes the individual to premature CHD.
   a. Metabolic syndrome is diagnosed when 3 or more of the following factors are present.
   b. Abdominal obesity, elevated triglycerides, low HDL cholesterol, high blood pressure (≥130/≥85 mm Hg), or fasting glucose ≥110 mg/dL.
2. Metabolic abnormalities include defective glucose uptake by the skeletal muscle, increased release of free fatty acids by adipose tissue, over production of glucose by the liver, and hypersecretion of insulin by pancreatic beta-cells.
3. The Framingham Study did not contain all of the risk determinants used to diagnose the metabolic syndrome. The importance of metabolic syndrome as a risk factor may be underestimated.

Divalent Cations

1. Sodium
   a. For the general population, the AHA recommends eating less than 6 grams of salt or 2,400 mg. of sodium per day
   b. Lower sodium guidelines may be recommended for patients with HTN and heart failure.
2. Potassium, calcium, and magnesium
   a. Low calcium consumption (300 to 600 mg per day) is associated with HTN.
   b. High potassium consumption is associated with lower blood pressure in people with HTN.
3. DASH — **D**ietary **A**pproaches to **S**top **H**ypertension — manipulated dietary intake of potassium, calcium, and magnesium while holding sodium intake constant.
   a. A diet rich in fruits, vegetables, and low-fat dairy products significantly reduced systolic and diastolic pressure in comparison with a "normal" diet.
   b. The DASH diet has recently been shown to reduce homocysteine levels also.

Alcohol Use

1. Urban residents tend to have more education beyond high school, higher alcohol use, and engage in more cigarette smoking, and have higher medical specialist usage than rural populations.
2. There is a J-shaped relationship between alcohol consumption and blood pressure. Light drinkers have lower BP than both those who abstain and those who drink more heavily.
3. There is evidence from observational studies that red wine reduces risk of heart attack.
4. AHA recommends moderate alcohol consumption in appropriate individuals.
   a. Not more than one alcoholic beverage for women and two for men per day.
   b. An alcoholic beverage is defined as 12 oz. of beer, 4 oz. of wine, 1-1/2 oz. of 80-proof liquor, or 1 oz. of 100 proof liquor.

Tobacco Use and Exposure

Physiologic Effects

1. Cigarette smoking is a powerful risk factor for developing CVD.
2. Smoking accelerates the rate of coronary plaque development.
3. Facts from the Framingham study indicate that smoking may destabilize coronary plaques and promote plaque rupture and therefore myocardial infarction.
4. Smoking is the major cause of peripheral arterial disease and doubles the risk of ischemic stroke.
5. The longer and the more packs per day smoked the greater the risk of developing CVD.

Cessation Techniques and Guidelines

1. Smoking intervention systems increase the proportion of smokers who are identified, counseled about cessation, referred to cessation programs, and supported in their efforts to quit.
2. Cessation of smoking may reduce mortality and reinfarction rates by 50%.
3. Cessation techniques may include temptation management, cue extinction, contingency management, persuasive techniques, pharmacologic agents, and behavior modification.

Cardiac Rehabilitation

First developed in the 1960s cardiac rehabilitation programs are designed to take advantage of the benefits of walking during prolonged hospitalization and promote secondary prevention in a formal, structured program.

1. Cardiac rehabilitation involves medical supervision and electrographic monitoring of patients post cardiac event while they follow an exercise prescription over a period of 4 to 12 weeks.
2. A medical referral is necessary to enroll in outpatient cardiac rehabilitation.
3. Base line exercise stress test is done to determine if exertional ischemia or dysrhthymia is present.
4. The exercise prescription is followed under medical supervision, with nurse monitoring and input by exercise physiologists on exercise activities and progression of exercise intensity.
5. Aerobic exercise, resistance training, and work capacity are included in rehabilitation.
6. Health insurance may require a co-payment paid per visit or program.

Expected Benefits

1. The expected benefits of cardiac rehabilitation include reduced CVD morbidity and mortality, increased functional capacity and exercise tolerance, as well as improvement in patient-reported ability to perform activities of daily living.
2. Cardiac rehabilitation has been shown to increase HDL cholesterol levels and modestly reduce triglycerides that are above 200 mg/dL.
3. The minimal effect of cardiac rehabilitation on low-density LDL cholesterol suggests a need for concurrent nutritional counseling and drug therapy.
4. Oral hypoglycemic agents or insulin may need to be adjusted downward in response to increased sensitivity to insulin caused by exercise.

Content

Cardiac rehabilitation includes nutritional counseling, smoking cessation, review of medications, dietary modification, and exercise prescriptions to reduce modifiable risk factors, subsequent coronary events, and rehospitalization.

1. Cardiac rehabilitation may be covered by health insurance for a specific number of visits (12 to 36 per single cardiac event), after MI, PTCA, chronic stable angina, or open heart surgery.
2. Visits may be 2 or 3 times a week.
3. Cardiac rehabilitation is also appropriate for patients with chronic heart failure and cardiac transplantation.
4. Only 10% to 20% of appropriate cardiac candidates participate in outpatient cardiac rehabilitation.

Programs

Cardiac rehabilitation provides structured programs to reduce cardiovascular risk for patients with established CVD who are at risk for recurrent cardiac events and death from cardiac causes.

1. More than 50% of patients in cardiac rehabilitation are 65 years or older.
2. Preventing and minimizing disability is of prime concern in this age group.

CHAPTER 9

Hypertension Management

Normal Blood Pressure

1. Normal blood pressure (BP) for adults over 18 years is <120 mm Hg systolic and <80 mm Hg diastolic.
2. BP is the force exerted by the blood against the walls of the blood vessel and is a function of cardiac output (CO) and systemic vascular resistance (SVR).
   a. BP = CO X SVR
3. CO is the volume of blood ejected from the heart per minute and is a function of heart rate (HR) and stroke volume (SV).
4. SV is the amount of blood ejected from the heart with each contraction; the normal volume at rest is approximately 75 ml.
   a. CO = HR X SV
   b. Pulse pressure (the difference between SBP and DBP) is an indirect estimate of SV.
5. SVR (sometimes referred to as peripheral vascular resistance) is the force within the vascular bed that opposes ejection of blood from the left ventricle.
   a. SVR is the major variable determining afterload.
   b. Vessel radius is the primary determinant of resistance and the primary sites for SVR are the small arteries and arterioles.

Regulation of BP

BP is regulated through the interaction of nervous, cardiovascular, renal and endocrine functions. Actions of the nervous system and the vascular endothelium are rapid (seconds) and short-term (days), while renal and endocrine actions contribute to long-term (days to weeks) regulation.

Autonomic Nervous System Effects

1. Baroreceptors located in the aortic arch and carotid sinus sense change in BP and send either inhibitory or excitatory impulses to the vasomotor control centers in the medulla.

a. When increased BP is sensed, inhibition of sympathetic nervous system (SNS) activity results directly in decreased HR, decreased cardiac contractility, and increased peripheral vasodilation. Also, increased parasympathetic activity, mediated through the vagus nerve, reduces HR. The net effect of SNS inhibition is to decrease BP.

b. When decreased BP is sensed, excitatory impulses are generated. Afferent SNS nerves release the neurotransmitter norepinephrine (NE) into the neuroeffector junction. NE stimulates adrenoreceptors.

c. Adrenoreceptors have been classified into two general groups: α-adrenergic and β-adrenergic. The net effect of SNS activity is determined by the distribution of sympathetic nerve endings and adrenoreceptors in body tissues.

   1) β_1 adrenoreceptors in the heart increase HR (positive chronotropic effect), contractility (positive inotropic effect), and conductivity (positive dromotropic effect).
   2) β_2 adrenoreceptors in coronary arteries and peripheral arterioles of skeletal muscles produce vasodilation and decrease SVR. β_2 adrenoreceptors in the lungs produce bronchodilation.
   3) Decreased BP in the renal afferent arterioles, decreased sodium chloride concentration in the distal convuluted tubule, and stimulation of b-adrenoreceptors on the juxtaglomerular apparatus (JGA) stimulate renin release. See discussion of Renin-Angiotensin-Aldosterone (RAA) on page 111.
   4) α_1 adrenoreceptors in vascular smooth muscle produce vasoconstriction (increase SVR).

2. Cardiopulmonary baroreceptors (also called mechanoreceptors or stretch receptors) are low-pressure receptors located in the heart and pulmonary circulation. Cardiopulmonary baroreceptors sense small changes in cardiac filling pressure and volume. Small increases in cardiac filling pressure and volume inhibit SNS and neurohormonal (RAA) activity — reducing BP and intravascular volume. Small decreases, on the other hand, stimulate SNS and RAA activity — increasing BP and intravascular volume.
3. Chemoreceptors, located in the carotid and aortic bodies, when stimulated by hypoxia, excite the SNS producing increased ventilation and venous resistance without significantly altering HR.
4. Epinephrine, secreted by the adrenal medulla in response to physical or emotional stress, can activate the SNS also.

   a. β_1 receptors in the heart increase HR and cardiac contractility (increased CO).

b. β_2 receptors in skeletal and splanchnic arterioles produce vasodilation.
   1) Vasodilation of these large beds may decrease SVR.
c. In pharmacological doses (which are higher than physiologic concentrations), epinephrine stimulates a receptors in vascular smooth muscle producing systemic vasoconstriction (but coronary vasodilation) and increasing SVR.

Renal Effects

1. The Renin-Angiotensin-Aldosterone (RAA) system regulates BP directly and also through a long-term effect on fluid balance.
   a. Renin is released from the JGA of the kidney in response to increased SNS activity, decreased renal perfusion pressure, or decreased sodium concentration in the early distal tubule.
   b. Renin acts on angiotensinogen to produce Angiotensin I (A-I), an inactive peptide.
   c. A-I is converted to Angiotensin II (A-II), a potent vasoconstrictor, through the action of angiotensin-converting enzyme (ACE).
      1) A-II produces generalized vasoconstriction (increases SVR).
      2) A-II potentiates SNS effects (increases SVR and HR).
      3) A-II stimulates release of aldosterone from the adrenal cortex.
   d. Aldosterone inhibits sodium excretion causing water retention and increased blood volume.
2. Arginine Vasopressin (Antidiuretic Hormone, ADH) is released from the posterior pituitary gland.
   a. Increased plasma osmolality is the primary stimulus for ADH release but it may be released also in response to low blood volume and pressure (for example, hemorrhage).
   b. ADH enhances water absorption at the distal and collecting tubules of the kidney.

Local Vascular Effects

1. Vascular endothelium effects SVR and BP by secreting vasodilator and vasoconstrictor substances.
   a. Vasodilating substances include nitric oxide (NO), endothelium-derived relaxing factor, prostacyclin, endothelium-derived hyperpolarizing factor, and bradykinin.
   b. Vasoconstricting substances include endothelium-derived contracting factor, Endothelin–1, prostanoids, and superoxide anions.

2. Certain vascular beds (for example the heart, brain, kidney and skeletal muscle) alter local vascular resistance to maintain perfusion (autoregulation). The mechanism is unknown but three hypotheses have been proposed.
   a. The myogenic hypothesis proposes that increased arterial pressure stimulates contraction of vascular smooth muscle, which increases vascular resistance. Increased resistance in response to increased pressure maintains constant flow.
   b. The metabolic hypothesis proposes that metabolic substances liberated from the tissues exert a local vasodilator effect.
   c. The tissue pressure hypothesis proposes that increased interstitial pressure passively decreases vessel diameter and flow.

Intravascular Fluid Volume

1. Changes in intravascular fluid volume do not directly affect arterial BP but do affect venous pressure and cardiac contractility. The Frank-Starling law of the heart states that stretching of myocardial fibers during diastole increases the force of contraction during systole.
   a. Within limits, hypervolemia increases cardiac filling and contractility thereby increasing CO. If SVR remains constant, increased CO will produce increased BP.
   b. Hypovolemia decreases cardiac filling and contractility decreasing CO. If SVR remains constant, decreased CO will produce decreased BP.

Hypertension

Hypertension (HTN) in adults over 18 years is defined as sustained SBP of 140 mm Hg or greater, DBP of 90 mm Hg or greater in individuals who are not taking antihypertensive medication. This definition is based on the average of 2 or more readings taken at each of 2 or more visits after an initial BP screening. HTN has been classified by the Joint National Committee on Detection, Evaluation, and Treatment of High BP (JNC-VII) as Stage 1 and Stage 2. (See Table 9–1.)

Primary HTN

1. Primary (essential) HTN is elevated BP without a known cause. Primary HTN accounts for 90% to 95% of HTN in adults.
2. Most cases of primary HTN result from a complex interaction of genetic, environmental, and demographic factors. Factors associated with primary HTN include:

a. Excessive salt and water retention.
b. Increased SNS activity. Circulating NE levels are usually higher in individuals with HTN than in those with normal or optimal BP.
c. Increased vasoconstrictive response to SNS activity and circulating catecholamines.
d. Decreased production of NO, a potent vasodilator released from the vascular endothelium.
e. Inherited cardiovascular risk factors. HTN coexists with hypercholesterolemia and with diabetes. HTN, insulin resistance, dyslipidemia and obesity occur concomitantly and multiply the risk of cardiac and vascular disease.

Secondary HTN

1. Secondary HTN is elevated BP with a specific cause that can be identified and corrected.
2. Secondary HTN accounts for 5% to 10% of HTN in adults but more than 80% of HTN in children. (Table 9–2 lists common correctable causes of secondary HTN.)
   a. Onset of HTN in an individual less than age 20 or over age 50 suggests secondary HTN.
      1) In children, the most common causes of secondary HTN are renal disease and vascular problems.
      2) In adults, chronic renal disease, renovascular disease, primary aldosteronism, and the use of oral contraceptives are the most common causes of secondary HTN.

TABLE 9–1.
Classification of Blood Pressure for Adults 18 Years of Age and Older

Category	Systolic (mm Hg)	Diastolic (mm Hg)
Normal	<120	<80
Prehypertension	120–139	80–89
Hypertension, Stage 1	140–159	90–99
Hypertension, Stage 2	160	100

Adapted from The Seventh Report of the Joint National Committee on Prevention, Detection, Evaluation, and Treatment of High Blood Pressure, NIH Pub. No. 04–5230, 08/04

b. Clinical findings suggestive of secondary HTN include:
   1) Unexplained hypokalemia suggests primary aldosteronism.
   2) Abdominal or renal bruits suggest renovascular disease.
   3) Labile BP with a history of palpitations, sweating and tremor suggest pheochromocytoma.
   4) Family history of renal disease suggests renovascular disease.
   5) Decreased BP in the legs in comparison with the arms suggests aortic coarctation.

Incidence and Demographics

1. HTN is common to all human populations (except a few thousand, culturally isolated individuals) and accounts for 6% of deaths in adults worldwide.

TABLE 9–2
Selected Causes of Secondary Hypertension

Kidney	**Drugs and Chemicals**
Renal parenchymal disease	Cyclosporin
Chronic nephritis	Alcohol
Polycystic kidneys	Sympathomimetics
Diabetic nephropathy	Some cold remedies
Acute glomerulonephritis	Cocaine, crack
Renal vascular disease	Some appetite suppressants
Renal transplant	Tyramine with monoamine oxidase inhibitors
Renin-secreting tumors	Nonsteroidal antiinflammatory drugs
Endocrine	Oral contraceptives
Adrenal	**Vascular**
Primary aldosteronism	Coarctation of the aorta
Cushing syndrome	Anemia
Pheochromocytoma	Aortic valvular insufficiency
Hyperparathyroidism	**Neurological**
Thyrotoxicosis	Increased intracranial pressure
Paget disease of bone	Obstructive sleep apnea
Pregnancy	Quadriplegia
Preeclampsia	
Eclampsia	

2. About 1 in 4 American adults have HTN. Of those with HTN, 31.6% are unaware of the condition, 27.4% are on medication and have it controlled, 26.2% are on medication but do not have their blood pressure controlled, and 14.8% aren't on medication.
3. Ethnicity is related to the prevalence of HTN.
   a. The prevalence of HTN is higher in African-American and American-Indian men and women than in Caucasian-American men and women.
      1) Blacks develop HTN earlier and their average BPs are higher than whites at all ages.
      2) Blacks have a greater rate of stroke (fatal and nonfatal), death from heart disease, and end-stage kidney disease than whites.
   b. In comparison with Caucasian-American men and women, the prevalence of HTN in Mexican-Americans is slightly lower for men and slightly higher for women.
4. The prevalence of HTN increases with age, but systolic and diastolic pressures behave differently over time. These differences account for the high prevalence of isolated systolic HTN (SBP >140 mm Hg with DBP <90 mm Hg) in older adults.
   a. SBP rises slowly beginning in the early adult years and continuing into old age.
   b. DBP rises steadily in early adulthood, but begins to decline at about age 60.
   c. Among Americans 60 years and older, HTN was found in 60% of non-Hispanic whites, 71% of non-Hispanic blacks, and 61% of Mexican-Americans.
   d. Isolated systolic HTN may account for 65–75% of HTN in the elderly.
5. Individuals with lower educational and income levels tend to have higher BP.

Risk for Cardiac and Vascular Disease

1. HTN is a major modifiable risk factor for vascular disease affecting the brain, heart, peripheral vessels, and kidneys.
2. Not only the level of BP but also the presence or absence of target-organ damage (TOD) and other risk factors determine the overall risk for cardiac and vascular disease.
   a. The presence of TOD or clinical cardiovascular diseases (CVD) increases the risk associated with HTN and modifies treatment recommendations.

b. TOD and CVD associated with HTN include:
   1) Heart diseases: left ventricular hypertrophy, angina or prior myocardial infarction, prior coronary revascularization, and heart failure
   2) Stroke or transient ischemic attacks
   3) Nephropathy
   4) Peripheral arterial disease
   5) Hypertensive retinopathy

c. The presence of other major risk factors increases the risk associated with HTN and modifies treatment recommendations. Major risk factors include:
   1) Smoking
   2) Dyslipidemia
   3) Diabetes mellitus
   4) Age more than 60 years
   5) Gender (men and postmenopausal women)
   6) Family history of cardiovascular disease in women before age 65 years and in men before age 55 years

Sequelae and Complications

1. Target organ damage
   a. Cardiac effects
      1) HTN is a major risk factor for coronary heart disease — angina pectoris, myocardial infarction and sudden death.
      2) Sustained HTN increases cardiac work resulting in concentric left ventricular hypertrophy (LVH) and increased wall thickness.
      3) LVH is initially compensatory, but eventually the ventricle dilates and symptoms of heart failure appear.
   b. Neurologic effects
      1) Retinal effects: Increasing severity of HTN is associated with focal spasm and progressive, general narrowing of the arterioles. Retinal hemorrhage, exudate, and disc edema may be seen on fundoscopic examination.
      2) Central nervous system effects
         a) Cerebral infarction due to atherosclerosis (i.e., stroke)
         b) Cerebral hemorrhage due to HTN and development of cerebrovascular microaneurysms
         c) Hypertensive encephalopathy is characterized by severe HTN (often 250/150 mm Hg), headache that is sometimes accompanied by restlessness and confusion, and resolution of symptoms with BP reduction.

1. Nausea, projectile vomiting, and visual blurring may occur.
2. Optic disc edema with retinal hemorrhages and exudates may be observed.

c. Renal effects
   1) Decreased glomerular filtration rate and tubular dysfunction due to arteriosclerotic lesions of the afferent and efferent renal arterioles.
   2) Proteinuria and microscopic hematuria due to glomerular lesions.

d. Peripheral vascular effects
   1) HTN enhances atherosclerosis in the peripheral blood vessels, leading to the development of aortic aneurysm, aortic dissection, and peripheral vascular disease.

2. Hypertensive crises are rare situations that require immediate BP reduction to prevent or limit TOD. Examples of TOD associated with hypertensive crisis are hypertensive encephalopathy, intracranial hemorrhage, unstable angina, acute myocardial infarction, dissecting aortic aneurysm, and eclampsia.
   a. Hypertensive emergencies are defined as SBP greater than 220 mm Hg and DBP greater than 120 mm Hg.
      1) Patients require admission to intensive care for intravenous vasodilator therapy and monitoring.
      2) Initial goal is to reduce mean arterial BP no more than 25% within several minutes to 2 hours. BP is reduced toward 160/100 mm Hg over next 2 to 6 hours.
      3) Past practice of administering sublingual nifedipine to rapidly lower pressure is not recommended.
   b. Hypertensive urgencies are situations in which it is desirable to reduce BP within a few hours. Examples are upper level stage 3 HTN (SBP >180 or DBP >110 mm Hg), HTN with optic disc edema, progressive target organ complications, and severe perioperative HTN.

Clinical Assessment

1. The purpose of clinical assessment in HTN is to determine risk for cardiac and vascular disease.
   a. To accurately measure BP
   b. To identify the presence of TOD
   c. To identify the presence of other cardiovascular risk factors
   d. To identify the presence of cardiac or vascular disease
   e. To identify secondary causes of HTN when present

f. To identify coexisting conditions that affect diagnosis, prognosis or treatment, such as:
   1) Sleep apnea
   2) Pregnancy
   3) Substances that may cause HTN
      a) Oral contraceptives
      b) Sympathomimetics — including cocaine
      c) Adrenal steroids
      d) Alcohol
      e) Excessive salt intake
      f) Herbal weight loss agents containing ephedra.

2. HTN causes no symptoms until it has become severe and TOD is present.
   a. Symptoms related to TOD include fatigue, headache, transient weakness or blindness, loss of visual acuity, chest pain, dyspnea, and claudication.
   b. Headache is characteristic of severe HTN only. Nosebleed, blurring of vision due to retinal changes, and TIAs are symptoms of associated vascular disease.
   c. Symptoms related to secondary causes of HTN include muscle weakness, episodes of tachycardia, sweating and tremor, thinning of the skin, and flank pain.
3. HTN is easily detected, but can not be diagnosed from a single BP measurement.
   a. BP varies markedly related to time of day, body position, activity, and physical and emotional state
   b. Diagnosis and classification of HTN is based on an average of 2 or more BPs taken on 2 or more occasions after an initial screening. (See Table 9–1)
   c. BP should be measured in a standard fashion using equipment that meets certification criteria.

Physical Examination

1. Physical examination of the individual with HTN includes:
   a. Vital signs: variable BP, tachycardia, or bradycardia,
   b. Heart: size, rhythm, sounds, murmurs,
   c. Neck: jugular venous pressure, carotid pulses and bruit, thyromegaly,
   d. Vascular: renal, or femoral bruits, anklebrachial systolic pressure index,
   e. Lungs: respiratory rate, rhythm, and presence of adventitious sounds (rales or wheezes),
   f. Eyes: retinal hemorrhages, exudates, and disc edema,

g. Neuro: decreased visual acuity, focal neurological deficits associated with past stroke,
h. Abdomen: waist circumference, aortic and renal masses or bruits.

Obesity

1. Body mass index (BMI) of 27 or greater is closely correlated with HTN. Obesity is defined as BMI of 30 or greater.
   a. BMI = weight in Kg divided by height in meters squared
   b. BMI = weight in pounds divided by height in inches squared multiplied by 704.5
2. Abdominal obesity (waist circumference greater than 40 inches in men and greater than 35 inches in women) is closely correlated with risk for HTN, cardiovascular disease, type II diabetes, and dyslipidemia.
3. Signs of secondary causes of HTN include abdominal bruit, truncal obesity, excessive hair growth, abdominal striae, and buffalo hump.

Diagnostic Studies

1. Diagnostic studies may be done to determine TOD, risk factors, and secondary HTN, or to establish base line function before initiating therapy.
2. Routine tests include urinalysis, complete blood cell count, serum electrolytes, fasting glucose, total and high-density lipoprotein cholesterol, and 12-lead electrocardiogram.
3. Additional tests that may be indicated in some patients include creatinine clearance, 24-hour urine for protein and microalbumin, blood calcium, uric acid, fasting triglycerides, glycosolated hemoglobin, thyroid-stimulating hormone, renal or carotid artery doppler studies, and echocardiography.
4. Some clinicians recommend measuring plasma catecholamine and aldosterone level, 24-hour urine for metanephrine, and dexamethasone suppression test.

Management of HTN

The goal of treatment for patients with HTN is to prevent TOD and the progression of atherosclerosis by the least intrusive means possible.

1. Treatment of HTN is based on individual risk. (See Table 9–3. Risk Stratification and Treatment.)
2. Non-pharmacological management of HTN consists of lifestyle modification.

Four lifestyle interventions have been shown in clinical trials to delay or prevent the onset of HTN. These interventions are used in the non-pharmacological management of HTN.

1. Weight reduction
2. Sodium restriction
3. Reduced alcohol intake
4. Physical activity

Lifestyle Interventions

All patients with HTN should be encouraged to adopt lifestyle interventions. Even when lifestyle interventions alone do not control HTN, they may reduce the number and dosage of antihypertensive medications needed. There is some evidence that lifestyle interventions can prevent or delay the onset of HTN.

1. **Weight reduction.** Weight-loss has been shown to reduce BP more effectively than any other lifestyle measure.

TABLE 9–3.
Risk Stratification and Treatment

Blood Pressure Stages (mm Hg)	Risk Group A (No risk factors; No TOD/CCD)	Risk Group B (At least 1 risk factor, not including diabetes; No TOD/CCD)	Risk Group C (TOD/CCD and/or diabetes with or without other risk factors)
High normal (130–139/85–89)	Lifestyle modification	Lifestyle modification	Drug therapy*
Stage 1 (140–159/90–99)	Lifestyle modification (up to 12 mo.)	Lifestyle modification (up to 6 mo.)	Drug therapy
Stages 2 and 3 (≥160/≥100)	Drug therapy	Drug therapy	Drug therapy

Note: For example, a patient with diabetes and a blood pressure of 142/94 plus left ventricular hypertrophy should be classified as having stage 1 hypertension with target organ disease and another major risk factor (diabetes). This patient would be categorized as "Stage 1, Risk Group C" and recommended for immediate initiation of pharmacologic treatment. Lifestyle modification should be adjunctive therapy for all patients recommended for drug therapy.

TOD/CCD indicates target organ disease/clinical cardiovascular disease

*For those with heart failure, renal insufficiency, or diabetes.

   a. Loss of 10 pounds reduces BP in a large proportion of overweight individuals with HTN.
   b. Weight loss complements pharmacological management of BP.
   c. Overweight individuals should be counseled about calorie restriction and increased activity.
   d. Sustaining weight loss is difficult; documented reduction in BP and other cardiovascular risk factors may reward persistence.
2. **Moderate alcohol use.** Excessive alcohol intake is an important risk factor for HTN, can cause resistance to HTN therapy, and increases risk for stroke.
   a. Men who drink alcohol should be advised to consume not more than two alchohol-containing beverages a day.
      1) One alcohol-containing beverage is defined as 12 oz. of beer, 4 oz. of wine, 1-1/2 oz. of 80-proof liquor, or 1 oz. of 100 proof liquor.
   b. Women and lighter-weight men who drink alcohol should be advised to consume not more than one alcohol-containing beverage per day.
3. **Reduced sodium.** Clinical trials have shown that reduction of sodium intake lowers BP is some salt-sensitive people with HTN. There is no clinical test to determine which individuals are salt-sensitive.
   a. JNC-VII recommends sodium intake of not more than 6 gms of sodium chloride or 2.4 gms of sodium per day.
   b. 75% of sodium intake is derived from processed foods. Population-level reduction of sodium in processed food may be more effective than intervention with individuals.
4. **Diet high in fruits and vegetables.** The Dietary Approaches to Stop Hypertension (DASH) Trial found that a diet high in fruits, vegetables, and low-fat dairy products and low in saturated and total fat resulted in a marked decline in both SBP and DBP.
5. **Physical activity.** Regular, moderately intense activity (such as brisk walking) for 30 to 45 minutes on most days of the week has been shown to lower BP.
   a. Most people can safely increase their level of activity without extensive medical evaluation.
   b. Patients with family history of cardiac disease or other risk factors should be instructed in signs and symptoms of heart attack and stroke and action to take if symptoms occur.
   c. Patients with cardiac or other serious disease and those with major risk factors may need a more through evaluation or referral to a medically supervised exercise program.
   d. Increased activity increases weight loss and improves lipid-profile.

6. **Control of other risk factors.** Although smoking cessation and improving lipid-profile do not improve a patient's BP, they reduce overall risk of morbidity and mortality from atherosclerotic disease.

Pharmacological Management

1. The decision to initiate pharmacological therapy is based on the degree of BP elevation, presence of TOD, and the presence of other clinical risk factors. (See Table 9–3.)
2. Reducing BP with drugs has been shown to protect against stroke, coronary events, heart failure, progression of renal disease, more severe BP elevation, and all cause mortality.
3. The beneficial effect of drug therapy has been seen across age, gender, race, BP level, and socioeconomic status.
4. Six classes of drugs are used in managing HTN. (Drugs are discussed in Chapter 15.)
   a. Diuretics
   b. Adrenergic inhibitors
      1) α-Adrenergic blockers
      2) Centrally acting inhibitors
      3) Central α-adrenergic agonists
      4) β-Adrenergic blockers
      5) Combined α- and β-adrenergic blockers
   c. Vasodilators
   d. Calcium channel blocking agents
   e. ACE inhibitors
   f. Angiotensin II receptor blockers
5. If there are no indications for another class of drug, a diuretic or β-adrenergic blocker is recommended for initial treatment of uncomplicated HTN. In clinical trials, diuretics and β-blockers have been shown to reduce morbidity and mortality in patients with HTN.
6. Other classes of drugs are recommended for initial treatment when specific indications exist.
   a. For patients with HTN and insulin-dependent diabetes mellitus and proteinuria, ACE inhibitors are recommended (instead of diuretic and β-blockers) for initial therapy.
   b. For patients with HTN and heart failure, ACE inhibitors and diuretics are recommended.
   c. In older adult patients with isolated systolic hypertension, diuretics and long-acting dihydropyridine calcium antagonists are recommended.

   d. For patients with myocardial infarction and HTN, β-blockers (non-intrinsic sympathomimetic activity) and ACE inhibitors (with systolic dysfunction) are recommended.
7. For most patients with HTN, an initial trial of lifestyle modification followed by initiation of low-dose drug therapy is appropriate. If necessary, dose of the initial drug can be increased and other agents with different mechanism of action can be added.
8. In high-risk patients (stage 3 HTN or risk group C), drug therapy is started without delay.
   a. Patients with an average SBP of 200 mm Hg or higher require immediate therapy, as do those with average DBP of 120 mm Hg or higher. If symptomatic TOD is present, these patients may require hospitalization and the use of parenteral antihypertensive agents.
9. Management of HTN is modified by individual patient characteristics including membership in specific groups.
   a. HTN in women
      1) Women taking oral contraceptives experience a small but detectable increase in SBP and DBP.
      2) Clinical HTN is 2 to 3 times more prevalent in women taking oral contraceptives than among those not taking these drugs.
      3) HTN that occurs in nonpregnant women and HTN that occurs before the 20th week of gestation or persists more than 6 weeks after delivery are considered chronic.
      4) Gestational HTN occurs in the third trimester and is not associated with signs of eclampsia.
         a) Preeclampsia is elevated BP associated with proteinuria and edema
         b) Eclampsia is a HTN emergency that occurs during pregnancy.
         c) Neither ACE inhibitors nor angiotensin II blockers should be used. A central α-agonist (eg, methyldopa) is the drug of choice.
   b. HTN in older adults
      1) Isolated systolic hypertension (SBP >140 mm Hg with DBP <90 mm Hg) is common in older adults.
      2) Target BP is the same as for younger adults (less than 140/90 mm Hg) although an interim goal of 160/90 mm Hg may be necessary.
      3) Among older adults, SBP is a better predictor of events (CHD, CVD, heart failure, stroke, end-stage renal disease and all cause mortality) than DBP.

4) Treatment includes lifestyle modification and drugs. Diuretics are the preferred first-line drug therapy unless there is specific indication for another drug.
   a) Treatment reduces stroke, CCD, CVD, heart failure, and mortality.
5) Pseudohypertension (falsely high BP readings) may occur due to excessive vascular stiffness. Signs of pseudohypertension include high BP without TOD and lack of response to treatment.
6) High risk of orthostatic HTN exists among older adults. Always measure BP and pulse while standing, as well as while sitting or supine.

c. HTN and coexisting disease
   1) Reduce BP gradually in people with cerebrovascular disease to avoid orthostatic hypotension.
   2) HTN is major risk factor for carotid atherosclerosis, peripheral artery disease, and aneurysm. Data are not available to determine if treatment of HTN reduces the risk of these processes. Data show reduced risk of death from aortic dissection.
   3) In individuals with diabetes mellitus and HTN, the goal is to reduce BP below 130/85 mm Hg.
      a) Lifestyle modification — especially weight loss and exercise
      b) ACE inhibitors, α blockers, calcium channel antagonists, or low dose diuretics are preferred agents.
   4) In individuals with renal disease and HTN, control of HTN (<130/85 mm Hg) slows the progression of renal failure.
      a) Lifestyle modification — especially sodium restriction.
      b) ACE inhibitor is the preferred drug class.
   5) Lower target BP may be desired in patients with existing coronary heart disease or heart failure.
      a) After MI, β-blocker is the preferred drug class.
      b) For patients with heart failure, ACE inhibitors and combined α–β-blockers are preferred.

10. After BP has been controlled on drug therapy for one year, an attempt to reduce drug dosage should be made.

Nurses' Role

1. Nurses' role in managing HTN depends on the individual nurse's preparation, work experience, and clinical setting.

2. Nursing diagnoses are derived from the comprehensive assessment. High frequency diagnoses among patients with HTN include:
   a. Deficient knowledge about disease process and management
   b. Ineffective therapeutic regimen management
   c. Noncompliance (specify)
   d. Deficient fluid volume related to diuretic therapy
3. General therapeutic goals for individuals with HTN include:
   a. Achieve and maintain individually determined target BP
      1) In individuals with average risk, SBP less than 140 mm Hg and DBP less than 90 mm Hg.
      2) If tolerated, further lowering of BP may prevent stroke, preserve renal function, and prevent or slow the progression of heart failure.
      3) Lower target BP (130/85) has been established for individuals with diabetes, renal disease, or heart disease.
   b. Understand and implement lifestyle interventions.
   c. Comply with therapeutic regimen.
4. Frequently used nursing interventions when caring for patients with HTN include:
   a. Exercise promotion
   b. Nutritional counseling
   c. Teaching: Diet, Disease process, Health behaviors, Medication, Prescribed activity, Treatment regimen
   d. Weight reduction assistance
   e. Patient contracting
   f. Smoking cessation assistance
5. Dependent upon individual patient assessment and practice setting the following indicators of nursing outcomes may be appropriate.
   a. Compliance behavior
   b. Circulation status
   c. Knowledge: Diet, Disease process, Health behaviors, Medication, Prescribed activity, Treatment regimen
   d. Neurological status
   e. Nutritional status
   f. Tissue perfusion: Abdominal organs, cardiac, cerebral, peripheral, pulmonary
   g. Vital signs status
6. Collaborative strategies to enhance adherence to HTN therapy
   a. Educate patients
      1) Assess understanding of diagnosis and treatment
      2) Discuss concerns and clarify misunderstandings — assess for unpleasant secondary drug effects
      3) Inform patient of actual and desired BP level

4) Provide specific written information
5) Emphasize that HTN is symptomless and the importance of continued therapy

b. Individualize treatment
1) Include patient in decision making
2) Simplify and minimize cost of treatment
3) Incorporate treatment into daily life
4) Encourage self-monitoring of BP
a) BP of individuals with HTN tends to be lower when measured at home.
b) Average readings of 135/85 mm Hg or greater are considered elevated.
5) When weight-loss is desired, discourage quick weight loss regimens, fasting, or unscientific methods.

c. Provide reinforcement
1) Trend BP over time
2) Give positive feedback for behavioral and BP improvement
3) Solicit questions and concerns
4) Use appointment reminders and contact patients to confirm
5) Schedule more frequent appointments with non-adherent patients. Consider nurse-initiated telephone follow-up.
6) Consider clinician-patient contracting.
7) Involve family member, if appropriate.

CHAPTER 10

Dyslipidemia Management

Management of dyslipidemia is essential to the prevention and treatment of atherosclerosis. High levels of low-density lipoprotein (LDL), low levels of high-density lipoprotein (HDL), and high levels of triglycerides increase the risk of developing this condition. The Adult Treatment Panel III (ATP III) contains the National Cholesterol Education Program's (NCEP) evidence-based clinical guidelines for lipid testing and management. This chapter presents screening guidelines for CHD risk and the metabolic syndrome, the ATP III guidelines for primary and secondary prevention of atherosclerosis, and the implications of dyslipidemia management for nursing practice.

Metabolic Syndrome

The metabolic syndrome consists of dyslipidemia (triglyceride ≥150 mg/dL and HDL cholesterol <40 mg/dL in men and <50 mg/dL in women), abdominal obesity (waist circumference >40 inches in men and >35 inches in women), elevated BP (≥130/85), and glucose intolerance (fasting blood glucose >110 mg/dL).

Metabolic syndrome is present in approximately 22% of the adult (≥20 years) population.

Individuals with the metabolic syndrome have an increased risk of developing atherosclerosis and a higher incidence of cardiac events than those without this syndrome.

Treatment of metabolic syndrome is a secondary target in managing dyslipidemia. That is, after LDL cholesterol is reduced further risk reduction can be achieved by treating the metabolic syndrome.

Screening for Atherosclerosis Risk

In all adults (≥20 years), a fasting lipoprotein profile (total cholesterol, LDL cholesterol, HDL cholesterol and triglyceride) should be obtained once every 5 years.

Assessment of other atherosclerosis risk factors should be done also. (Assessment and management of cardiac and vascular risk is discussed in Chapters 7 and 8 of this manual.)

1. Modifiable risk factors
   a. Cigarette smoking
   b. Uncontrolled diabetes mellitus (Hemoglobin A1C >6%)
   c. Uncontrolled hypertension
   d. Obesity
   e. Sedentary lifestyle
   f. Atheroslerotic dyslipidemia
      1) Low HDL cholesterol (<40 mg/dL)
      2) High LDL cholesterol (>160 gm/dL)
      3) High triglycerides (≥200 mg/dL)
2. Non-modifiable risk factors
   a. Family history of early MI or sudden death (1st degree male <55 years or 1st degree female <65 years)
   b. Increased age — men >45 years and women >55 years
   c. Early onset of menopause due to total abdominal hysterectomy
3. Individuals with multiple risk factors should be screened more frequently than every 5 years, regardless of gender or race.6
   a. Rapid result machines can give an entire lipid panel from a drop of blood within 5 minutes.
4. Risk reduction is an important component of prevention and treatment of atherosclerosis and CHD.
5. The presence of risk factors determines the acceptable level of blood lipids and the level at which pharmacological reduction should be initiated.

ATP III Guidelines

The purpose of the guidelines is to provide direction to health care providers in the prevention and treatment of dyslipidemia in people with and without CHD.

ATP III Classification

1. For the general adult population, ATP III classification of LDL, Total, and HDL Cholesterol (mg/dL) is the following:
   a. LDL cholesterol
      1) <100 is optimal
      2) 100 to 129 is near but above optimal
      3) 130 to 159 is borderline high
      4) 160 to 189 is high
      5) ≥190 is very high
   b. Total cholesterol
      1) <200 is desirable
      2) 200 to 239 is borderline high
      3) ≥240 is high

c. HDL cholesterol
    1) <40 is low
    2) ≥60 is high (desirable)
2. Major risk factors (exclusive of LDL choleterol) that modify LDL treatment goals.
    a. Cigarette smoking
    b. Hypertension
    c. Low HDL cholesterol
    d. Positive family history of premature CHD
    e. Age (men ≥45 years; women ≥55 years)
3. LDL treatment goals related to risk:
    a. For individuals with clinical CHD or CHD risk equivalents, the LDL goal is <100 mg/dL.
    b. For individuals with >2 major risk factors, the LDL goal is <130 mg/dL.
    c. For individuals with ≤1 major risk factor, the LDL goal is <160 mg/dL.

CHD Risk Equivalents

1. CHD risk equivalents include:
    a. Other forms of clinical atherosclerotic disease (ie, peripheral arterial disease, abdominal aortic aneurysm, and symptomatic carotid artery disease)
    b. Diabetes
    c. Multiple risk factors that confer a 10-year risk for CHD >20%
        1) For individuals with ≥2 risk factors, data from the Framingham study are used to estimate the 10-year risk of CHD.
        2) Points are assigned by gender for age, total cholesterol, HDL cholesterol, smoking, and blood pressure.
            a) Point total predicts 10-year risk for CHD
            b) 10-year risk for CHD ≥20% is a CHD equivalent and reason for more intensive lowering of LDL cholesterol
        3) The Framingham scoring method is included in the ATP III guidelines that can be downloaded from the website of the National Heart Lung and Blood Institute (www.nhlbi.gov).

Therapeutic Lifestyle Changes

1. ATP-III recommends a multifaceted approach to CHD risk reduction designated "therapeutic lifestyle changes (TLC)."
    a. Reduced intake of saturated fats (<7% of total calories) and cholesterol (<200 mg per day)

b. Use of plant stanols/sterols (2 g/day) and increased soluble fiber (20 to 30 g/day)
    1) Plant stanols/sterols are naturally occurring food substances that are combined with small amount of canola oil and added to food substances.
    2) Currently, regular and 'light' spreads fortified with plant stanols/sterols are available comercially.
    3) Soluble fiber is found in oats, legumes, grains, vegetables, and fruits.

c. Weight reduction

d. Increased physical exercise

Implications for Nursing Practice

1. Nurses screen, monitor, and teach individuals and groups about the management of dyslipidemia and atherosclerotic risk.
    a. Screening occurs in community and acute care settings.
        1) Patients admitted to the hospital with a cardiovascular event should be screened within 24 hours of admission.
    b. Individual risk assessment and modification is essential.
    c. Routine monitoring of the lipid profile allows the individual to observe improvement and reinforces behavior change.
        1) Providing laboratory results, together with target goals, in writing enables the individual to monitor his or her progress over time.
2. Nurses and dietitians are responsible for teaching people about therapeutic lifestyle changes.
3. Nurses monitor the therapeutic and side effects of pharmacotherapy and promote patient adherence.

Treatment of Dyslipidemia

Primary Prevention

1. Primary prevention consists of screening and therapeutic lifestyle changes (TLC).
2. TLC dietary recommendations include:
    a. Total fat (saturated, polyunsaturated, and monounsaturated) should not exceed 25% to 30% of total calories.
        1) Saturated fat <7% of total calories
        2) Polyunsaturated fats may be up to 10% of total calories
        3) Monounsaturated fats may be up to 20% of total calories
    b. Carbohydrates (primarily whole grains, fruits and vegetables) may be up to 50% to 60% of total calories.

c. Fiber 20 to 30 grams per day
d. Protein approximately 15% of total calories
e. Cholesterol less than 200 mg per day
f. Total calories consumed should be balanced with energy expended to achieve and maintain desirable body weight.

3. If the target lipid levels are not achieved after 6 weeks with the TLC diet, plant stanols/sterols are added.
4. If target lipid levels are not achieved after 12 week, pharmacotherapy is initiated. LDL-lowering drugs reduce the risk for major coronary events and coronary death.
5. At each visit, TLC are reviewed and reinforced, even after drug treatment is begun.

Secondary Prevention

1. Cholesterol treatment goals for individuals with clinical CHD or CHD equivalents are more stringent.
   a. LDL cholesterol should be <100 mg/dl.
2. Lipid profile should be obtained within 24 hours of hospital admission for an acute coronary event and therapy should be initiated before discharge.
   a. ATP-III guidelines recommend starting a bile acid sequestrant or nicotinic acid, if appropriate.
   b. Many clinical experts recommend starting HMG CoA reductase inhibitors (statins).
3. Lipid profile should be reevaluated in 6 and 12 weeks after initiating drug treatment.
4. Therapeutic lifestyle changes and reduction of other risk factor reduction should be encouraged also.

Drug Therapy

1. Drugs used to treat dyslipidemia are described in detail in Chapter 15.
2. HMG CoA reductase inhibitors, also known as statins, decrease mortality, reduce the risk of major coronary events by 30%, and stimulate plaque regression in coronary heart disease.
   a. Statins are most effective when taken at bedtime.
   b. Statins decrease LDL (18% to 55%), increase HDL (5% to 15%), and decreased triglycerides (7% to 30%).
   c. Statins can be combined with nicotinic or fibric acids if necessary.
   d. Statins are contraindicated in individuals with active or chronic liver disease.

   e. Liver enzymes are assessed after 6 weeks and every 6 months during treatment.
   f. Patients must be taught to report symptoms of muscle aches or weakness.
3. Bile acid sequestrants
   a. Decrease LDL (15% to 30%) and increase HDL (3% to 5%) without affecting triglycerides.
   b. May be added to statin therapy in individuals who do not reach target levels on statins alone.
   c. Side effects include GI distress and constipation.
   d. May interfere with absorption of other drugs.
4. Nicotinic acid
   a. Decreases LDL (5% to 25%) and triglyceride (20% to 50%) and increases HDL (15% to 35%).
   b. Side effects include flushing, hyperglycemia, hyperuricemia (gout), upper gastrointestinal distress, and hepatotoxicity.
5. Fibric acids (Gemfibrozil, fenofibrate, clofibrate)
   a. Decrease LDL (5% to 20%) and triglyceride (20% to 50%) and increase HDL (10% to 20%).
   b. Side effects include dyspepsia, gallstone, and myopathy. Unexplained, non-CHD deaths were seen in clinical trials.
   c. Contraindicated in severe renal or hepatic disease.

CHAPTER 11

Pathophysiologic Processes

Pathophysiology is the study of disrupted function and the mechanisms of disease. Pathophysiologic processes interfere with the provision of basic cellular survival needs (oxygen, nutrients, waste removal, electrolyte and acid-base balance) and cause cellular injury and death. Cellular injury and death disrupt tissue, organ, and system function. This chapter review the pathophysiology of major cardiac and vascular conditions.

Pathophysiologic Stimuli

Stimuli

1. Hypoxia, lack of sufficient oxygen to maintain aerobic metabolism, is the most common cause of cellular injury.
2. Ischemia, lack of sufficient blood supply to tissues, is the most common cause of cellular hypoxia. Ischemia injures tissues faster than hypoxia does because insufficient nutrients are supplied to tissues (restricting anaerobic metabolism) and lactic acid builds up also.
3. Physical agents — mechanical trauma, pressure or temperature gradients and irradiation
4. Chemical agents — drugs and poisons (alcohol)
5. Microorganisms and their toxins
6. Genetic defects
7. Nutritional imbalances — protein, vitamin or mineral deficiency
8. Cellular and chemical components of the immune and inflammatory response

Response

Cellular response to pathophysiologic stimuli occurs along a continuum from adaptation through injury to death. Cellular structure and function is disturbed or destroyed.

Cellular Structure and Function

Cytoplasm, the internal compartment of the cell, contains organelles and cytosol.

Organelles

1. Organelles (little organs) are membrane bound compartments within the cell that have specialized functions.
   a. Mitochondria generate cellular energy through aerobic metabolism.
   b. Endoplasmic reticulum (ER) provides a large surface within the cell on which chemical reactions can occur.
   c. Ribosomes synthesize protein.
   d. Golgi apparatus (GA) processes and packages chemicals for transport to more distant cells. The GA also produces polysaccharides, modifies some activating enzymes, and produces lysosomes.
   e. Lysosomes contain digestive enzymes and peroxisomes contain oxidative enzymes. Peroxisomes play a major role in lipid metabolism.
   f. Nucleus contains large quantities of deoxyribonucleic acid (DNA), which forms the genes that regulate and differentiate cell function.
2. Cytosol is the fluid medium in which the organelles are suspended.

Plasma and Intracellular Membranes

1. Plasma membrane surrounds the entire cell and separates intracellular and extracellular fluid compartments. Characteristics of the plasma membrane include the following:
   a. Consists of a double layer of lipid molecules (the lipid bilayer).
   b. Proteins, which are anchored on or in the lipid bilayer, transport and exchange material between the cell and its environment.
   c. Damage to or altered function of the plasma membrane is a common, early response to pathophysiologic stimuli.
2. Cell junctions are specialized regions on the plasma membrane that link individual cells into tissues and allow small molecules to pass from cell to cell. Three kinds of junctions have been identified.
   a. Desmosomes hold cells together and maintain structural stability.
      1) Cardiac intercalated discs maintain the functional integration of myocardial cells.
   b. Tight junctions prevent the leakage of small molecules between adjacent cells.

c. Gap junctions coordinate the activity of adjacent cells.
   1) Synchronize contraction of myocardial cells
   2) Facilitate the rapid spread of action potentials in neural tissues
d. Opening or loosening of cell junctions allows potassium to leak out of and water to move into injured cells.

3. Intracellular membranes surround the organelles and allow specific functions to occur within each.
4. Substances can move across the plasma and intracellular membranes by passive or active processes.
   a. Passive movement does not require cell energy
      1) Diffusion is the movement of a substance from a region of higher concentration to a region of lower concentration down a concentration gradient.
      2) Osmosis is the net movement of water across a semipermeable membrane, which separates compartments with different solute concentrations. Water moves into the compartment with the higher solute concentration.
      3) Filtration is the net movement of water due to a pressure gradient. Water moves from an area of higher pressure to one of lower pressure.
      4) Facilitated diffusion uses a carrier protein to move a substance across a semipermeable membrane. Glucose uses insulin (carrier protein) to move into cells.
   b. Active movement is energy dependent. When pathophysiologic processes interfere with energy production (ATP), active movement slows or ceases.
      1) The sodium-potassium pump (Na+-K+–ATPase) maintains fluid and electrolyte balance between extracellular and intracellular fluid (cytosol).
         a) Failure of the sodium-potassium pump produces cellular swelling — intracellular sodium concentration increases and draws water into the cell (osmosis).
      2) An active calcium transport system (Ca++–ATPase) maintains differential calcium concentrations in the cytosol and organelles.
         a) Failure of the calcium transport system interferes with muscle contraction, cell signaling and plasma membrane function.
         b) Calcium ions are important in the regulation of cardiac muscle contraction.
            1. Calcium is released from the sarcoplasmic reticulum and transverse tubules.

2. Calcium is required for actin and myosin filaments to contract.

3) An active hydrogen transport system (H+–ATPase) is one mechanism used to maintain acid-base balance.

Electrical Properties of Cells

1. An electrical gradient (membrane potential) exists across the plasma membrane of all living cells.
   a. The electrical charge within resting cells is more negative than the charge outside cells.
   b. Cardiac, skeletal muscle, and nerve cells are excitable cells. Excitable cells are capable of generating and propelling an action potential along the plasma membrane.
      1) Resting membrane potential in excitable cells is minus 70 to minus 90 mV. Excitable cells are polarized when at their resting potential.
      2) In resting cardiac cells there is a slow inward flow of positively charged ions. When the membrane potential reaches threshold (minus 60 to minus 70 mV), specialized channels open in the plasma membrane and positively charged ions rush into the cell.
         a) Reduction of cell membrane potential to a less negative value is depolarization.
         b) Restoration of the cell to its resting membrane potential is repolarization.

Cardiac Action Potential (AP)

1. Myocardial cells
   a. Phase O — depolarization — is characterized by the rapid upstroke.
      1) Membrane channels open and sodium ions rush into the cell.
      2) Membrane potential changes from approximately -90 millivolts (mv) at rest to + 20 mv.
   b. Phase 1 represents a brief period of repolarization.
      1) Inward sodium movement slows and slow inward calcium movement begins.
      2) Membrane potential changes from approximately + 20 mv to + 5 mv.
   c. Phase 2 is the plateau phase during which cardiac contraction occurs.
      1) Slow inward calcium current

        2) Slow downward drift of membrane potential from approximately + 5 to -5 mv
    d. Phase 3 is repolarization.
        1) Potassium moves out of cell.
        2) Membrane potential changes from approximately -5 to -80 mv.
    e. Phase 4 is the resting membrane potential
        1) Corresponds to diastole
        2) Approximately -80 to -90 mv
2. Specialized conduction cells — sinoatrial (SA) and atrioventricular (AV) nodes
    a. Slow spontaneous rise in resting membrane potential due to a slow inward sodium leak (Phase 4).
        1) Catecholamines increase heart rate (HR) by increasing rate of rise to threshold.
        2) Acetylcholine (vagal neurotransmitter) reduces rate of rise and slows HR
    b. When membrane reaches threshold (approximately -55 mv) rapid depolarization (Phase 0) occurs.
    c. No plateau phase; immediate repolarization (Phase 3).
3. Pathophysiologic processes that interfere with plasma membrane permeability or deplete cellular energy affect the electrical properties of cells.
    a. Cardiac dysrhythmia results from interference with the generation or proagation of cardiac APs.
4. Antidysrhythmic drugs are grouped according to their effects on the cardiac AP. (See Chapter 15.)

Cellular Energy Metabolism

1. Adenosine triphosphate (ATP), the major carrier of cellular energy, is required for many cellular processes — muscle contraction, active transport, and biochemical synthesis, for example.
2. ATP is generated from chemical processes during the metabolism of food (carbohydrates, fats and proteins).
    a. Aerobic metabolism and energy generation occur in the mitochondria.
        1) Fats, proteins and carbohydrates are broken down and combined with molecular oxygen to form carbon dioxide and water.
        2) Kreb's cycle (also called the citric acid or the tricarboxylic acid cycle) is the final common pathway for metabolism of pyruvate (from glucose), amino acids (from proteins), and fatty acids (from fat).

3) Oxidative phosphorylation is the process in which inorganic phosphate couples with adenosine diphosphate (ADP) to form ATP.
4) The net gain of energy from aerobic metabolism of one mole of glucose is 38 moles of ATP.

b. Anaerobic metabolism occurs in the cytoplasm
   1) Glucose is converted to pyruvate and ADP is converted to ATP in the process — glycolysis.
   2) The net gain of energy from anaerobic metabolism of one mole of glucose is two moles of ATP and two moles of pyruvate.
      a) If oxygen is present, pyruvate moves into the Kreb's cycle.
      b) In the absence of oxygen, pyruvate is converted to lactic acid, builds up and stops the metabolic process.
   3) Anaerobic metabolism generates much less energy (1 mole of glucose yields 2 moles of ATP) than aerobic metabolism (1 mole of glocose yields 38 moles of ATP)
   4) Despite inefficient energy production, anaerobic metabolism prevents cell injury for a few minutes under hypoxic conditions.

Cellular Reproduction/Regeneration

1. Most cells have the ability to reproduce through mitosis.
2. Labile cells (for example, vascular endothelial cells and platelets) regenerate frequently and have a short life span.
3. Stable cells (for example, osteophytes) retain the ability to regenerate but do so only under special circumstances.
4. Permanent cells do not regenerate (for example, nerve and muscle cells).

Cellular Communication

1. Receptors on the plasma membrane bind with messenger molecules to produce a specific response.
   a. Primary messengers include hormones, neurotransmitters, and local mediators
   b. When messengers and receptor bind, 4 types of cellular response may occur.
      1) Change in membrane permeability and the electrical properties of cells
      2) Alter contraction of muscle cells
      3) Alter secretion
      4) Alter cellular metabolism

2. Other receptors, when activated, regulate intracellular responses through the release of secondary messengers.
   a. G-protein linked receptors increase the intracellular concentration of cyclic adeno-sine monophosphate (AMP)
      1) β_1 receptors in the plasma membrane of myocardial cells bind with nor-epinephrine and activate cyclic AMP to increase the force of contraction.
   b. Inositol-phospholipid (IP_3) linked receptors increase intracellular calcium and activate protein kinase C, which activates other intracellular proteins.
      1) Muscarinic receptors of myocardial cells may act by way of the IP_3 system.
3. Autonomic nervous system regulates cardiovascular function.
   a. Sympathetic nervous system (SNS)
      1) Preganglionic SNS neurons release the neurotransmitter acetylcholine (Ach).
      2) Postganglionic SNS neurons release norepinephrine (NE) at the effector site.
      3) Receptors are present on the target cells — $alpha_1$, $alpha_2$, $beta_1$ and $beta_2$
         a) Myocardial cells have $beta_1$ receptors that, when stimulated, increase HR, contractile force, and conduction velocity.
         b) Arterioles, including coronary arteries, have alpha and $beta_2$ receptors.
            1. When stimulated, alpha receptors produce vasoconstriction.
            2. When stimulated, $beta_2$ receptors produce vasodilation.
      4) The number or density of receptors activated determines the intensity of response.
         a) $Beta_1$ receptors in cardiac tissue can be up or down regulated. That is, the number of receptors can be increased or decreased.
         b) Distribution of receptors in vascular beds is variable — for example, skin, mucosa, and cerebral arterioles have primarily alpha receptors.
   b. Parasympathetic nervous system
      1) Parasympathetic postganglionic neurons release the neurotransmitter Ach, which acts on muscarinic receptors.
         a) Myocardial cells have muscarinic receptors that, when stimulated, decrease HR, contractile force and conduction velocity.

Cellular Injury and Death

Apoptosis

Apoptosis, programmed cell death, is designed to eliminate unwanted cells through an internally programmed series of events. It can be a normal process during embryologic development or can be initiated by toxins.

1. Stimuli of apoptosis include injurious agents, withdrawal of growth factors or hormones, and the action of specific death substances (eg, tissue necrosis factor).
2. Intracellular proteins can inhibit or promote the cell's death.
3. Execution enzymes (capsases) initiate a cascade of cellular degradation that results in the formation of apoptotic bodies that contain organelles and cytosol.
4. Phagocytes devour the apoptotic bodies. The dead cells leave without a trace — little or no inflammation occurs.

Necrosis

Necrosis refers to cell or tissue death characterized by cellular swelling and the breakdown of proteins and organelles. General mechanisms include the following:

1. Energy depletion and decreased ATP generation
2. Formation of toxic oxygen-derived free radicals (OFR)
3. Disruption of calcium homeostasis and increased calcium concentration in the cytosol
4. Defects in plasma membrane permeability
5. Irreversible damage to mitochondria

Vascular Structure and Function

Wall Structure

1. Basic constituents of vascular wall are endothelium, smooth muscle, and the extracellular matrix, which is made up of elastic elements and collagen.
2. Endothelial cells (vascular endothelium) have multiple functions.
   a. Maintain vessel permeability
   b. Elaborate anticoagulant substances — prostacyclin, thrombomodulin
   c. Elaborate a balance of antithrombotic (plasminogen activator) and prothrombotic (von Willibrand factor, tissue factor, plasminogen activator inhibitor) substances

d. Modulate vascular tone and blood flow
e. Regulate immune and inflammatory reactions by controlling leukocyte interaction with the vessel wall
f. Modify lipoprotein deposit and metabolism within the vessel wall
g. Regulate growth of smooth muscle cells in the vessel wall

3. Smooth muscle cells determine lumen size and vascular resistance, ie, vasoconstriction and dilation. Smooth muscle cells may also:
   a. Synthesize collagen and elastin
   b. Elaborate growth factors and cytokines
   c. Migrate to the intima and proliferate

Arteries

1. Arteries have three concentric layers:
   a. Intima — closest to the lumen, made up of vascular endothelial cells
   b. Media — middle layer of smooth muscle encased in the internal and external elastic lamina
   c. Adventitia — outer layer made up of connective tissue and encasing nerve fibers and the vasa vasorum
2. Vasa vasorum (vessels of the vessel) perforates the adventitia and external elastic lamina to nourish the media. The intima obtains oxygen and nutrients directly from circulating blood.

Small Vessels

1. Arterioles, the smallest branches of the arterial tree, are the principal source of vascular resistance and convert blood flow from pulsatile to steady.
2. Capillaries have thin walls primarily made up of endothelium supported by a thin basement membrane.
3. Post-capillary venules

Veins

1. Veins are large caliber, thin-walled vessels.
   a. Large capacity — approximately 2/3 of circulating blood is in the veins.
   b. Relatively little support and easily compressed.
   c. Valves prevent reverse flow — particularly in the extremities.

Lymphatics

Lymphatics are thin-walled, endothelium-lined channels that drain interstitial fluid to the blood.

Vascular Cells Response to Injury

Injurious Stimuli

1. Cytokines and inflammatory products
2. Hemodynamic stress and lipids
3. Microorganisms
4. Components of the complement cascade
5. Hypoxia

Endothelial Cell Response

1. Endothelial cells are activated by vascular injury and may:
   a. Elaborate adhesion molecules and other inflammatory mediators
   b. Elaborate growth factors that contribute to vascular stenosis
   c. Elaborate vasoactive substances that produce vasoconstriction or vasodilation
   d. Elaborate pro- or anticoagulant substances
2. Endothelial functions and response to injury is an area of active research.

Smooth Muscle Cell Response

1. Vascular injury stimulates smooth muscle cell growth by disrupting the balance between inhibition and stimulation.
   a. Intimal thickening is an exaggerated healing response that can cause stenosis or occlusion of small vessels.

Hypoxia and Ischemia

1. Hypoxia, lack of sufficient oxygen at the tissue level, is the most common cause of cellular injury.
   a. Molecular oxygen must be present for aerobic metabolism to occur.
   b. As cellular oxygen tension decreases mitochondrial energy production is reduced.
   c. At a critical level, the cell shifts to anaerobic metabolism.
2. Ischemia, lack of sufficient blood supply accelerates tissue damage from hypoxia because of lack of fuel for anaerobic metabolism and the accumulation of metabolic waste products. Under resting conditions, tissues extract differential amounts of oxygen from the blood. For example, myocardial cells extract 70% to 75% of the available oxygen, whereas peripheral muscle cells extract 30%. When stressed, peripheral cells increase oxygen extraction but myocardial cells cannot.

Causes of Hypoxia and Ischemia

1. Decreased oxygen carrying capacity (decreased amount or altered function of red blood cells and hemoglobin)
2. Decreased oxygen saturation (due to pulmonary disease, fever or acidosis)
3. Impaired oxygen delivery (hypoperfusion or ischemia)
   a. Stenosis or narrowing of blood vessels due to plaque formation
   b. Thrombosis or embolism occluding vessels
   c. Weakening and rupture of vessels
   d. Decreased force of cardiac contraction

Effects of Hypoxia and Ischemia

1. Energy depletion and decreased ATP synthesis due to shift to anaerobic metabolism
2. Anaerobic metabolism leads to accumulation of lactic acid and cellular acidosis
3. Reduced activity of Na^+-K^+ pump produces cellular swelling
4. Reduced protein synthesis and lipid deposition
5. End result is cellular necrosis

Functional Impact

1. Coronary occlusion
   a. Myocardial cells cease to contract within 60 seconds
   b. Continued energy depletion leads to plasma and intracellular membrane damage
   c. Irreversible injury to heart muscle occurs after 30 to 40 minutes
2. Cerebral ischemia
   a. Irreversible injury to brain cells by hypoxia occurs after 4 to 6 minutes.
   b. Survival of brain cells depends, in part, on duration of ischemia, presence of collateral circulation, and the magnitude and rapidity of flow reduction.

Clinical Manifestations

1. Cardiac dysfunction — dysrhythmia, decreased contractility
2. Cerebral dysfunction — decreased level of consciousness, aphasia, motor deficits
3. Pain — intermittent claudication, angina

Reperfusion Injury

1. Reperfusion injury is cell damage that occurs after blood flow is returned to ischemic tissue. Reperfusion injury may be clinically significant in MI, after thrombolytic or angioplastic procedures, and stroke.
   a. Reperfusion results in production of OFRs (oxygen-derived free radicals).
      1) OFRs are highly toxic to vascular endothelium and to mitochondria.
      2) OFRs damage the myocardial or brain cell and also the microvasculature.
   b. Cytokines and adhesion molecules produced by ischemic cells initiate inflammation and further cell injury.
   c. Reperfusion dysrhythmia may be due to increased calcium load or to OFRs.

Inflammation

Inflammation is a defensive response of the body to cellular injury.

Causes of Inflammation

1. Microorganisms
2. Physical trauma with the release of blood into tissues
3. Direct irritation due to physical, mechanical or chemical injury
4. Immune reaction, including autoimmune

Phases of Inflammation

1. Purpose of inflammation is to rid the body of the causative agent and reduce injury.
2. Acute inflammation begins immediately after cell injury and lasts a few minutes to several days.
   a. Vascular phase
      1) Neural reflex produces vasoconstriction of arterioles near site of injury.
      2) Vasodilation (hyperemia) and increased blood flow follow vasoconstriction.
      3) Plasma proteins leak into tissues and generate an osmotic pull that causes edema (swelling).
      4) Movement of fluid into tissues (extravasation) increases red blood cell concentration and slows capillary circulation.
      5) Endothelial cells lining capillaries and venules retract producing spaces between cells (vascular permeability).

b. Cellular phase
   1) Slowed capillary circulation and fluid extravasation cause white cells to line up along the vascular endothelium.
   2) Adhesion molecules under the influence of inflammatory mediators cause the white cells to adhere to the vascular endothelium.
   3) Lymphokines are released at the site of injury and attract white cells (chemotaxis).
   4) White cells (first neutrophils later macrophages) ingest invading organisms, dead cells, and cellular debris (phagocytosis).

Inflammatory Mediators

1. A large number of substances, some not yet discovered others not well characterized, mediate inflammation.
   a. Vasoactive proteins
      1) Histamine and serotonin, released from mast cells and platelets, cause arteriolar dilation and increase permeability of venules.
      2) Prostaglandins potentiate the vascular action of histamine and serotonin and are involved in pain and fever response.
      3) Platelet activating factor (PAF) increases vascular permeability, activates platelets and increases leukocyte aggregation and adhesion.
   b. Cytokines, produced by many cell types, modulate the function of other cells. Interleukin-1 (IL–1) and TNF are major inflammatory cytokines.
      1) IL-1 and TNF induce the synthesis of adhesion molecules and growth factors. They increase the thrombogenicity of the endothelial surface.
      2) IL-1 and TNF induce systemic responses including fever, loss of appetite, sleepiness, and the release of corticosteroids.
      3) TNF is a primary mediator of the hemodynamic effects of septic shock.
   c. Nitric oxide (NO) is a potent vasodilator, which is released from vascular endothelium.
   d. Intermediary substances in the complement cascade increase vascular permeability and vasodilation, white cell adhesion, and chemotaxis and enhance phagocytosis. Terminal elements of the complement cascade breakdown plasma and intracellular membranes and cause cell lysis.
   e. The clotting system forms a fibrinous mesh at the site of inflammation, which traps microorganisms and prevents the

spread of infection. Fibrin forms a clot that stops bleeding and provides a framework for healing and repair.

f. Kinins (especially bradykinin) promote vasodilation, vascular permeability, and contribute to the pain response.

Resolution

1. Acute inflammation resolves through cell regeneration and scarring or becomes chronic.
2. Chronic inflammation may follow acute inflammation or may occur as a distinct process.
   a. Dense infiltration of lymphocytes and macrophages
   b. Macrophages may wall-off an infected site producing a granuloma

Functional Impact

1. Vasculitis is a general term for inflammation of blood vessels.
   a. Arteritis or angiitis are terms for inflammation of an artery.
   b. Phlebitis is inflammation of a vein.
2. Myocarditis, pericarditis, and endocarditis are inflammatory processes affecting cardiac function.
3. Atherosclerosis is viewed currently as a chronic inflammatory process.

Atherosclerosis

Definition

1. Atherosclerosis is the process of lipid deposition within the intimal layer of large and medium sized arteries.
2. Arteriosclerosis involves deterioration of the intima and media of smaller arteries and arterioles.

Lesion Progression

1. Fatty streak is an early, detectable lesion that can occur within first decade of life.
   a. Mainly intracellular lipid accumulation
   b. No obstruction to blood flow; clinically silent
2. Atheromatous plaque develops from:
   a. Extracellular lipid accumulation within the intima
   b. Fibrous cap made up of smooth muscle cells encapsulates the lipid deposits

c. Shoulder of the cap is common site of rupture
   1) Macrophages are active at the shoulder
d. May be clinically silent or symptomatic

3. Fibroatheroma
   a. Lipid core and fibrotic layers
   b. May be mainly calcified or mainly fibrotic
   c. May be clinically silent or symptomatic
4. Complicated lesions culminate in:
   a. Calcification that leads to arterial stiffness and reduces accommodation to pulsatile flow.
   b. Areas of rupture and ulceration that may dislodge debris and cause embolization.
   c. Hemorrhage into the plaque that may produce hematoma, which impinges on the vessel lumen.
   d. Superimposed thrombosis at the site of injury may occlude the vessel lumen.
   e. Complicated lesions may be clinically silent or symptomatic.

Inflammatory Response Hypothesis

1. Damage to vascular endothelium by established and emerging cardiovascular risk factors, eg, hyperlipidemia, hypertension, increased homocysteinuria.
2. Chronic inflammatory response of the arterial wall
   a. Increased endothelial permeability that allows low density lipoprotcin cholesterol (LDL) to move into the intimal layer.
   b. LDL is oxidized and attracts macrophages.
   c. Macrophages take up LDL and become foam cells.
   d. Enzymes are released that weaken the fibrotic cap.
3. Progressive development of plaque is associated with continuation of the inflammatory response.

Location of Lesions

Atheromatous plaque can occur in any artery; however, certain sites are affected more commonly.

1. Lower abdominal aorta is most common
2. Other sites in descending order of frequency
   a. Coronary arteries
   b. Popliteal arteries
   c. Descending thoracic aorta
   d. Internal carotid arteries
   e. Vessels of the circle of Willis

Functional Impact

1. Atheromatous plaque protrudes into vessel lumen and decreases blood flow.
2. Plaque encroaches on the medial layer and weakens the vessel wall leading to aneurysm, vessel rupture or thrombosis.
3. Complicated lesions become friable and embolize, occlude vessel lumen, or thrombus develops at the site.

Thrombosis and Embolism

1. Thombosis is the formation of blood clot within the vasculature.
2. An embolus is a piece of thrombus that breaks off and travels within the blood stream.
   a. Other substances (eg, fat or air) may enter the blood stream, travel as a bolus and occlude smaller vessels.
3. Thrombosis depends on 3 general components
   a. Endothelial injury
   b. Platelet adhesion
   c. Activation of the coagulation cascade

Causes of Thrombosis and Embolism

1. Triad ofVirchow — 3 factors that increase the risk of thrombosis
   a. Injury to the vessel wall
   b. Decreased blood flow
   c. Hypercoagulability
2. Elevated plasma homocysteine is toxic to the vascular endothelium, promotes thrombosis, increases collagen production, and decreases availability of NO.
   a. Nutritional deficiency of B vitamins is associated with high homocysteine level.

Effects of Thrombosis and Embolism

1. Thrombus narrows vessel lumen and reduces blood flow producing distal hypoperfusion and ischemia.
2. Embolism travels through the blood stream and occludes more distal vessels.
   a. Venous embolism travels to the pulmonary vasculature where it becomes trapped.
   b. Arterial embolism reduces or blocks arterial blood supply distal to its origin.
3. Thrombus within a vessel produces a local inflammatory reaction.

Functional Impact

1. MI
2. Ischemic and thrombotic stroke
3. Deep vein thrombosis (DVT)
4. Acute arterial insufficiency
5. Pulmonary embolism

Altered Vascular Function

Arterial

1. Coronary Heart Disease (CHD)
    a. Atherosclerosis of the coronary arteries is the primary mechanism.
    b. Plaque or atheroma partially occludes the vessel lumen.
        1) Asymptomatic until occluding 75% or more of blood supply
            a) Initially myocardial cells avoid ischemia through autoregulation of coronary blood flow.
            b) Collateral circulation develops among smaller arteries and may adequately nourish myocardium under non-stress conditions.
    c. Pathophysiology of myocardial ischemia
        1) Myocardial ischemia results when myocardial oxygen demand exceeds supply.
        2) Factors that increase oxygen demand
            a) Increased heart rate
            b) Increased systolic wall tension
            c) Increased contractility
        3) Myocardial cells shift to anaerobic metabolism and the resulting accumulation of lactic acid impairs cardiac contractility.
        4) Ischemia is reversible if the oxygen imbalance is corrected.
    d. Pathophysiology of MI
        1) Infarction results from prolonged ischemia. Cell death characterizes MI.
        2) Infarction is irreversible and the necrotic cells are replaced by scar tissue.
        3) Replacement of myocardial cells with scar tissue impairs cardiac function.
            a) Reduced contractility and abnormal wall motion
            b) Increased ventricular compliance (stiffening), which impedes diastolic filling

c) Reduced stroke volume and ejection fraction
d) Increased left ventricular end diastolic pressure
4) Acute MI has a central area of necrosis that is surrounded by an area of injury; an area of ischemia surrounds the area of injury.
a) Signs of infarction, injury and ischemia may be observed on the electrocardiogram.
b) When myocardial cells die, they liberate intracellular proteins (troponin and myosin) and enzymes (lactic dehydrogenase and creatine kinase) that can be used diagnostically.

2. Cerebrovascular Insufficiency
a. Transient ischemic attacks (TIA) result in temporary neurologic dysfunction.
1) Duration 15 minutes to 24 hours
2) Due to thrombosis that narrows an atherosclerotic cerebral vessel
3) Major risk factor for subsequent ischemic stroke
b. Stroke results from the occlusion of cerebral arteries by thrombosis or embolism or from hemorrhage.
c. Ischemic stroke is due to thrombosis or embolism. Ischemia is the etiology of 84% of strokes.
1) The central ischemic core is surrounded by a larger area called the ischemic penumbra.
2) Oxygen to the core is depleted within 10 seconds of occlusion and irreversible neuron damage occurs within 2 to 4 minutes.
3) The ischemic penumbra remains potentially viable for longer periods.
d. Pathophysiology of ischemic stroke
1) Mitochondria in ischemic cells are unable to generate sufficient ATP; there is a shift to anaerobic metabolism with accumulation of lactic acid and OFR.
a) Within the ischemic core, cellular acidosis leads to cell death.
2) Within the ischemic penumbra, cellular ionic gradients are disrupted leading to cellular swelling, a shift in electrolyte balance, and the accumulation of glutamate, the major excitatory neurotransmitter.
a) Excitotoxicity (accumulation of glutamate in ischemic tissue) causes cell damage by over stimulation and persistent opening of calcium channels producing toxic intracellular calcium concentration.

3) Increased intracellular calcium concentration activates prostaglandins, cytokines, leukotrienes, and NO.
4) Cell products destroy plasma and intracellular membranes and cause breakdown of the blood—brain barrier, increased vascular permeability and edema, and cell death.

e. Thrombotic stroke
   1) Thrombus forms on atherosclerotic plaque and occludes the blood vessel; occurs most commonly at curves and bifurcations
      a) Vessels affected commonly include the internal carotid artery, vertebral and basilar arteries, the middle cerebral artery (MCA), the posterior cerebral artery (PCA), and the anterior cerebral artery (ACA).
   2) Site of occlusion determines the clinical manifestations.
      a) Collateral circulation may compensate for obstruction proximal to the circle of Willis; obstruction distal to the circle of Willis results in infarction.
      b) Thrombotic stroke may progress to cerebral infarction.
      c) Location and amount of intracerebral damage determines recovery.

f. Embolic stroke
   1) Heart is the main source of emboli; less common sources include fat, air or tumor emboli.
   2) Embolus lodges most frequently in the MCA.
   3) A large embolus may break into smaller ones that occlude smaller, more distal branches.

g. Hemorrhagic stroke
   1) Intracerebral hemorrhage is caused most frequently by hypertension (HTN).
      a) Elevated BP weakens the vessel and leads to rupture
      b) Charcot-Buchard aneurysms that form at the bifurcation of small intracerebral arteries in individuals with HTN are a frequent source of bleeding.
      c) In large bleeds, the blood forms a mass that compresses and disrupts surrounding brain tissue.
      d) Blood in the parenchyma of the brain causes extensive neuronal destruction.
         1. Blood is reabsorbed eventually.
         2. Remaining area is filled with connective (scar) tissue.

h. Subarachnoid hemorrhage — bleeding into the subarachnoid space
   1) Most result from congenital malformation of cerebrovascular beds

      2) May accompany cerebral tumor, trauma, atherosclerosis or infection
   i. Cerebral aneurysm — a congenital weakness in the middle layer of the vessel results in a saccular out-pouching at the weakened area.
      1) Fusiform cerebral aneurysms result from weakening of the middle layer of the vessel due to atherosclerosis.
   j. Arteriovenous malformations (AVM) are developmental defects of cerebral vasculature.
      1) Veins connect with the artery without an intermediate capillary bed.
      2) Higher pressure in the arterial circulation is transmitted to the weaker venous system and causes rupture.
3. Occlusive disease of extremities produces ischemia in distal tissues.
   a. Iliac bifurcation of the aorta and the femoral popliteal narrowing are the most common sites.
   b. Gradual occlusion results in development of collateral circulation that prevents symptoms for a variable period of time.
      1) Collateral circulation is native, undeveloped blood vessels that enlarge and develop in response to inflammatory mediators of ischemia.
4. Aortic and large artery aneurysm
   a. Fusiform aneurysm is a circumferential arterial dilation usually related to atherosclerosis and weakening of the middle layer of the arterial wall.
      1) Abdominal aortic aneurysms arise below the renal arteries and may extend to include the iliac arteries.
      2) Thoracic aneurysms are located in the ascending aorta, aortic arch, or descending segment of the thoracic aorta.
   b. Aortic dissection occurs when tearing and degeneration of the medial layer allow blood to separate the aorta's intimal layer from the adventitial layer.
      1) Hematoma forms in the area of separation.
      2) Aortic dissection is associated with HTN and with Marfan syndrome.
   c. Saccular aneurysms are outpouching on one side of aorta.
      1) Saccular aneurysms are associated with syphilis and congenital malformations.
      2) Risk of rupture
5. Raynaud phenomenon
   a. Episodic constriction of the small arteries or arterioles of the extremities, causing intermittent pallor and cyanosis of the skin of the fingers, toes, ears or nose.

1) Pallor is caused by spasm of the arterioles and possibly the venules that produces decreased or absent capillary flow.
2) Cyanosis results from capillary dilation and slow blood flow.
3) Vasoconstriction may be followed by hyperemia due to a reactive vasodilation.

6. Vasculitis is inflammation of the vessel wall. Two most common mechanisms are immune-mediated inflammation and direct invasion of the vessel wall by infectious pathogens.
   a. Large vessels — may involve medium-sized arteries also
      1) Infective aortitis — invasion of the aortic wall by blood-borne pathogens
      2) Takayasu disease — inflammation of the aorta and its upper branches
         a) Ischemic symptoms involving the upper extremities and central nervous system may occur.
         b) Etiology is unknown.
      3) Giant cell arteritis occurs mainly in the cerebral arteries (especially the temporal artery) but may affect the aorta.
         a) The affected artery is infiltrated with granulomatous inflammations that contain giant cells. (Giant cells are fused epithelial cells.)
         b) Granulomas become foci for necrosis in the vessel wall.
         c) The affected artery becomes swollen, nodular and tender.
   b. Medium vessels
      1) Polyarteritis nodosa
         a) Inflammation may lead to weakening of vessel wall and aneurysm formation.
         b) Etiology unknown
      2) Kawasaki disease
         a) Usually occurs in children before age 12 years
         b) Coronary arteries often affected
      3) Thromboangiitis obliterans (Buerger Disease)
         a) Segmental thrombosing inflammation of medium-sized and small arteries
         b) Principally affects the tibial and radial arteries; may extend to veins and nerves of the extremities
         c) Strong association with cigarette smoking
         d) Clinical manifestations: cold sensitivity, instep claudication, chronic ulcers, and pain at rest
   c. Small vessels: arterioles, venules and capillaries
      1) Wegener granulomatosis
      2) Churg-Strauss syndrome
      3) Microscopic polyarteritis
      4) Hypersensitivity drug reactions

Venous

1. Venous thrombosis — thrombotic occlusion of vein or venule
   a. Thrombus develops as a result of endothelial dysfunction, which causes imbalance of the pro-coagulant and anticoagulant substances, and slowed blood flow.
   b. Venous thrombosis obstructs venous blood flow from distal tissues.
      1) Collateral circulation may partially compensate.
      2) Venous pressure distal to the occlusion rises and produces edema.
      3) Cellulitis, a diffuse infection of the skin and soft tissues, may occur.
   c. Thrombus may completely and permanently occlude the vessel or it may resolve.
2. Venous insufficiency and stasis occur when something, usually incompetent venous valves, interferes with blood flow against gravity.
   a. Elevated venous pressure produces edema, hyperpigmentation, dermatitis, induration, stasis cellulitis and venostasis ulcers.
   b. Venous insufficiency may develop after venous thrombosis.
3. Varicose veins are dilated, elongated and tortuous superficial veins of the lower extremities.
   a. Incompetent valves and increased venous pressure produce varicose veins.
   b. Varicose veins can lead to chronic venous insufficiency.

Cardiac Structure and Function

Cardiac muscle cells (myocytes) have 5 major components:
1. Cell membrane (sarcolemma) and T tubules — for conduction
2. Sarcoplasmic reticulum — a calcium reservoir for excitation-contraction coupling
3 Contractile elements
4. Mitochondria
5. Nucleus

Sarcomere

Sarcomere, the contractile unit of cardiac muscle, is an orderly arrangement of actin and myosin together with the regulatory proteins, troponin and tropomyosin.

Intercalated Discs

1. Intercalated discs that permit both mechanical and ionic coupling promote functional integration of myocytes.
   a. Gap junctions, plasma membrane channels, directly link the cytoplasmic components of neighboring cardiac cells.

Conduction System

1. Specialized excitatory and conducting myocytes within the cardiac conduction system regulate cardiac rate and rhythm.
   a. Sinoatrial (SA) node is the pacemaker of the heart.
   b. Atrioventricular (AV) node regulates impulse conduction from atria to ventricles.
   c. Bundle of HIS is the conduction pathway from the right atrium to the ventricular septum that divides into the bundle branches.
   d. Bundle branches arborize (Purkinje fibers) ventricular muscle

Circulation

1. Coronary arteries run along external surface of the heart and feed smaller vessels (intramural arteries that penetrate the myocardium).
   a. Left anterior descending artery supplies the apex of the heart, the anterior left ventricular wall, and the anterior 2/3 of the ventricular septum
   b. Left circumflex artery supplies the lateral wall of the left ventricle in most people.
   c. Right coronary artery supplies the right ventricular wall and the posterobasal wall of the left ventricle and the posterior third of the ventricular septum in most people.

Valves

Cardiac valves function to maintain unidirectional blood flow.

Altered Cardiac Function

Dysrhythmia

1. Cardiac dysrhythmia disrupts the orderly sequence of cardiac contraction.
2. Mechanism of cardiac dysrhythmia
   a. Enhanced automaticity — increased rate of depolarization of cardiac muscle cells.

b. Depressed automaticity — decreased rate of depolarization of cardiac muscle cells.
c. Reentry occurs when an impulse is able to excite previously depolarized cardiac tissue through anatomic or functional circuits.

Valvular Heart Disease (VHD)

Interferes with normal forward flow of blood by reduced opening (stenosis) or inadequate closing (insufficiency) of the valves.

1. Stenosis — valve orifice narrows and valve leaflets fuse thereby obstructing blood flow.
   a. Pressure rises in the chamber behind the stenotic valve.
   b. Myocardial fibers hypertrophy to generate more force to push blood through the stenotic valve.
2. Insufficiency — valve can not close completely due to scarring and retraction of the valve leaflets.
   a. Blood flows backward (regurgitation) through the insufficient valve.
   b. The chamber that receives the regurgitant flow must pump an increased blood volume (normal filling volume plus regurgitant volume).
   c. Myocardial fibers hypertrophy and the chamber dilates.
3. Mixed lesions — both stenosis and insufficiency occur in the same valve.
   a. Usually signifies advanced disease
4. Rheumatic fever is the most common cause of VHD worldwide.

Pump Failure

1. Damaged cardiac muscle contracts weakly and the chambers do not empty properly.
2. Heart failure (HF) is a clinical syndrome that results from the heart's inability to pump enough blood to meet the body's metabolic demand.
   a. As contractility and cardiac output (CO) decline, venous return to the ventricles remains the same or increases.
3. Systemic responses to decreased CO include:
   a. Increased sympathetic activity
      1) Increased HR and contractile force
      2) Systemic vasoconstriction
   b. Renin release from the kidney
      1) Renin converts angiotensinogen to angiotensin I (A-I).

2) Angiotensin converting enzyme (ACE) converts A-I to angiotensin II (A-II), a potent vasoconstrictor.
3) A-II stimulates release of aldosterone from the adrenal cortex.
   a) Aldosterone promotes sodium and water reabsorption in the kidney tubule, producing increased blood volume.
4) Increased circulating level of A-II acts in conjunction with signals from the atrial baroreceptors to release antidiuretic hormone (ADH) from the posterior pituitary.
   a) ADH promotes water reabsorption through the distal tubule of the kidney.

c. Myocardial oxygen balance
   1) Oxygen demand is increased due to increased HR, force of contraction, and muscle wall stress.
   2) Oxygen supply is reduced because of decreased CO.
d. Atrial and ventricular tissues release respectively atrial natriuretic peptide (ANP) and brain natriuretic peptide (BNP).
   1) ANP and BNP promote diuresis through a direct effect on the kidney.
   2) ANP also suppresses aldosterone, renin, and ADH release.
   3) The effect of ANP and BNP is small and probably overwhelmed by factors that promote sodium and water retention and vasoconstriction.

4. Cardiac responses to increased blood volume are initially compensatory but beyond a critical point contribute to inadequate systemic perfusion.
   a. Starling's Law of the Heart states within normal limits the more the heart is filled during diastole, the greater the force of contraction during systole.
      1) This mechanism enhances CO up to a critical point beyond which further stretch on myocardial fibers increases cardiac energy requirements beyond that which can be supplied.
      2) Beyond this critical point, increased volume and pressure are transmitted in a retrograde fashion to the pulmonary circulation and may result in pulmonary congestion and edema.
   b. Dilation of cardiac chambers (acute response)
      1) Ventricles dilate in acute HF
      2) Dilation increases myocardial oxygen demand and decreases the effectiveness of cardiac contraction.

c. Myocardial hypertrophy (chronic response)
   1) Hypertrophy results from increased cardiac workload, commonly HTN.
   2) Hypertrophy increases myocardial oxygen demand. When oxygen supply to the hypertrophied muscle is inadequate, ischemia and cardiac dysfunction result.

5. Cardiomyopathy — primary abnormality of the myocardium
   a. Dilated cardiomyopathy (DCM) — progressive cardiac hypertrophy, dilation, and contractile dysfunction
      1) Etiology: viral, alcohol or other toxicity, pregnancy-associated, genetic influences
      2) Clinical features
         a) May occur at any age, commonly affects those 20–60 years old
         b) Slowly progressive HF
         c) Mortality without transplant: 50% within 2 years, 75% within 5 years
         d) Embolism and dysrhythmia are common complications
   b. Hypertrophic cardiomyopathy (HCM) — myocardial hypertrophy, abnormal diastolic filling, and intermittent left ventricular outflow obstruction
      1) Etiology: strong genetic basis
      2) Clinical features
         a) Reduced CO and increased ventricular pressure cause a secondary increase in pulmonary venous pressure
         b) Focal myocardial ischemia occurs as muscle hypertrophy exceeds intramural arterial blood supply
         c) Atrial fibrillation with mural thombosis and possible embolization
         d) Ventricular dysrhythmia and sudden death
   c. Restrictive cardiomyopathy (RCM) — decreased ventricular compliance resulting in impaired filling
      1) May be idiopathic or associated with radiation fibrosis, amyloidosis, sarcoidosis, or metastatic tumor
      2) Clinical features similar to HCM

Inflammatory Heart Disease

1. Infective endocarditis occurs when microorganisms invade the lining of the heart.
   a. Causative agents include bacteria, fungi, rickettsiae, and virus or parasites.
   b. May be acute (ABE) or subacute (SBE)

1) ABE occurs most commonly in intravenous drug users. Most common causative organism is Staphylococcus aureus.
2) SBE is caused by organisms of low virulence. The most common causative organism is Streptococcus viridans. It usually affects a damaged heart (eg, congenital or acquired valvular disease).

c. Bloodborne organisms attach to the endocardial lining of the heart and become enmeshed in fibrin and platelets (vegetations). Vegetations lodge on valve cusps and may embolize throughout the vasculature.
d. Clinical features
   1) Fever most consistent sign — may be accompanied by chills, lassitude, and weakness.
   2) Complications
      a) Cardiac: valvular insufficiency or stenosis and HF; with artificial valves partial disruption with paravalvular leak may occur.
      b) Embolic: cerebral infarct or abscess, MI, spleen or kidney abscess
      c) Renal: embolic infarction, glomerulonephritis, due to trapping of antigen-antibody complexes, leading to renal failure

2. Myocarditis — inflammatory processes that result in injury to myocardial cells.
   a. Viral infection — Coxsackie virus most common; Cytomegalic virus (CMV) and human immunodeficiency virus (HIV) less common
   b. Occurs in approximately 2/3 of patients with Lyme disease
   c. Allergic and immune process
   d. Clinical features
      1) Variable presentation: may be asymptomatic or present with sudden HF and dysrhythmias
      2) Usually self-limited but may progress to DCM
3. Pericarditis may be secondary to physical trauma (after heart surgery), infection (viral or bacterial), or immune-mediated inflammation (eg, Post-MI, drug hypersensitivity).
   a. Fluid (blood, effusion, or pus) accumulates in the pericardial sac and interferes with cardiac filling.
   b. With slow accumulation pericardial sac may accommodate up to 500 ml without symptoms. If rapid accumulation, collections of 200 ml may impair cardiac filling and produce potentially fatal cardiac tamponade.

CHAPTER 12

Cardiac and Vascular Assessment

Information included in this chapter relates to the patient with cardiac or vascular disease. The chapter focuses on key symptoms of cardiac and vascular disease and examination of body systems directly related to these symptoms. Excellent health assessment textbooks are available to readers requiring a more comprehensive or more basic review.

Basic Principles

Assessment is the process of data collection and interpretation. Sources of data include the history, physical examination, laboratory testing and diagnostic imaging.

1. Historical (subjective) information and physical (objective) findings direct appropriate laboratory and diagnostic testing.
2. Assessment data are used to formulate clinical diagnoses (both nursing and medical), establish patient goals, plan care, and evaluate outcomes.
3. Patient condition (stage of illness) and the purpose of the encounter determine areas that are included in an assessment.
4. Elements of the history and physical examination are the same whether performed by a physician, nurse, or other clinician.

Data Quality

Quality of the data obtained through assessment is related to the rapport established between the clinician and patient.

1. Create a comfortable environment
   a. Ensure privacy
   b. Comfortable temperature, sufficient lighting, minimal noise
2. Focus on the patient as a unique individual
   a. Refuse interruptions
   b. Review available records before the encounter; avoid repeating elements obtained by other clinicians
   c. Be aware of cultural needs; avoid stereotypes
   d. Attend to both verbal and nonverbal cues
   e. Establish equal-status seating (ie, both comfortably seated at eye-level)

Subjective Information (History)

Subjective information is usually obtained through patient interview. The patient is the expert on his experience. Secondary sources of data include family interview and record review. Secondary data sources may be needed during periods of acute illness, when the complaint is syncope, or whenever the patient is unable to provide information.

Symptom Analysis

For each symptom presented by the patient, the clinician attempts to determine the following characteristics. Pain is used as an example.

1. Quality: Describes the character of the symptom
   a. Dull, sharp, squeezing or aching pain
2. Quantity: Describes the severity, intensity or amount of the symptom in measurable terms
   a. Pain rated on an 11-point scale
   b. 0 — pain free; 10 — worst possible pain
   c. Documented as fraction or ratio (ie, 6/10)
3. Location: Describes the specific bodily location where the symptom is experienced; includes any area of radiation
   a. Substernal chest pain radiating to the left arm, jaw, throat, or back
   b. Have patient point to area(s) of pain
4. Timing: Describes the evolution of the symptom over time; includes onset, frequency, and duration
   a. Timing for each episode: For example, "sudden onset of chest pain rapidly reaching maximal intensity (6/10) and resolving over approximately 10 minutes."
      1) Discrete, intermittent episodes versus sustained pain that waxes and wanes
   b. Course of disease: For example, "Initially experienced occasional episodes of chest pain 4 years ago, over the last 6 months has experienced chest pain more frequently (2 or 3 times per week)."
5. Precipitating factors: Describes events that initiate the symptom, such as activity or emotional upset
6. Aggravating factors: Describes that which makes the symptom worse, such as position change or jarring
   a. Pain associated with acute pericarditis may be exacerbated by lying down or by movement; sitting up and leaning forward may alleviate it.
   b. Angina is usually worse with activity.

7. Alleviating factors: Describes that which relieves the symptom, such as medications or heat; may include past treatments, such as angioplasty or surgery
8. Associated symptoms: Symptoms rarely occur in isolation; recognition of patterns of symptoms leads to clinical diagnoses

Key Symptoms of Cardiac Disease

A full description is elicited for each symptom that is present.

1. Chest pain
   a. Visceral pain is deep, diffuse, and poorly localized
      1) Cardiac: angina, myocardial infarction, and acute pericarditis
      2) Esophageal: spasm, gastroesophageal reflux
      3) Pulmonary embolism and infarction
      4) Vascular: dissecting aortic aneurysm
   b. Chest wall pain is reproduced or intensified by palpation
      1) Skin and subcutaneous structures: herpes zoster
      2) Muscular skeletal: costochondritis, strain of pectoral muscle
2. Cough may be productive or nonproductive
3. Shortness of breath or breathlessness is an abnormal awareness of breathing
   a. Dyspnea on exertion: The clinician attempts to quantify the degree of exertion that reliably induces dyspnea. For example, dyspnea with climbing 10 steps at moderate pace.
   b. Orthopnea is breathlessness that occurs in a supine position and prompts the patient to elevate the head and thorax.
      1) Orthopnea is suggestive of left ventricular failure
      2) The clinician may quantify the orthopnea by the number of pillows used, for example two-pillow orthopnea.
   c. Paroxysmal nocturnal dyspnea is breathlessness that occurs after a period of recumbence and usually sleep. The patient reports being awakened with a suffocating sensation necessitating assuming an upright position. Sometimes patients report that they need to go to an open window or exit the building for relief.
4. Palpitations describes abnormal awareness of the heart beat; may be related to rapid rate or irregular rhythm.
5. Cyanosis is a bluish discoloration of the skin caused by the presence of 5 or more grams of reduced (unoxygenated) hemoglobin in 100 ml of blood.
   a. Central cyanosis is present in high bloodflow areas, such as the tongue and soft palate. Central cyanosis is usually associated with inadequate oxygenation.

b. Peripheral cyanosis occurs in low or slow blood flow areas, such as the fingers, toes, and lips. Peripheral cyanosis may be present in normal individuals due to vasoconstriction as well as in patients with low cardiac output.

6. Nocturia is increased urine formation during sleep and recumbency. In general, awakening once per night to void is within normal limits awakening two or more times per night is abnormal.
7. Fatigue is a sense of weariness or mental exhaustion. Fatigue is a nonspecific but worrisome symptom. It may be present in cardiac patients with heart failure, myocardial ischemia, and sleep apnea. It is the seventh most common complaint in primary care practices and may be unrelated to cardiac or vascular disease.
8. Syncope is sudden loss of consciousness associated with muscle weakness (faint).
   a. True syncope has three stages.
      1) The prodromal stage usually begins in the erect position and the patient feels weak and unsteady; dimming of the vision, nausea, vomiting, and pallor are common.
      2) The syncopal stage consists of muscle weakness and impaired consciousness. The patient usually falls to the ground, but it is a gradual fall and usually does not result in serious injury.
      3) Recovery stage occurs while the patient is in the horizontal position. Gradually color comes back and the patient awakens with an immediate awareness of the surroundings, but muscle weakness persists.
   b. Syncope must be differentiated from "nearsyncope" in which the patient does not experience loss of consciousness.
   c. Patients may experience light-headedness and muscle weakness before losing consciousness from myocardial ischemia, transient ischemic attacks, cerebrovascular accidents, or cardiac dysrhythmia.

Key Symptoms of Vascular Disease

There is considerable overlap among symptoms of cardiac and vascular disease. This is explained, in part, by the overlap of pathophysiological processes. While the following symptoms may be seen in patients with cardiac disease, they are more commonly observed among those with vascular disease.

1. Pallor is an absence of normal coloration, may be localized or generalized. When localized it reflects vascular disease. There are many causes of generalized pallor.
2. Swelling of feet or ankles results from an abnormal accumulation of fluid in the interstitial tissue. It may reflect systemic illnesses,

such as heart failure or cirrhosis, or vascular diseases, such as acute or chronic thrombophlebitis and chronic venous insufficiency.
   a. A weight gain of 10 lb, which is indicative of approximately 5 L of fluid, precedes visible edema in most patients.
   b. Bilateral edema is associated with systemic process; unilateral edema is associated with localized process.
3. Amaurosis fugax is monocular blindness of less than 10-minute duration. Patients may describe a sensation that a blind is falling over their field of vision. This is a symptom of reduced cerebral circulation.
4. Intermittent claudication is pain or weakness in the muscle of one or both legs that occurs after walking a fixed distance.
   a. If the patient stops walking, the pain or weakness resolves only to recur after walking a similar distance.
   b. If the patient continues walking, intense muscle cramping occurs.
   c. There are no symptoms at rest.
5. Raynaud phenomenon is a syndrome of peripheral vasospasm with intermittent cutaneous pallor or cyanosis. Precipitating factor is usually exposure to cold.
6. Gangrene is death of tissue due to severe hypoxia that may occur due to blockage of major arteries or severe peripheral vasospasm.
   a. Gas gangrene is due to infection by a species of Clostridium.
7. Acute epigastric abdominal pain can have many causes including dissecting aneurysm and mesenteric ischemia.

Review of Systems (ROS)

A systematic review of symptoms associated with all body systems. Major health assessment textbooks include lists of major symptoms associated with each body system.

1. Cardiac ROS: heart trouble, high blood pressure, rheumatic fever, heart murmurs, chest pain or discomfort, palpitations, dyspnea, orthopnea, paroxysmal nocturnal dyspnea, edema, past electrocardiogram or other heart test results.
2. Vascular ROS: Intermittent claudication, leg cramps, varicose veins, past clots in veins.

Functional Assessment

Nurses collect data about functional patterns also. For each pattern the nurse elicits information about usual pattern and recent changes. Assessment aids in the identification of strengths and resources, as well as problems and symptoms.

1. Health perception — Health management: Includes patient perceptions and concerns about current health and activities used to manage and maintain health
2. Nutrition — Metabolism: Includes information about food consumption, preparation, and preferences
3. Elimination — Includes patterns of urination and defecation; may include urinary incontinence, constipation, etc.
4. Activity — Exercise: Includes current level of activity, as well as recent changes due to symptoms or treatment
5. Cognitive — Perceptual: Includes the special senses — hearing, seeing — as well as memory, thinking, and judgement. Affect (eg, depression) may be included in this pattern. May include information about preferred learning style.
6. Sleep/Rest — Includes symptoms of sleep apnea such as snoring and early morning headache
7. Self-perception–Self-concept — Includes thoughts and feelings associated with self-evaluation and general satisfaction with body image and personality
8. Roles and Relationships — Includes family structures, work role, and changes related to illness
9. Sexuality — Includes function and satisfaction. Many drugs as well as cardiac and vascular illnesses and emotional response have a negative effect on sexual function. Patients may be reluctant to discuss concerns unless the nurse asks these questions.
10. Coping–Stress — Includes usual ways of coping; may include affect (eg, depression)
11. Values–Beliefs — Includes religious and spiritual beliefs and practices

Cardiac and Vascular Risk Factors

The presence of atherosclerosis risk factors is included in the history.

Medications

1. Include all medications currently taken — prescribed and over-the-counter, herbs and supplements.
2. Note allergies and sensitivities.
   a. Allergy to iodine (shellfish or previous contrast medium) should be specifically elicited.

Physical Examination

Basic Principles

1. Organization of the examination
   a. Systematic head-to-toe sequence assures completeness.
   b. Side-to-side comparison helps to evaluated normality. In some situations (eg, muscle strength, range of motion), patient-to-examiner comparison helps evaluate normality.
   c. The usual sequence of examination techniques is inspection, palpation, percussion, and auscultation.
      1) Abdominal exam sequence is inspection, auscultation, palpation, and percussion.
      2) Not all techniques are used for all systems — for example, skin examination uses inspection and palpation only.
2. Comfort of the patient and clinician
   a. Clinician usually stands on the patient's right side
   b. Privacy and draping to assure comfort and dignity

Special Equipment

1. Stethoscope is essential for auscultation.
   a. Double tubing no more than 30 to 40 cm long and 4 mm in diameter. (Longer and wider tubing may distort sounds.)
   b. Ear pieces fit snugly, but comfortably in the ear canals. Ear piece opening is directed toward the ear canal.
   c. Use the diaphragm to detect high-pitched sounds (eg, breath sounds, bowel sounds, some cardiac sounds). Use the bell to detect low-pitched sounds (eg, bruits, some cardiac sounds).
2. Sphygmomanometer must fit properly to give accurate readings
   a. The inflatable bladder should have a width of about 40% and a length of about 80% of the upper arm circumference.
   b. Cuffs are generally available in adult, obese, and child sizes.
   c. Cuffs that are too short or too narrow may give falsely high readings.
3. An ophthalmoscope is a light source with lens and mirrors, which is used to examine internal eye structures. Examination of the undilated pupil may be difficult. In general, nurses do not use drugs to dilate the pupil for fundoscopic examination.
4. Pulse oximeter is a photoelectric device that noninvasively measures arterial oxygen saturation.

General Survey

1. Includes height, weight, body mass index (BMI), and vital signs — T, P, R and BP
   a. Ideal body weight (IBW) ranges can be read from standardized tables
      1) General rule for women: IBW = 100 lb for first 5 feet plus 5 lb per inch above 5 feet
      2) General rule for men: IBW = 105 lb for first 5 feet and 6 lb per inch above 5 feet
   b. BMI describes relationship between height and weight
      1) BMI = weight (in kg) divided by height (in meters squared)
      2) BMI = weight (in lb) divided by height (in inches squared) multiplied by 704.5
      3) BMI values of 20–25 are optimal; 25 to 29 are overweight and ≥30 is obese
   c. Accurate blood pressure (BP) and pulse is fundamental to the physical examination of the cardiac and vascular patient. The following steps will help to assure accuracy.
      1) Patients should be seated in a chair with their backs supported. Arms should be bared and supported at heart level.
      2) Patients should refrain from smoking and caffeine ingestion for 30 minutes prior to measurement.
      3) Measurement should begin after at least 5 minutes of rest.
      4) The bladder within the cuff should encircle at least 80% of the arm. Cuff width should be at least 40% of arm circumference.
      5) Mercury sphygmomanometer measurements are the gold standard. A recently calibrated aneroid manometer or a validated electronic device can be used.
      6) Both systolic (first appearance of sound) and diastolic (disappearance of sound) pressure should be recorded.
         a) Auscultatory gap, a period of silence that occurs during Korotkoff sounds, is of no clinical importance — except that if you miss it's existence you may report an erroneously low (or normal) systolic pressure.
         b) Auscultatory gaps have been reported in patients with hypertension, aortic valve disease, bradycardia and heart failure.
         c) To be sure you have inflated the cuff above systolic pressure, keep your finger on the pulse while you are inflating the cuff the first time. When you reach systolic pressure the pulse disappears.

7) BP should be measured in both arms initially. The arm with the higher reading should be used for subsequent measurements.
8) Two or more readings separated by 2 minutes should be averaged. If the readings differ by more than 5 mm Hg, additional readings should be obtained and averaged.
9) Patient should be informed of the reading and advised of the need for periodic reassessment.

d. Arterial pulses are palpated in the radial, brachial, femoral, carotid, posterior tibialis and dorsalis pedis arteries.
1) Assess and compare characteristics of arterial pulses on the right and left side of the body
2) A 4-point scale is used to communicate pulse volume and amplitude. Pulses are described as 0 — absent, 1+ — weak or thready, 2+ — normal, and 3+ — full and bounding.
3) Abnormal arterial pulses
a) Water hammer (Corrigan) pulse is a rapidly rising and falling pulse associated with aortic insufficiency. It transmits a tapping sensation to the palpating fingers.
b) Pulsus parvus is a low amplitude pulse associated with stenosis of any of the heart valves and any form of low-output heart failure.
c) Pulsus tardus is a slow-rising pulse associated with aortic stenosis
d) Unequal right and left carotid and radial pulses may be seen in aortic dissection. Other causes of unequal pulses (right to left) include supravalvular aortic stenosis, thoracic outlet syndrome, and local occlusive disease of the peripheral artery.
e) Pulsus alternans is the alternation of stronger and weaker beats in a regular rhythm associated with severe heart failure.
1. Regular rhythm differentiates pulsus alternans from atrial or ventricular bigeminal rhythms.
f) Pulse deficit is the difference between apical and radial artery pulse rate associated with atrial fibrillation and non-perfusing ectopic impulses.

e. Allen test is a special examination technique used to determine patency of the palmar arch in the hand. Adequacy of the ulnar artery and palmar arch is assessed before puncturing the radial artery for blood samples.
1) The patient is asked to make a tight fist with one hand.
2) The examiner occludes both the radial and ulnar arteries.

3) The patient is asked to release the fist while the examiner maintains arterial occlusion– the palm is pale.
4) The examiner releases pressure over the ulnar artery. If the artery and arch are patent the palm flushes within 3 to 5 seconds.

f. Pulse pressure, the difference between systolic and diastolic pressure in mm Hg, is an indirect indicator of stroke volume. Pulse pressure is normally approximately 1/3 of systolic pressure.
   1) May be increased during exercise and in people with valvular heart disease (aortic insufficiency).
   2) May be decreased in people with heart failure or intravascular volume deficits.
g. Mean arterial pressure (MAP) is the diastolic BP plus 1/3 of the pulse pressure. MAP represents average pressure within the vessels throughout the cardiac cycle.
h. Postural (orthostatic) hypotension occurs when blood pressure drops on standing and compensatory mechanisms are insufficient to prevent symptoms.
   1) Postural change in BP and pulse should be assessed in elderly patients, those with diabetes mellitus, those taking antihypertensive medications including diuretics, and anyone complaining of dizziness or syncope.
   2) Attention to the following points will assure accuracy and allow meaningful interpretation of results.
      a) Have patient rest in a recumbent position for at least 10 minutes before the initial measurement of BP and pulse.
      b) Check supine pressure and pulse before upright measurement. Always check both BP and pulse in each position. Do not remove the cuff between measurements.
      c) Have the patient assume an upright position. (In some cases BP may be measured in a seated position, although standing is preferred.)
         1. Measure BP and pulse immediately and after 2 minutes.
         2. If orthostasis is strongly suspected and not immediately apparent, take the BP and pulse every 2 minutes times 5 while the patient remains standing.
      d) Be alert for signs or symptoms of patient distress, including dizziness, weakness, blurred vision and syncope.
   3) Normal postural response on standing:
      a) Transient increase in pulse (5 to 20 beats per minute)
      b) Decrease in systolic BP (<10 mm Hg)
      c) Increase in diastolic BP (approximately 5 mm Hg)

4) The pattern of postural change consisting of increased pulse, decreased systolic BP (≥15 mm Hg), and decreased diastolic BP suggests intravascular volume depletion.
5) Orthostatic hypotension must be differentiated from autonomic insufficiency. Constant pulse rate when the patient's position changes from supine to standing suggests autonomic insufficiency.

i. Paradoxical pulse is an exaggeration of the normal decrease in systolic BP during inspiration.
   1) Steps to assess paradoxical pulse
      a) Have patient comfortable and breathing normally
      b) Inflate and gradually deflate the cuff until the first Korotkoff sound is heard during expiration.
      c) Continue slowly deflating the cuff until sounds are heard during both inspiration and expiration.
   2) Normal pressure differential from expiration to inspiration is less than 10 mm Hg.
   3) Paradoxical pressures should be measured on all patients in the cardiac care unit and in those with pericarditis or a temporary pacing wire.

j. Ankle-Brachial Index (ABI) is the ratio of systolic BP measured in the lower leg (ankle) to that measured in the arm (brachial).
   1) Normal ABI is ≥0.95
   2) ABI ≤0.80 is abnormal
   3) Abnormal ABI is seen with arterial insufficiency

Skin, Hair, and Nails

Inspection and palpation of the skin, hair and nails may reveal abnormalities associated with specific cardiac and vascular conditions.

1. Capillary refill: pressure-induced blanching of the nail is used to assess peripheral blood flow. After blanching the nail bed should resume its normal color within 2 seconds of pressure release. Capillary refill is slowed in low flow states.
2. Quinke pulsation: Visible pulsation seen at the pink-white junction with pressure-induced blanching of the fingernail. Associated with aortic insufficiency may be accompanied by involuntary head bobbing.
3. Splinter hemorrhages under the nails, purpura and ecchymoses, Janeway lesions, and petechiae are skin signs that may be seen with infective endocarditis.
   a. Janeway lesions are painless, circular or oval, non-tender macules that appear and fade over a week or two.

4. Clubbing is enlargement of the connective tissue in the terminal phalanges of the fingers and toes.
   a. Clubbing is often associated with cyanosis
   b. Hypoxia does not explain its occurrence in many conditions
5. With arterial insufficiency, skin of the lower legs may appear pale, shiny and relatively hairless. Pulses may be diminished or absent. Postural change in skin color may be observed.
   a. With the patient recumbent, raise both legs to about 60 degrees until maximal pallor develops (approximately one minute).
   b. Have the patient sit up with legs dependent. Normally color returns within 10 seconds and veins fill within 15 seconds. When arterial flow is insufficient:
      1) Pallor may persist for more than 10 seconds, or
      2) Dusky redness (rubor) may develop.
6. Hemosiderin (brown) staining may be seen over the lower legs in the presence of chronic venous insufficiency.

Head, Eyes, Ears, Nose and Throat

1. Examination of the eyes and ears
   a. Inspection
      1) Corneal arcus: a thin grayish-white circle around the iris, may be a sign of hyperlipidemia and precocious atherosclerosis in white people under age 50 years. After age 50, loses significance.
      2) Xanthelasma: slightly raised, yellowish plaques of cholesterol in the skin that appear along the eyelids. May be associated with hyperlipidemia but may be a normal variant.
      3) A deep, diagonal crease running across the ear lobe may be associated with coronary heart disease. This does not apply to Native American Indians.
   b. Examination of the retinal circulation is the only opportunity for direct visualization of blood vessels.
      1) Normal retinal arteries and veins appear to arise from the optic disc.
         a) Arteries are lighter in color than veins and have a more prominent light reflex.
         b) Vein-to-artery ratio is 3:2
         c) Retinal background is a uniform reddish-orange color
         d) The macula is located directly temporal to the optic disc and appears darker than the surrounding retina.

2) Diabetic retinopathy

a) Nonproliferative diabetic retinopathy (NPDR) occurs early and produces microaneurysms, dot-and-blot hemorrhages, hard exudates and macular edema.

b) Proliferative diabetic retinopathy (PDR) is responsible for most of the visual loss from diabetes. In response to retinal ischemia, new vessels form (neovascularization) in the area of the optic disc. These new vessels are fragile and if untreated may bleed into the vitreous. Retinal detachment may occur.

3) Hypertensive retinopathy

a) Changes due to atherosclerosis

1. Arteriolar sclerosis causes thickening of the vessel wall, the central light reflex thickens. As sclerosis progresses, the light reflex occupies most of the vessel producing copper wire vessels.

2. There may be zones where the vein, passing beneath the thickened arterial wall, may be invisible producing A-V nicking. A-V nicking can lead to retinal venous occlusions and decreased central visual acuity.

b) Changes due to elevated BP

1. Moderate acute rise in BP results in arteriolar constriction. Severe acute elevation (diastolic pressure >120 mm Hg) causes necrosis of the vessel wall producing exudates, flame-shaped hemorrhages, and whitish swelling and edema of large areas of the retina.

2. In most severe BP elevation, optic disc swelling is seen.

c. Response of pupils to light and assessment of extra ocular movements are included in the examination of cranial nerves.

2. Examination of vascular structures in the neck

a. Carotid arteries

1) Inspection, palpation, and auscultation

a) Carotid pulsation may be visible and palpable in the neck just medial to the border of the sternomastoid muscle.

1. Abnormally vigorous pulsation may be seen and felt in aortic insufficiency and in high output states.

2. Carotid pulsation can be used to time intracardiac events, but there is a short time lag.

b) Palpate each carotid pulse in the lower third of the neck.
   1. Palpate low in the neck and singly to avoid carotid sinus stimulation and reflex slowing of the heart rate.

c) Auscultate each carotid artery for bruits, a swooshing sound made by turbulent blood flow due to carotid artery stenosis.
   1. Avoid excessive pressure with the stethoscope as external pressure may create turbulent flow.
   2. Bruits are usually low-pitched sounds best heard with the bell.
   3. Referred cardiac murmurs are more intense lower in the neck.

b. Jugular veins reflect intravascular volume and cardiac function.

1) Internal jugular venous pressure (JVP) reflects right atrial (central venous) pressure and volume.

a) Position patient comfortably with head slightly elevated and the sternomastoid muscle relaxed.
   1. Start with the head of the bed or table elevated to 30 degrees and adjust the angle to maximize visibility of jugular pulsation in the lower neck.
   2. The internal jugular vein lies deep to the sternomastoid muscle. The vein itself is not visible. A diffuse wavelike pulsation is seen in the soft tissue of the neck.

b) Measure the height of the highest pulsation seen with reference to the sternal angle.
   1. Normal venous pressure is 3 cm or less above the sternal angle.
   2. Increased JVP is seen in right-sided heart failure, constrictive pericarditis, tricuspid stenosis, and superior vena caval obstruction.
   3. Decreased JVP is seen in intravascular volume depletion (dehydration or over diuresis).

2) The amplitude and timing of the jugular venous pulsation reflect the phases of the cardiac cycle.

a) The *a* wave precedes S_1 and reflects atrial filling during diastole. Conditions that produce overloading of the right atrium (eg, tricuspid stenosis, pulmonary hypertension, or right heart failure) create giant a waves.
   1. Cannon *a* waves occur when the atria contracts against a closed A-V valve. Presence of cannon *a* waves can help differentiate ventricular tachycardia from supraventricular tachycardia.

b) The x descent follows S_1 and reflects early systole.
c) The v wave coincides with S_2 and the y descent marks early diastole.

3) Abdominojugular test (also known as hepatojugular reflux)
   a) Apply pressure with the palm of the hand over the abdomen for 30 to 60 seconds.
   b) Observe jugular venous pulsation
      1. Increase in the height of the jugular pulsation above the sternal angle associated with abdominal pressure is a positive test.
      2. There is a normal increase in the height of jugular pulsation during inspiration. This increase is augmented and sustained during expiration for a positive test.
   c) A positive test is associated with right-sided heart failure.

Chest and Thorax

The breast exam, in both males and females, is part of the examination of the chest and thorax. Readers are directed to one of the health assessment texts for information about the breast examination.

1. Cardiac exam
   a. Chest wall regions
      1) Aortic valve area — 2nd intercostal space (ICS) at the right sternal border
      2) Pulmonic valve area — 2nd ICS at the left sternal border (LSB)
      3) Second pulmonic area — 3rd ICS at the LSB
      4) Tricuspid valve area — 4th ICS along the lower LSB
      5) Mitral valve area (apical area) — 5th ICS at the left midclavicular line (MCL)
   b. Inspection and palpation
      1) Apical pulsation (also known as point of maximal impulse [PMI]) is the lowest and left-most visible (or palpable) pulsation on the precordium.
         a) Reflects contraction of the left ventricle and is the best guide to heart size.
         b) Normal apical pulsation is localized to the 4th or 5th ICS at or medial to the left MCL. The normal impulse is not larger than a nickel.
      2) Right ventricular pulsation may be visible or palpable in the lower sternal areas. This is most often due to right ventricular enlargement or hypertrophy.
      3) Visible or palpable pulsation in the epigastrium usually originates from the aorta, liver, or right ventricle.

c. Percussion was used in the past to assess heart size; rarely used today.

d. Auscultation of the precordium should be compulsively systematic.

  1) Begin at the mitral area (apex) or at the aortic area (base) and gradually move the stethoscope over the entire precordium listening attentively in each area.
  2) Examine all areas with both the bell and the diaphragm of the stethoscope.
  3) Listen with the patient in the recumbent and sitting position.
     a) Having the seated patient lean forward brings the heart closer to the chest wall and may bring out soft sounds (for example, pericardial friction rub or diastolic murmur of aortic insufficiency).
     b) Turning the recumbent patient to the left side brings the heart closer to the chest wall and may bring out left-sided events (for example S_3 or mitral clicks and murmurs).
  4) Audible sounds should be identified as occurring during systole or diastole.
     a) At normal heart rates, systole is shorter than diastole.
     b) S_1 marks the beginning of systole.
     c) S_2 marks the beginning of diastole.
     d) S_1 — systole — S_2 — diastole — S_1

e. Heart rate (HR) and rhythm are determined during cardiac auscultation.

  1) Normal HR is 60 to 100 beats per minute (BPM)
     a) Tachycardia is >100 BPM
     b) Bradycardia is <60 BPM
  2) Normal heart rhythm is regular.
     a) Minor variation in rate associated with respiratory phase may be normal (sinus dysrhythmia).
        1. HR increases during inspiration and decreases during expiration.
     b) Atrial or ventricular extrasystoles may cause sporadic irregularity.
     c) Atrial fibrillation may cause total irregularity (irregularly irregular).

f. Normal heart sounds (S_1 and S_2) coincide with closure of heart valves.

  1) S_1 coincides with closure of the mitral and tricuspid valves.
  2) S_2 coincides with closure of the aortic and pulmonic valves.

3) The valves may not close simultaneously and produce splitting of S_1 or S_2.
4) Splitting may be physiological (normal) or pathological (abnormal).
   a) Physiological splitting of S_2 is heard during inspiration, but not during expiration. Reversal of this normal pattern is associated with heart disease.
   b) Pathological splitting of S_1 is associated with right bundle branch block (RBBB) and ventricular extrasystoles.
   c) Pathological splitting of S_2 is associated with atrial septal defects, right and left bundle branch block, and pulmonary hypertension.
5) S_1 is lower pitched and of longer duration than S_2.
6) S_1 precedes the carotid pulsation and S_2 follow this pulse.
7) S_1 is loudest at the apex and is best heard with the diaphragm of the stethoscope. S_2 is loudest at the base and is best heard with the diaphragm.

f. Extra systolic sounds
   1) Transients
      a) Aortic or pulmonic ejection sounds may be heard with aortic or pulmonary valve stenosis. The sounds are best heard with the diaphragm at the base of the heart.
      b) Systolic click, associated with mitral valve prolapse, is heard during midtolate systole.
   2) Systolic murmurs
      a) Innocent systolic murmur is commonly heard in children and adolescents.
      b) Benign systolic murmurs are soft, short, and low-pitched. They have no hemodynamic significance.
      c) Loud systolic murmurs may be due to ventricular septal defect, pulmonary or aortic stenosis, or mitral or tricuspid insufficiency.

g. Extra diastolic sounds
   1) Transients — the third (S_3) and fourth (S_4) heart sounds
      a) S_3 and S_4 are low-pitched sounds best heard with the bell of the stethoscope.
      b) S_3 is normal when heard in children and young adults (<40 years).
      c) In individuals older than 40 years, S3 is abnormal. It is often heard in left-sided heart failure.
      d) S_4 is expected when ventricular filling is augmented by atrial contraction.

1. Ventricular filling may be augmented in hypertension, myocardial infarction, thyrotoxicosis, and anemia.
2. S_4 depends on atrial contraction and is never heard during atrial fibrillation.

2) Diastolic murmurs
   a) Always abnormal
   b) Aortic or pulmonary valve insufficiency
   c) Mitral or tricuspid valve stenosis

h. Pericardial rub, associated with pericarditis, is characteristically scratchy, creaking or grating.
   1) Triphasic associated with atrial systole, ventricular systole, and diastole
   2) Best heard with the diaphragm of the stethoscope along the LSB as the patient leans forward.
   3) Differentiate pericardial rub from pleural rub by asking patient to hold his breath. Pericardial rub persists; pleural rub is abolished by breath holding.

i. Heart murmurs represent turbulent flow and are frequently produced by abnormal heart valves. The following characteristics of murmurs should be assessed.
   1) Phase of the cardiac cycle — systole or diastole
      a) Diastolic murmurs are associated with disease.
      b) Systolic murmurs may be normal in some cases.
   2) Loudness or intensity is graded on 6-point scale. Systolic murmurs of grade III or more are usually hemodynamically and clinically significant.
      a) Grade I: Heard only with concentration; distinct but faint.
      b) Grade II: Faint but heard immediately.
      c) Grade III: Comparable loudness to heart sounds.
      d) Grade IV: Loud; may be associated with palpable thrill (buzzing sensation).
      e) Grade V: Very loud; may be heard with only one edge of the stethoscope in contact with the chest wall. Thrill often present.
      f) Grade VI: Very loud; may be heard with stethoscope off the chest. Thrill present.
   3) Location and radiation help determine the cause and significance of the murmur. Note the area where the murmur is loudest and any area of radiation.
      a) For example, Grade III/VI systolic murmur, loudest at the apex, and radiating to the left axilla.

2. Lung exam
   a. Inspection: Observe the rate, depth, and effort of breathing.
      1) Normal respiratory rate is 14 to 20 breaths per minute.
      2) Expiration is normally slightly longer than inspiration, but prolonged expiration signifies airway disease.
      3) Some abnormal respiratory patterns include the following:
         a) Tachypnea: respiratory rate >20
         b) Hyperpnea: abnormally deep, large volume breaths
         c) Bradypnea: respiratory rate <14
         d) Cheyne-Stokes breathing: periods of deep breathing alternate with periods of apnea. There is a waxing and waning to the cycle. May be seen in left heart failure.
         e) Biot breathing: unpredictable irregularity of respiratory rate and depth; usually associated with brain damage.
         f) Hyperventilation is the elimination of excessive CO_2. It is diagnosed by analysis of CO_2 content in the blood and not by observation of breathing pattern.
   b. Palpation: Palpate any areas of chest pain and tenderness. Check for vocal fremitus (vocal vibrations transmitted through the chest wall to the ball of the hand). Compare side to side.
      1) Fremitus is reduced when there is an obstructed bronchus, pleural effusion, pneumothorax, or a very thick chest wall.
      2) Fremitus is increased when lung tissue is consolidated (eg, pneumonia).
   c. Percussion: Direct or indirect percussion helps determine whether lung structures are air-filled, fluid-filled, or solid. Compare side to side. Normal, air-filled lung produces a resonant percussion note.
      1) Dull percussion note is heard when fluid or solid tissue replaces air-filled lung.
      2) Hyperresonance is heard with overinflated lungs (eg, emphysema).
   d. Auscultation: Normal lung sounds are normal when heard in normal places and abnormal when heard in abnormal places. Compare side to side.
      1) Vesicular sounds are soft, relatively low-pitched sounds heard over the lung periphery. Inspiratory phase sounds longer than expiratory phase.
      2) Bronchovesicular sounds are louder than vesicular sounds, normally heard in the region between the scapulae. Inspiratory and expiratory phases sound equal in duration.
         a) Bronchovesicular sounds heard in the periphery may represent pneumonia or tumor.

3) Bronchial breath sounds are loud, relatively high pitched and heard over the manubrium, if at all. Expiratory phase sounds longer than inspiratory phase. There may be a slight pause between the inspiratory and expiratory phases.
   a) Bronchial sounds that are heard in other locations might represent pneumonia or tumor.
4) Adventitious (ie, added) sounds are superimposed on normal lung sounds and are abnormal.
   a) Crackles (rales) are discontinuous sounds that are intermittent and brief. They may be heard during inspiration, expiration, or both.
      1. Note respiratory phase and lung region where heard.
      2. Crackles may clear with cough; have patient cough to see if they change.
      3. Crackles are abnormal and may be due to pneumonia, fibrosis, atelectasis, heart failure, or bronchitis.
   b) Wheezes are relatively high-pitched, continuous sounds. Wheezes suggest narrowed airways (eg, asthma, COPD, or bronchitis.)
   c) Rhonchi are relatively low pitched, continuous sounds. Rhonchi suggest the presence of secretions in the large airways.

Abdomen

1. Waist circumference is associated with increased risk for cardiovascular disease and diabetes.
   a. Waist circumference ≥40 inches in men and ≥35 inches in women indicates abdominal fat distribution and increased risk.
2. Listen for bruits over the aorta, iliac and femoral arteries and in each upper abdominal quadrant.
   a. Bruits with both systolic and diastolic components are associated with arterial stenosis.
   b. A systolic-phase bruit may be a normal finding.

Peripheral Circulation: Extremities

1. Compare arm-to-arm and leg-to-leg
   a. Observe and compare size, temperature, symmetry, pigmentation, scars and ulcers.
2. Edema: an abnormal accumulation of fluid in the interstitial space.
   a. Weight gain of 10 pounds, indicative of 5 L of fluid, precedes visible edema.
   b. Daily weights provide the best serial measure of edema.

c. Edema fluid accumulates in areas of dependency.
    1) For ambulatory or seated patients, edema accumulates in feet and lower legs.
    2) For bedridden patients, edema accumulates in the sacral or lumbar regions
d. Anasarca: generalized edema
e. Grading of edema — not all edema is pitting
    1) Edema causes swelling that may obscure the veins and bony prominences.
    2) To check for pitting edema, press firmly for at least 5 seconds
        a) Over the dorsum of each foot
        b) Behind each medial malleolus
        c) Over the shins
    3) Severity of edema can be graded on a 5-point scale from 0 — none to 4 — very severe.
    4) Leg circumference can be measured, compared side-to-side, and monitored over time to assess changes in the amount of edema.
f. Long-standing edema may induce pigmentation (brownish), inflammation (redness), induration, and fibrosis of the skin and subcutaneous tissues. Edema reduces skin mobility and resiliency.

3. Varicose veins are dilated, tortuous superficial veins with incompetent valves.
4. Thrombophlebitis is inflammation of the vein with associated thrombus.
    a. Homan sign is positive in about 35% of patients with deep venous thrombosis (DVT) of the lower legs.
        1) With the patient's knee flexed, the examiner abruptly dorsiflexes the ankle.
        2) Sign is positive if pain is experienced in the calf or popliteal region. May be positive also in people with lumbar-sacral disc pathology.
5. Venous insufficiency is a syndrome that involves destruction of the venous valves and obliteration of thrombosed veins.
    a. Pain, if present, is described as a dull ache or heaviness.
    b. Brownish discoloration of skin may occur.
    c. Edema that increases with dependency and decreases with elevation may be present.
    d. Chronic venous insufficiency (CVI) may cause ulceration of the lower leg around the ankle.
        1) Skin surrounding the ulcer may be pigmented (brownish) or inflamed (reddened) and edematous.

2) CVI ulcers may be very painful.
3) Ulcer may have irregular shape and uneven borders.
4) Venous ulcers are commonly located on the anterior or medial aspect of the lower leg.

6. Arterial insufficiency is a syndrome of hypoperfusion.
   a. Pain is present in the affected extremity.
      1) Intermittent claudication is relieved with rest.
      2) When pain is continuous, it is less severe with the affected extremity in the dependent position.
   b. Skin of the lower extremity is dry, thin, shiny and little hair is present.
   c. Toe nails are thick and brittle.
   d. Foot and extremity are cool and pale.
      1) Elevation pallor and dependent rubor (redness)
   e. Pulses are weak or absent.
      1) Iliac or femoral bruits may be present.
   f. Chronic arterial insufficiency may cause ulceration of the toes, feet or ankle.
      1) Skin surrounding the ulcer may be atrophic. The ulcer has smooth edges and a "punched out" appearance.
      2) Pain may be severe unless masked by neuropathy.
      3) Gangrene may be associated.

Neurological Exam

Neurological examination answers two important questions. Are right and left-sided findings symmetrical? And, if findings are abnormal, does the causative lesion lie in the central or peripheral nervous system?

1. Mental status and speech
   a. Altered mental status is associated with hypertensive encephalopathy, stroke, and multi-infarct and vascular dementia.
   b. Stroke most common cause of acquired speech defect in adults.
      1) Dysarthria: Defect in the muscular control of the speech apparatus
      2) Aphasia: Disorder in producing or understanding language
   c. Levels of consciousness
      1) Alert: When spoken to in a normal tone of voice, the patient opens his eyes and responds fully and appropriately to stimulus.
      2) Lethargic: When spoken to in a loud voice, the patient may open his eyes but falls back to sleep immediately.

3) Obtunded: When physically shaken, the patient opens his eyes, but responds slowly and is somewhat confused.
4) Stupor: Arouses only with application of a painful stimulus. Verbal response is slow or absent.
5) Coma: Eyes remain closed; no evidence of response to stimuli.

2. Cranial nerves
   a. CN II and III: Optic and oculomotor
      1) Observe pupil size and symmetry and test response to light (direct and consensual)
      2) Test visual acuity
   b. CN III, IV, and VI: Oculomotor, trochlear, and abducens
      1) Test extraocular movements in the six cardinal directions of gaze
      2) Identify nystagmus — rapid eye movements
      3) Look for ptosis and lid lag
   c. CN V: Trigeminal
      1) While palpating temporal and masseter muscles, have patient clench and unclench his or her teeth. Notice the strength of muscle contraction.
      2) Test for sensation of the forehead, cheek and chin area
      3) Test corneal reflex
   d. CN VII: Facial
      1) Observe the facial musculature at rest and during conversation for asymmetry
      2) Ask the patient to do the following maneuvers; notice any weakness or asymmetry.
         a) Smile and show his teeth
         b) Close his eyes tightly and don't let the examiner open them
         c) Puff out both cheeks
         d) Stick out his tongue
   e. CN VIII: Acoustic
      1) Assess hearing — whisper test or finger rub
      2) If hearing loss is present, test for lateralization and compare air and bone conduction
   f. CN IX and X: Glossopharyngeal and vagus
      1) Observe voice quality
      2) Observe swallowing
      3) Observe movement of the soft palate and the pharynx
      4) Test the gag reflex

g. CN XI: Spinal accessory
    1) Ask the patient to shrug both shoulders up against your hands. Observe the strength and contraction of the trapezius muscles.
h. CN XII: Hypoglossal
    1) Inspect the tongue for fasciculation
    2) Ask patient to protrude tongue and move it from side to side; look for asymmetry

3. Motor strength and function
    a. Observe for involuntary movements
    b. Observe muscle size and contours — look for symmetry and atrophy
    c. Check muscle strength and spontaneous movement
        1) Paresis — impaired strength or weakness
        2) Plegia — absence of strength or paralysis
4. Sensation
    a. Peripheral neuropathy — numbness in foot or leg
5. Reflexes
    a. Deep tendon reflexes are graded on a 5-point scale: 0 = no response, 1+ = diminished response, 2+ = normal or average response, 3+ = brisker than average response, and 4+ = very brisk hyperactive response with clonus.

Diagnostic Tests

Sensitivity and Specificity

An ideal diagnostic test would be 100% sensitive and 100% specific. No diagnostic test is ideal.

1. Sensitivity of a test is the ability of the test to detect patients with the disease in question (ie, how often false negatives occur). For example, Troponin I is 98% to 99% sensitive for MI, elevated troponin level is rarely seen in other conditions. (Clinical controversy suggests troponin may be elevated in patients after cardiac surgery or with end stage renal disease.)
2. Specificity of a test is how well test abnormality is restricted to those people who have the disease in question (ie, how often false positives occur). An ECG is 100% specific for MI. ECG changes associated with MI are only seen in patients who actually have MI.

Sensitivity and specificity are inversely correlated, thus increasing sensitivity decreases specificity and the opposite.

1. Combinations of tests are used to enhance sensitivity and specificity.
2. The combination of elevated Troponin I and characteristic ECG changes makes the diagnosis of MI.

Laboratory Tests Using Blood

Obtaining Venous Sample

To enhance the reliability of venous samples:

1. Avoid hemolysis
   a. Dry skin with gauze after antiseptic prep.
   b. Minimize duration of tourniquet.
   c. Use double needle and vacuum tube, if possible.
   d. Use appropriate size needle — small needle when drawing multiple samples increases risk of hemolysis.
   e. Remove needle from syringe, if used, before putting blood into tube.
2. Do not draw blood from an arm where a solution is infusing intravenously.
3. Color of the tube stopper reflects additives. Be sure to have "correct" tube for each test.

Reference Values are Laboratory Specific

Interpret test results in light of the range provided

1. Variables that affect test results
   a. Age and gender: There may be different ranges established for men and women or for age groups.
   b. Time of day: Most hormones show diurnal variation, so time of day affects results.
   c. Drug interference
   d. Time since food consumption: Some tests must be obtained with the patient in the fasting state.
2. Reference range is established by testing a large number of healthy people and ranking results.
   a. Values above a cutoff point (often 95%) are considered abnormal.
   b. Because all tests in the reference group were done on healthy people, 5 out of 100 healthy people will have an abnormal result and be considered unhealthy statistically.

Cardiac Markers

Enzymes are proteins that catalyze chemical reactions in cells. Some enzymes are present in nearly all cells; others are specific to cells of certain organs.

1. Cardiac Enzymes
   a. Creatine kinase (CK) is an enzyme present in brain, myocardial and skeletal muscle cells. It is released from cells after irreversible injury — the presence of CK in the blood indicates cardiac, cerebral, or skeletal muscle injury.
      1) CK isoenzymes are specific to each type of tissue.
         a) CK-MB (CK–2) is from myocardial cells
         b) CK-BB is from brain cells
         c) CK-MM is from myocardial and skeletal muscle cells
      2) Enzyme release and clearance follows a predictable pattern after injury, which can be used diagnostically.
         a) Reference range for Total CK is 30–180 IU/L
         b) Reference range for CK-MB is 0–5 IU/L or 0–5% of total CK.
         c) Total CK and CK-MB levels rise within 4 to 6 hours after a myocardial infarction (MI), peak within 12 to 24 hours and (if there is no further injury) return to normal within 3 to 4 days.
         d) Peak levels after a MI are more than 6 times the normal value. Smaller elevations may be seen after reperfusion by angioplasty or thrombolysis and after electrical cardioversion.
         e) Total CK and CK-MB are highly sensitive (93% to 100%) tests for MI. Total CK is a less specific (57% to 88%) test than CK-MB (specificity = 93% to 100%).
            1. Intramuscular injection and skeletal muscle injury elevate Total CK
      3) CK and CK-MB are repeated every 6 to 8 hours to establish the pattern.
2. Cardiac Proteins
   a. Myoglobin is a protein found in myocardial and skeletal muscle that is released into blood after cell injury. Blood levels elevate in 1 to 3 hours after MI, peak in 8 to 12 hours, and return to normal in 12 to 30 hours.
      1) Myoglobin is more sensitive than but not as specific as CK-MB for MI.
      2) Because of early elevation, myoglobin is used in conjunction with cardiac enzyme elevation or ECG changes to make decisions for thrombolysis or early angioplasty.

3) Reference range: Levels are undetectable in normals.

b. Troponin is found in both myocardial and skeletal muscle. Three isotopes have been identified. Troponin I and T are found in myocardium; levels elevate in 4 to 6 hours after MI and remain elevated for 5 to 7 days.
   1) Troponin I is 98% to 99% sensitive for MI
   2) Reference range: Levels are undetectable in normals.

Coagulation Tests

1. Platelets are elements of the blood that clump and stick to rough surfaces when clotting is necessary.
   a. Reference range: 150,000–400,000/mm^3
   b. Bleeding time (how long it takes blood to clot in the body) is a simple test of platelet funtion.
      1) Reference range: 3–7 minutes
      2) Aspirin therapy reduces platelet adhesion and prolongs bleeding time.
      3) Aspirin effect on platelets is not reversible (ie, lasts approximately 10 days).
      4) Bleeding test may not be reliable indicator of platelet function. Use varies by practice region.
2. Prothrombin time (PT) and international normalized ratio (INR) are used to initiate and maintain anticoagulation therapy with Coumadin.
   a. PT is used to initiate therapy; after a stable dose is achieved (approximately one week) the INR is used for monitoring.
   b. Reference range: PT 10–13 seconds or 70–100%
   c. Therapeutic range for PT is 2 to 2.5 times the control.
   d. In most cases, the therapeutic INR range extends from 2 to 3.5. Ranges have been established for specific conditions
      1) For DVT prophylaxis, INR range of 1.5 to 2.0
      2) For DVT treatment, INR range of 2.0 to 3.0
      3) For prevention of embolism in atrial fibrillation, INR range of 2.0 to 3.0
      4) For pulmonary embolism treatment, INR range of 3.0 to 4.0
      5) For mechanical valve prophylaxis, INR range of 2.5 to 3.5
   e. Most antibiotics taken with Coumadin enhance the effect on PT and INR.
      1) Aspirin and other antiplatelet medicines may be used with Coumadin.
      2) Caution patients about increased bleeding tendency with these combinations.
   f. Instruct patients to avoid variable intake of Vitamin K and to observe for and report signs of bleeding

3. Partial thromboplastin time (PTT) and activated PTT (aPTT) are used when patients receive unfractionated heparin.
   a. Reference range: PTT 60–70 seconds; aPTT 20–35 seconds
   b. The therapeutic range for both the PTT and aPTT is 1.5 to 2.5 times baseline.
   c. Laboratory monitoring is not required for patients receiving low molecular heparin.

Plasma Lipoproteins

1. Elevated total and LDL cholesterol increase atherosclerosis risk.
2. Elevated HDL cholesterol is protective (ie, associated with lower atherosclerosis risk.)
3. Classification of plasma cholesterol levels in the general adult population
   a. Total Cholesterol
      1) Desirable: <200 mg/dl
      2) Borderline high: 200–239 mg/dl
      3) High: ≥240 mg/dl
   b. LDL Cholesterol
      1) Optimal: <100 mg/dl
      2) Near optimal: 100–129 mg/dl
      3) Borderline high: 130–159 mg/dl
      4) High: 160–189 mg/dl
      5) Very high ≥190 mg/dl
   c. HDL Cholesterol
      1) Low: <40 mg/dl
      2) High: ≥60 mg/dl
4. When patients are hospitalized with acute coronary syndromes or coronary procedures, a lipid profile should be measured on admission or within the first 24 hours.9
   a. LDL-lowering therapy should be initiated before or on discharge.
   b. Therapy may need adjustment after 12 weeks.
5. Random total cholesterol may be used for screening; fasting specimen (12 hours) is needed for diagnosis and treatment monitoring.

Drug Levels

1. Drug levels are quantitative tests used to monitor the effectiveness of drug therapy.
2. Therapeutic drug monitoring is used when a drug has a low therapeutic to toxic dose range, such as digoxin and lithium.

3. Serum concentrations must be interpreted within the clinical context.
   a. Symptoms of digoxin toxicity can occur despite a therapeutic drug level if the patient has hypokalemia.
   b. Digoxin may control heart rate effectively at less than therapeutic levels.
4. To assure accurate interpretation of results, note the drug name and dosage, time of last dose, route of administration, time blood was drawn, patient's age and clinical characteristics (eg, creatinine clearance indicates renal function).

Non-invasive Diagnostic Testing

Chest X-ray

1. Two views of the chest, posterior to anterior (PA) and left lateral (LL)
2. Provides information about the heart, lungs, thoracic vascular and bony structures.
   a. Size and contour of cardiac chambers
   b. Presence of acute and chronic pulmonary disease
   c. Dilation and calcification of thoracic vessels
3. Correlation with clinical context and comparison with previous chest films provides the most useful information.
4. X-ray is used for screening purposes and followed by other extensive diagnostic tests
5. X-ray gives a two-dimensional view.

Computed Tomography (CT) Scan

1. A narrow x-ray beam examines body sections from many different angles to build up a 3-dimensional picture of the structures.
2. Performed with or without contrast dye. Contrast enhances tissue absorption and allows small defects to be seen.
3. Purpose: To examine for head, liver, and renal lesions; tumors; abscesses; vascular diseases; stroke; bone destruction; and coronary heart disease. Can be used to find foreign objects within soft tissues (eg, a bullet lodged in the chest or abdomen.)
4. General preparation: If contrast is not used, the CT scan is considered non-invasive.
   a. With contrast, patient is NPO (nothing by mouth) for at least 4 hours before the procedure. Patients who are sensitive to iodine or shellfish may be allergic to contrast dye.

b. Prescribed medications usually given with small amount of water
c. CT scanner is tubular with a circular opening. The camera rotates around the table while the patient lies motionless. Patient will hear the camera rotating and clicking.
d. If contrast dye is used, patient may experience warm flush or nausea at the time of injection.
e. If contrast dye is used, instruct patient to increase fluid intake after the scan.

Magnetic Resonance Imaging (MRI)

1. Uses radio waves and a magnetic field to create a computerized image of soft tissue structures. No ionizing radiation is used.
2. Purpose: To detect central nervous system lesions, vascular problems, perfusion problems, injury, tumor, or edema.
3. General preparation:
   a. Remove all metal objects and cosmetics that may contain metallic fragments.
      1) Individuals with pacemakers, some metallic heart valves, recent surgical clips, etc. may not be candidates for MRI
      2) Remove hearing aides and dentures. Patients with metallic fillings may experience a "tingling" sensation in teeth but fillings will not be pulled out.
   b. Contraindicated during pregnancy
   c. Patient must lie still on table within the scanner. Open scanners are available.
   d. MRI can disrupt the flow of intravenous fluid.
4. Contrast dye may be used with MRI to evaluate problems in the brain and spine. This dye is chemically unrelated to the contrast dye used in CT scan or arteriogram.
5. Resuscitation equipment can not be used in the MRI room.

Electrocardiogram (ECG)

Provides a graphic record of the electrical activity in the heart.

1. Cardiac electrical activity is recorded at standard speed (25 mm/sec) on special graph paper. The grid on the paper consists of small and large boxes, both horizontally and vertically.
   a. On the horizontal axis, one small box (1 mm) represents 0.04 seconds; on the vertical axis, one small box represents 0.1 mV.
   b. On the horizontal axis, one large box (5 mm) represents 0.20 seconds; on the vertical axis, one large box represents 0.5 mV.

c. ECG paper is marked with a vertical line in the top margin at 3-second intervals.

2. ECG waves, complexes, and intervals reflect electrical activity within the heart. Normal characteristics have been described for each wave, complex, and interval.
   a. P-wave represents atrial depolarization. It is normally no taller than 0.25 mV or wider than 0.11 second.
   b. PR interval, measured from the beginning of the P-wave to the beginning of the QRS complex, represents the time required for the impulse to travel through the atria, AV junction and Purkinje system. Normal duration is 0.12 to 0.20 second.
   c. QRS complex represents ventricular depolarization. Q is the initial negative deflection from baseline. R is the first positive deflection from baseline. S is a negative deflection that follows an R-wave. Normal QRS duration is 0.04 to 0.10 second.
   d. ST segment represents the time when the ventricles are depolarized. It begins at the end of the QRS and extends to the beginning of the T-wave. Normal ST segment should be a flat baseline and gently curve up to the T-wave.
   e. T-wave represents ventricular repolarization. It is normally in the same direction as the QRS complex. Normal T-waves are not taller than 5 mm in the limb leads or 10 mm in the precordial leads.
   f. QT interval represents ventricular depolarization and repolarization. It is measured from the beginning of the QRS complex to the end of the T-wave.
      1) Duration of the QT interval varies with HR.
      2) A nomogram is used to correct the observed QT interval to a rate of 60 bpm (QTc).
         a) Normal QTc is 0.42 second for men and 0.43 second for women.
   g. U-wave is a small wave that follows the T wave. It is not always visible.

3. Heart rate can be determined from an ECG strip.
   a. Count the number of R-R intervals in a 6-second strip (two 3-second markers in the top margin) and multiply by 10.
   b. If the rhythm is regular, count the number of small boxes between 2 R-waves and divide into 1500.

4. Uses/purpose
   a. To detect and evaluate coronary and valvular heart disease
   b. To detect cardiac dysrhythmia
   c. To identify electrolyte imbalance and drug effect
   d. To evaluate effects of anti-dysrhythmic drugs on ECG intervals

5. ECG signs of coronary heart disease
   a. Myocardial ischemia — classic pattern of ischemia is T-wave inversion. T-wave inversion is nonspecific. Other signs of myocardial ischemia include the following:
      1) ST segment depression of 0.5 mm or more below baseline
      2) An ST segment that remains at baseline longer than 0.12 second
      3) An ST segment that forms a sharp angle with the upright T wave
      4) Tall, wide-based T waves and inverted U waves
   b. Myocardial injury is most frequently indicated by ST segment elevation ≥1 mm above the baseline. Other signs of acute injury include the following:
      1) Straightening of the ST segment that slopes up to the peak of the T-wave without any time spent at baseline
      2) Tall, peaked T-waves
      3) Symmetric T-wave inversion
   c. Myocardial infarction: The classic pattern is development of new Q-waves in the leads reflecting the affected cardiac surface.
      1) Abnormal Q-waves are >0.03 second wide or >25% of the amplitude of the R-wave.
      2) Other signs include decreased R-wave amplitude, ST segment depression, and T-wave inversion.
6. Left ventricular hypertrophy is commonly associated with valvular heart disease and hypertension.
   a. Increased amplitude of R-waves in leads I, aVL, V_5, and V_6
   b. Increased amplitude of S-waves in leads V_1 and V_2
   c. R plus S wave amplitude in any precordial lead ≥45 mm
7. Selected drug and electrolyte effects
   a. Digoxin in therapeutic doses can produce sagging (cupping) of the ST segment with flattening of the T-waves, shortening of the QT interval, and prolongation of the PR interval.
   b. Digoxin toxicity causes conduction disturbances, extrasystoles, and tachycardia.
   c. Beta-blockers cause sinus bradycardia with slight prolongation of PR interval.
   d. Hyperkalemia (serum potassium ≥5 mEq/L):
      1) Tall peaked T waves and short QT interval
      2) PR interval >0.20 second
      3) With severe elevation, QRS becomes broad and bizarre and ventricular fibrillation may occur

e. Hypokalemia (serum potassium <3 mEq/L) and hypomagnesemia increase risk of dysrhythmia and digoxin toxicity.

Ambulatory ECG

Ambulatory ECG (Holter monitor) records cardiac electrical activity continuously for a period of time (eg, 12 or 24 hours) during unrestricted activity, rest and sleep.

1. Used in the diagnostic investigation of dizzness, syncope, and palpitations and to monitor effect of antidysrhythmic drugs. Can document silent ischemia.
2. Patients are instructed to mark and describe symptoms occurring during the monitoring period (eg, palpitations, rapid heart rate, or light-headedness).
   a. Monitor should not get wet. Avoid bathing and showering while monitoring.
   b. Avoid use of electric razor or toothbrush to avoid ECG artifacts.
3. An intermittent monitoring device, called a King of Hearts, may be used
   a. The patient activates the recorder only when he or she experiences symptoms.
   b. The recording can be sent over the telephone to the physician's office.

Exercise ECG

Exercise ECG identifies exercise-induced myocardial ischemia and evaluates cardiac dysrhythmia.

1. ECG is monitored and recorded while patient exercises under gradually increasing workload.
   a. Treadmill or exercise bicycle with predetermined levels of increasing speed, grade, or resistance is used (eg, the Bruce protocol).
2. BP is obtained in the arm for evaluation of cardiovascular exercise response. Expired gases may be collected to evaluate pulmonary function (eg, screening tool used to evaluate patients before heart transplant).
3. Clinicians assess for symptoms and ECG indications to stop the test:
   a. Severe angina
   b. Marked ST segment depression
   c. Ventricular or atrial tachycardia, atrial fibrillation or high degree A-V block
4. Patients exercise to reach capacity for their age and gender. The goal is to exercise at 85% of maximal heart rate for 3 minutes.

Head-up Tilt-Table Test

Head-up tilt-table test is used to evaluate vasodepressor syncope and near-syncope.

1. Patient is placed on a table and is tilted to an upright position.
2. ECG and BP are monitored to evaluate the relative contribution of bradycardia and hypotension to syncope.

Electron Beam Tomography

Electron beam tomography is a high-speed electron beam that images the heart (and other structures) in 3 dimensions.

1. Calcification of coronary or carotid arteries can be determined and scored.
2. This test is used to quantify risk in younger patients (30–50 years old) with a family history of early heart disease.

Diagnostic Ultrasonography

Principles

1. High frequency (above that which can be detected by the human ear) sound waves are sent through body structures by a transducer.
   a. Sound waves can not be heard or felt by the patient
   b. No known damage to tissues from clinical use of sound waves
2. The transducer also receives returning sound waves, which are deflected back as they bounce off bodily structures.
3. Sound waves reflected from a moving substance are changed in a predictable way (ie, Doppler effect). When the substance is moving toward the detector, the frequency increases; when the substance is moving away from the detector the frequency decreases.
   a. In clinical applications, high frequency sound waves are reflected off red blood cells and transformed into audible sound waves.
   b. Color Doppler assigns a different color to the image of the blood in relationship to its speed and direction
4. Ultrasound does not penetrate air or bone.
   a. Use coupling gel between transducer and skin
   b. Ultrasound techniques are not as useful for detecting thoracic as abdominal disease.
5. Real-time imaging refers to the use of rapid scanners that are able to display motion.
6. Duplex scans use both real-time imaging and Doppler flow imaging.

Echocardiography (ECHO)

ECHO uses high frequency sound waves and the Doppler effect to evaluate the size, shape and motion of cardiac structures and the direction and velocity of blood flow through the heart.

1. Transthoracic ECHO uses a transducer on the chest wall
    a. Stress ECHO helps identify silent and exercise-induced ischemia. Ventricular wall motion and thickness are evaluated at rest and at peak exercise (just as the patient comes off the treadmill).
        1) Exercise (bicycle ergometer or treadmill) or drugs (dobutamine or dipyridamole) are used to stress the cardiovascular system.
        2) Used in diagnosis of coronary heart disease, valvular heart disease, cardiomyopathy, and intracardiac masses or clots.
2. Transesophageal ECHO: A transducer, mounted on a flexible endoscope is introduced into the stomach to obtain clearer visualization and greater anatomic detail than transthoracic ECHO.

Venous and Arterial Duplex

Use sound waves and the Doppler principle to determine and evaluate blood flow in specific vascular structures.

1. Used to evaluate carotid stenosis in those with cervical bruit or transient ischemic attack (TIA) and to follow-up after carotid endarterectomy (CEA).
    a. Patients with TIA and more than 70% stenosis or ulcerated plaques are usually advised to have CEA.
2. Used to evaluate renal and peripheral artery stenosis
3. Venous duplex is a primary tool used to diagnose DVT
4. Arterial duplex is used to rule out pseudoaneurysm of the femoral artery after cardiac catheterization.

Transcranial Doppler

1. Uses sound waves and the Doppler principle to evaluate blood flow in selected intracranial blood vessels.
    a. Bone is not penetrated by ultrasound
    b. Acoustic windows allow evaluation of the middle cerebral, anterior communicating, posterior communicating, ophthalmic, distal internal carotid, vertebral and basilar arteries.
2. Used to evaluate subarachnoid hemorrhage, vertebrobasilar insufficiency, and collateral circulation in people with ICA lesions

Diagnostic Testing Using Radionuclides

Blood Pool Imaging

A scintillation camera obtains images as a bolus of radioactive tracer (technetium 99) mixed with blood passes through the heart.

1. Assesses cardiac function (ie, ejection fraction and wall motion)
2. Normal ejection fraction is ≥55%

Myocardial Perfusion Imaging

A radioactive tracer (thallium 201 or technetium 99m sestamibi) accumulates in the myocardium in proportion to myocardial blood flow and the extraction of the radionuclide by myocardial cells.

1. Need viable myocardial cell for tracer to accumulate
2. Areas of scar tissue and areas that are hypoperfused do not take up the tracer.
3. Can be combined with exercise to increase sensitivity and specificity of the test
4. Dipyridamole and adenosine may be infused intravenously to dilate coronary arteries and increase myocardial blood flow.
   a. Severely narrowed coronary arteries do not dilate and blood flow is not increased.

Invasive Diagnostic Testing

Cardiac catheterization or coronary angiography is an invasive test that delineates coronary anatomy. The test is the "gold standard" to diagnose coronary heart disease.

1. Indications include patients with acute coronary syndrome (symptoms and ECG pattern of ischemia or injury) and those who have been evaluated with noninvasive tests that suggest myocardial ischemia.
2. Patients may undergo right or left heart catheterization or both.
3. Right-heart catheterization
   a. In the catheterization lab under fluoroscopy, a specially designed catheter is placed through a peripheral (often the femoral) vein and threaded into the right side of the heart.
   b. Sensors on the catheter tip read chamber pressures and monitor blood flow rates.
   c. The catheter is floated into the pulmonary artery and pressures reflected from the left side of the heart are assessed.
      1) Pulmonary artery pressures and cardiac output are measured
      2) Left ventricular end diastolic pressure (pulmonary artery wedge or capillary pressure) is measured

4. Left-heart catheterization
   a. A second catheter is threaded in a retrograde direction from the femoral artery into the left side of the heart.
   b. Radio opaque dye is injected into the coronary arteries to evaluate patency of the arteries and myocardial perfusion.
   c. Radio opaque dye is injected into the left ventricle to assess ventricular function (ejection fraction)
5. The patient is on a cardiac monitor throughout the procedure because the catheter or the dye may irritate the heart and cause cardiac dysrhythmia.
6. Data recorded from the catheters and from fluoroscopic imaging can provide information about the following:
   a. Coronary circulation and areas of stenosis
   b. Pressures in each chamber of the heart
   c. Cardiac output and ejection fraction
   d. Cardiac size and malformations
   e. Aortic and mitral valvular stenosis and regurgitation (velocity and flow)
7. Post-procedure patients may be on bed rest and monitored for 1 to 12 hours depending on the size of the catheters and the type of antiplatelet medicines used.
   a. Precautions are taken to prevent bleeding at the arterial puncture site.
      1) Angioseals such as Perclose™ may be placed in the catheterization laboratory to establish immediate hemostasis. These patients may be ambulatory after catheterization.
   b. Puncture site and distal circulation is assessed frequently.
      1) Assess site for visible bleeding, swelling or tenderness
      2) Monitor circulatory parameters — pulse, limb temperature, capillary refill — distal to the puncture site
         a) Diminished or absent pulse and circulation may signify arterial occlusion.
      3) Auscultate the femoral artery puncture site
         a) Presence of a bruit suggests pseudoaneurysm
         b) Arterial duplex confirms pseudoaneurysm
   c. BP is monitored; cardiac rhythm may be monitored
   d. The contrast dye used in the procedure acts as an osmotic diuretic and patients require a large amount of fluids to facilitate excretion of the dye.
      1) Encourage patients to drink at least 4 glasses of water or juice if not contraindicated (eg, severe cardiomyopathy or renal disease).
      2) Monitor urine output for several hours after procedure.

e. Other potential problems after cardiac catheterization include MI, stroke and heart failure may occur.

Electrophysiology Studies (EPS)

Used to assess the diagnosis and mechanism of cardiac dysrhythmia

1. Indications: cardiac arrest survivors, differential diagnosis of wide complex tachycardia (ventrcular or supraventricular tachycardia), syncope when believed due to dysrhythmia, and the diagnosis and treatment of accessory pathways.
2. Procedure
   a. Specialty catheters with multiple electrodes are threaded into the heart from the periphery under fluoroscopy.
   b. Timing and sequence of cardiac activation is recorded
   c. Attempts are made to induce dysrhythmia and to relate it to clinical symptoms
   d. If the patient is hemodynamically stable in the induced dysrhythmia, attempts are made to find the ectopic site or pathway that corresponds to the ECG signal
3. Therapeutic radio-frequency ablation may be done on fast or slow conduction pathways, atrial flutter zones, the atrial-ventricular node or dysrhythmogenic foci
4. Post procedure patients require monitoring of the catheter site for bleeding or compromised distal perfusion as outlined above for patients undergoing cardiac catheterization.
   a. Intensive monitoring of cardiac rhythm may be required
   b. Laboratory studies including electrolytes and renal function tests may be required

Angiograms and Venograms

Angiograms: X-ray procedure used to examine the arterial supply of a specific region.

1. Contrast medium is injected through a selectively placed catheter.
2. Catheters are often placed under fluroscopy. Procedure is done in x-ray suite.
3. Angiograms are more sensitive and specific that ultrasound and Doppler studies, but they carry higher risk of harm than noninvasive studies.

Venograms: X-ray procedure that uses contrast medium to visualize venous system of a region. Procedure is done in x-ray suite. Usually an ambulatory patient procedure

CHAPTER 13

Cardiac and Vascular Disease Manifestations

Angina Pectoris

Description

Chest pain or discomfort from myocardial ischemia is due to inadequate coronary blood flow to the heart muscle. Angina pectoris is usually transient and reversible.

Etiology

Angina pectoris is usually from an atherosclerotic lesion. Other conditions include spasm and anomalies of the coronary artery.

Incidence and Demographics

Angina pectoris affects approximately 6,400,000 people in the US. More women (4,000,000) than men (2,300,000) have this health problem. In 1998, 36,000 men and 49,000 women were discharged from hospitals with this diagnosis.

Risk Factors

Non-modifiable risk factors for coronary heart disease (CHD) include increasing age, male gender, heredity, and race (African-American, Hispanic-American, Native-American).

Modifiable risk factors include tobacco smoking, hypertension (HTN), high serum cholesterol with elevated serum low-density lipoprotein cholesterol (LDL-C) and low serum high-density lipoprotein cholesterol (HDL-C), diabetes mellitus, stress, excess alcohol consumption, physical inactivity, and overweight/obesity.

Assessment

1. History
   a. Typical chest pain is substernal and may radiate to the arm or jaw.
   b. Atypical chest pain includes symptoms such as dyspnea, nausea, vomiting, and fatigue.
   c. Chronic stable angina from transient myocardial ischemia is stimulated by a predictable amount of physical exertion or fatigue.
   d. Unstable angina has a similar pattern of symptoms but the occurrences become more frequent, severe, or prolonged and may not have a specific triggering mechanism.
   e. Noncardiac problems such as pleurisy or costochrondritis may mimic some of these symptoms.
   f. Risk factors for CHD
2. Physical findings may be present at rest or only during pain
   a. S_4 heart sound
   b. Cardiac murmur
   c. Dysrhythmia
   d. Tachycardia
   e. HTN or hypotension
3. Diagnostic Tests
   a. Nitroglycerin test dose to determine if there is relief of symptoms.
   b. Electrocardiogram (ECG) may show ST segment depression or T wave inversion during pain.
   c. Exercise tolerance test to assess left ventricular function and evidence of ischemia
   d. Echocardiogram to determine if there are ventricular wall motion abnormalities

Management

1. Pharmacologic Management
   a. Aspirin is used as an antiplatelet agent.
   b. Beta adrenergic blockers are used to decrease cardiac workload and myocardial oxygen demand.
   c. Cholesterol lowering drugs are used to slow the progression of atherosclerosis.
   d. Nitrates are used for systemic vasodilation to decrease myocardial preload and coronary artery dilation to increase blood flow.
   e. Calcium channel blockers are used for vasodilation and to reduce myocardial contractility.

2. Patient/Family Education
   a. Teach patients and their families about the etiology, risk factors, and course of CHD.
   b. Educate them about risk factor modification including diet, exercise, weight reduction, smoking cessation, stress reduction, and pharmacologic interventions including actions, dosage, and side effects of medications.
   c. Discuss with them the acute symptoms associated with unstable angina and MI.
   d. Family members of people with cardiac disease should learn cardiopulmonary resuscitation (CPR) and how to activate the Emergency Medical System (EMS) in the event of cardiac arrest.

Outcomes and Follow-up

1. Patients and their families will be knowledgeable about angina pectoris and its treatment.
2. Patients will not experience any complications such as myocardial infarction.
3. Patients will follow-up as indicated with their health providers after diagnostic testing.

Myocardial Infarction (MI)

Description

1. Acute coronary syndrome (ACS) includes unstable angina, non-ST elevation MI (NSTMI), and ST-elevation MI (STEMI).
2. ACS involves imbalance between myocardial oxygen supply and demand (myocardial ischemia).
3. In unstable angina, the oxygen imbalance resolves within 20 minutes, without permanent damage to myocardium.
4. In MI, prolonged myocardial ischemia results in necrosis of myocardial tissue.

Etiology

1. Myocardial ischemia may result from:
   a. Thrombus formation on preexisting plaque,
   b. Coronary vasospasm,
   c. Atherosclerotic occlusion in the absence of clot or vasospasm,
   d. Inflammation or infection, or
   e. Ischemia secondary to decreased oxygen supply (anemia, acute blood loss or hypoxemia), or secondary to increased demand (metabolic disorders such as thyrotoxicosis).

2. The predominant cause of ACS is acute coronary thrombosis resulting from platelet adherence to a disrupted atherosclerotic plaque.

Incidence and Demographics

1. Two million Americans are diagnosed with ACS annually, of these 1 million will be diagnosed with unstable angina and 1 million with acute myocardial infarction (AMI).
2. Half of the people with AMI will die, about half within the first hour after onset of symptoms, most as a result of ventricular fibrillation.

Risk Factors

Presence of modifiable and non-modifiable risk factors for CHD.

Assessment

1. History
   a. Onset of symptoms (time, associated activity, or event), location of pain, and radiation (arm(s), jaw, or back), duration (constant or intermittent), character (squeezing, sharp, or dull), associated symptoms (fatigue, dyspnea, diaphoresis, nausea, vomiting, confusion, and syncope), relieved by (rest or nitroglycerin), treatments attempted by patient and their effect (rest, nitroglycerin, NSAIDS, or antacids).
   b. Presence of modifiable and non-modifiable risk factors
   c. Previous medical history (PMH) such as angina, MI, dysrhythmia (atrial fibrillation, heart block), stroke or transient ischemic attack (TIA), rheumatic heart disease, or diabetes
   d. Previous cardiovascular procedures including coronary artery bypass grafting (CABG), angioplasty, stent placement, carotid endarterectomy, pacemaker, or recent surgical procedures
   e. Smoking, alcohol, cocaine, or other illicit drug use
2. Physical Findings
   a. S_3 and S_4 heart sounds
   b. Dysrhythmia
   c. Tachycardia or bradycardia
   d. HTN or hypotension
   e. Cardiac murmurs
   f. Pericardial friction rub
   g. Pulmonary congestion (eg, rales and productive cough of pink, frothy sputum)

h. Jugular venous distention
i. Hepatomegaly or splenomegaly
j. Peripheral edema

3. Diagnostic Tests
   a. ECG for patients with ongoing chest pain, and as soon as possible in patients with chest pain consistent with ACS but whose pain has resolved by the time of evaluation. ECG should be compared to previous ECG if available.
   b. Laboratory tests
      1) Creatine kinase (CK) isoenzymes: CK-MB greater than 3% of total CK is considered positive for MI.
      2) Troponin (Tn) and myoglobin: Tn is undetectable in healthy people, and levels greater than 0.01 ng/ml are considered elevated; and levels greater than 0.1 mg/ml greatly elevated and indicative of high risk of cardiac death.
      3) Other tests include a complete blood count (CBC), basic metabolic panel, prothrombin time (PT) and activated partial thromboplastin time (APTT), and blood type and screen. Patients admitted with ACS should also have a lipid profile within the first 24 hours.
   c. Chest roentgenogram (x-ray) to evaluate for pulmonary edema, cardiomegaly, and other noncardiac etiologies for dyspnea or chest pain (pneumonia, rib fractures, etc.)
   d. Echocardiogram to evaluate left ventricular EF, cardiac wall motion abnormalities, and to identify pericardial effusions.

Management

1. ACS risk categories: The results of history, physical examination, ECG, and cardiac markers are used to assign patients to one of 4 ACS risk categories.
   a. High risk: ST-segment elevation. Patients with ST-segment elevation or with left bundle branch block (LBBB) should be treated immediately with either fibrinolytic therapy or primary angioplasty, depending upon time since onset of symptoms as well as relative or absolute contraindications for surgery or fibrinolytics. Glycoprotein (GP) IIb/IIIa inhibitors are recommended for patients to undergo percutaneous coronary intervention (PCI).
   b. High risk: non-ST-segment elevation. Patients with continuing ischemic symptoms, elevated cardiac markers, and ST-segment depression or elevation of less than 1 mm, or T-wave inversion should be treated medically with IV nitroglycerin

(NTG), heparin, and GP IIb/IIIa inhibitors. ECG should be repeated in 12 hours and enzymes should be repeated (after 6–8 hours).

c. Intermediate risk: non-ST-segment elevation. Patients with typical or atypical chest pain lasting longer than 20 minutes, with a known or possible history of CHD, with T-wave inversion or nonspecific ECG changes, and with negative or only slightly elevated cardiac markers should be treated medically with intravenous NTG, heparin, and GP IIb/IIIa inhibitors. ECG and enzymes should be repeated as indicated above.

d. Low risk: non-ST-segment elevation. Patients with typical or atypical chest pain that is new, intermittent in duration, and with normal ECG or nonspecific ECG changes, and with negative cardiac enzymes should be admitted for observation and treated medically with NTG (either SL, by nasal spray, or topical paste) and a beta-blocker.

2. Invasive Management
   a. PCI with primary angioplasty, with or without placement of a stent.
   b. Coronary stenting combined with GP IIb/IIIa inhibitors shown to result in better myocardial preservation and reduced need for late revascularization compared to fibrinolysis.
   c. Coronary artery bypass surgery
3. Pharmacologic Management
   a. Aspirin: All patients with ACS should receive aspirin (ASA), 160 to 325 mg po, with the first dose chewed and swallowed for immediate antiplatelet effect, followed by daily doses of 75 to 325 mg. ASA is contraindicated for patients with allergy (manifested as asthma), active gastrointestinal, genitourinary, retinal, or other bleeding, or severe untreated HTN. Patients allergic to ASA should receive either clopidogrel or ticlopidine, with clopidogrel preferred over ticlopidine.
   b. Unfractionated heparin (UFH): Use an initial bolus of 60 to 80 units/kg IV, followed by a continuous infusion at 1,000 units/hour. Assess aPTT every 6 hours and adjust infusion rate to achieve an aPTT 1.5–2.0 times control. After two therapeutic aPTT levels have been obtained, the aPTT is monitored at least daily.
   c. Low molecular weight heparin (LMWH) 1 mg/kg every 12 hours subcutaneously may be used for patients with unstable angina and non-ST-segment elevation MI. Advantages of LMWH over UFH include subcutaneous route of administra-

tion and elimination of aPTT monitoring. Irreversibility of effect of LMWH is a disadvantage.

d. Fibrinolytics are indicated for ST-segment-elevation ACS if treatment can be administered within 6–12 hours of onset of symptoms. Streptokinase and tissue plasminogen activator (tPA) are the most frequently used fibrinolytics. Third generation fibrinolytics include rPA, lanoteplase (nPA), and TNK-tPA.

e. Beta-adrenergic antagonists (beta-blockers): All patients with ACS should receive beta-blockers to achieve a heart rate of 60 beats per minute with systolic blood pressure greater than 90 mm Hg. For patients presenting with AMI, metoprolol 5 mg is given intravenously (IV) over 1 to 2 minutes and is repeated every 5 minutes for a total dose of 15 mg IV. Oral metoprolol 25 to 50 mg every 6 hours is started 15 minutes after the last IV dose and is followed by a maintenance dose of 100 mg twice daily.

f. GP IIb/IIIa inhibitors include abciximab, eptifibatide, and tirofiban.

g. Nitroglycerin (NTG) sublingual (SL), 3 doses of 0.4 mg, taken 5 minutes apart, is recommended for relief of angina. NTG may be started IV at a rate of 10 micrograms per minute and titrated to achieve symptom relief, in the absence of hypotension.

h. Morphine may be administered to patients whose pain is not resolved by 3 doses of NTG SL, at a dose of 1 to 5 mg IV, and repeated every 5 to 30 minutes, as needed to relieve pain.

i. HMG-CoA reductase inhibitors (statins)

j. Angiotensin converting enzyme (ACE) inhibitors have been shown to reduce morbidity and mortality when given to patients with recent MI. They are of particular benefit to patients with left ventricular dysfunction, diabetes, or with HTN that is not controlled with nitrates and beta-blockers.

k. Antidysrythmics are used according to the specific rhythm and ACLS protocols.

4. Patient/Family Education

a. Patients and families should be taught to recognize the symptoms of MI and complications such as dysrhythmias or heart failure.

b. Family members of people with cardiac disease should learn CPR and how to activate the EMS in the event of cardiac arrest.

c. Risk factors for CHD should be reviewed with patients and families, and they should be instructed about diet, medications, and lifestyle changes, including weight management, exercise, smoking cessation, and stress management to promote optimum heart health.

d. Patients who require invasive cardiovascular interventions should receive specific instruction concerning risks and benefits.

Outcomes and Follow-up

1. Patients and their families will be knowledgeable about MI and its treatment.
2. Patients will not experience any complications from this health problem or the associated treatment.
3. Patients will follow-up as indicated with their health providers after noninvasive and invasive therapies.
4. Cardiac rehabilitation is appropriate for patients after MI, cardiac revascularization, cardiac transplant, and for patients with stable angina and chronic HF. Specific exercise recommendations will be based upon age, risk factors, and functional status. Comprehensive cardiac rehabilitation programs include exercise, nutritional counseling, behavioral interventions, and monitoring of drug therapy.

Mitral Stenosis (MS)

Description

MS is the result of fusion of the valve apparatus so that the orifice is constricted or narrowed during diastole.

Etiology

1. The most common causes are rheumatic heart disease and infective endocarditis.
2. Less frequently occurring causes are congenital defects and systemic diseases such as systemic lupus erythematosus and amyloidosis.

Incidence and Demographics

1. 25% of patients with rheumatic heart disease have MS
2. Two-thirds of these patients are female.

Risk Factors

1. Infectious processes such as group A streptococcal infection (GAS)
2. Congenital heart disease
3. Systemic diseases

Assessment

1. History
   a. Rheumatic heart disease or other associated condition
   b. Shortness of breath, dyspnea, or productive cough
   c. Chest pain due to right ventricular hypertension and/or coronary artery atherosclerosis
   d. Thromboembolism from atrial fibrillation
2. Physical Findings
   a. Right ventricular lift from pulmonary hypertension
   b. Displacement of the left ventricular posteriorly because of right ventricular enlargement
   c Decrescendo, diastolic murmur with accentuated first heart sound and opening snap may radiate to the axilla or left sternal area
   d. Hemoptysis, productive cough, and inspiratory crackles from pulmonary edema and/or pulmonary infarction
3. Diagnostic Tests
   a. ECG to identify the presence of atrial fibrillation and left atrial enlargement
   b. Chest x-ray to detect pulmonary edema and left atrial enlargement
   c. Echocardiography to evaluate mitral valve function
   d. Angiography

Management

1. Invasive Management
   a. Balloon valvuloplasty
   b. Mitral valve surgery
      1) Closed mitral valvulotomy
      2) Open mitral valvulotomy
      3) Mitral valve replacement
2. Pharmacologic Management
   a. Endocarditis prophylaxis for surgical and dental procedures
   b. Diuretics and restriction of sodium intake for symptomatic patients
   c. Digitalis to slow the ventricular rate in atrial fibrillation and to treat ventricular failure
   d. Antidysrhythmics for the treatment of atrial fibrillation and other dysrhythmia
   e. Consider anticoagulant therapy for patients with atrial fibrillation

3. Patient/Family Education
   a. Teach patients and their families about the etiology, course of their disease, and preventive care prior to dental and surgical procedures.
   b. Educate them about pharmacological interventions to treat this health problem.
   c. Discuss with them the symptoms associated with acute mitral valve dysfunction. Family members of people with cardiac disease should learn CPR and how to activate the EMS in the event of cardiac arrest.
   d. If surgery is indicated, teach patients about preoperative preparation along with postoperative and discharge care before leaving the hospital.

Outcomes and Follow-up

1. Patients and their families will be knowledgeable about MS and its treatment.
2. Patients will not experience any complications from this health problem or its treatment.
3. Patients will follow-up as indicated with their health providers after noninvasive and invasive therapies.

Mitral Regurgitation (MR)

Description

Abnormalities of the mitral valve apparatus, leaflets, chordae tendineae, papillary muscles, and annulus, may cause MR whereby the valve leaflets do not close completely during ventricular systole.

Etiology

1. Rheumatic heart disease
2. Infectious endocarditis
3. Trauma
4. Congenital defect
5. Myxomatous degeneration (eg, mitral valve prolapse, Marfan syndrome)
6. Papillary muscle disorders

Incidence and Demographics

1. More common in men than women

Risk Factors

1. Infectious process such as GAS
2. Congenital heart disease
3. Cardiac injury
4. CHD

Assessment

1. History
   a. Patients may be asymptomatic for years.
   b. History of associated diseases or conditions
   c. Development of symptoms is longer than in MS.
   d. Pulmonary symptoms and embolization occur less frequently than in MS.
2. Physical Findings
   a. Pansystolic murmur best heard at the apex
   b. Radiation of murmur to the axilla
   c. Thrill palpated at the apex
   d. Hemoptysis, inspiratory crackles, productive cough
3. Diagnostic Tests
   a. ECG to identify left ventricular hypertrophy (LVH) and left atrial enlargement
   b. Chest x-ray to detect enlarged heart, left atrial hypertrophy, or pulmonary edema
   c. Echocardiography to evaluate mitral valve function
   d. Angiography

Management

1. Invasive Management
   a. Annuloplasty and/or reconstruction of the valve
   b. Mitral valve replacement
2. Pharmacologic Management
   a. Endocarditis prophylaxis
   b. Treatment of heart failure with vasodilators and diuretics.
3. Patient/Family Education
   a. Teach patients and their families about the etiology, risk factors, and course of their disease.
   b. Educate them about pharmacological interventions including actions, dosages, and side effects of medications.
   c. Discuss with them the symptoms associated with acute mitral valve dysfunction. Family members of people with cardiac

disease should learn CPR and how to activate the EMS in the event of cardiac arrest.

d. If surgery is indicated, teach patients about preoperative preparation along with postoperative and discharge care before leaving the hospital.

Outcomes and Follow-up

1. Patient and their families will be knowledgeable about MR and its treatment.
2. Patients will not experience any complications from this health problem or its treatment.
3. Patients will follow-up as indicated with their health providers after noninvasive and invasive therapies.

Aortic Stenosis (AS)

Description

AS is a valvular defect that results in left ventricular outflow obstruction because the leaflets do not open completely during systole.

Etiology

1. Congenital malformations of the aortic valve
2. Rheumatic AS results in adhesions and fusions of the commissures and cusps
3. Degenerative calcific AS
4, Atherosclerotic AS

Incidence and Demographics

1. Incidence of AS due to rheumatic fever is decreasing in industrialized countries.
2. Older adults have higher frequency of AS than younger adults.
3. More men than women develop AS.

Risk Factors

1. Atherosclerosis risk factors are diabetes mellitus, hypercholesterolemia, and Type II hyperlipoproteinemia
2. Calcified AS (Paget disease, end stage renal failure)
3. Advancing age

Assessment

1. History
   a. Most patients become symptomatic in the sixth decade of life because of the long period of latency for this disease.
   b. Cardinal manifestations are angina pectoris, syncope, and heart failure.
2. Physical Findings
   a. Systolic ejection murmur crescendo-decrescendo heard at the base of the heart
   b. Thrill may be present at the base
   c. Radiation to base of heart occasionally to the apex
   d. Inspiratory crackles and productive cough related to pulmonary congestion
3. Diagnostic Tests
   a. ECG shows LVH with ST changes
   b. Chest x-ray either normal heart size or LVH
   c. Echocardiography to evaluate aortic valve function
   d. Angiography

Management

1. Invasive Management
   a. Balloon valvuloplasty
   b. Aortic valve replacement
2. Pharmacologic Management
   a. Endocarditis prophylaxis
   b. Cardiac glycosides such as digoxin
   c. Diuretics used with caution to avoid hypovolemia
   d. Beta blockers used with great caution because of myocardial depression and potential for left ventricular failure
   e. Antidysrhythmics for treatment of dysrhythmia such as atrial fibrillation or atrial flutter
3. Patient/Family Education
   a. Teach patients and their families about the etiology, risk factors, and course of their disease.
   b. Educate them about pharmacological interventions including actions, dosages, and side effects of medications.
   c. Discuss with them the symptoms associated with acute aortic valve dysfunction. Family members of people with cardiac disease should learn CPR and how to activate the EMS in the event of cardiac arrest.
   d. If surgery is indicated, teach patients about preoperative preparation along with postoperative and discharge care before leaving the hospital.

Outcomes and Follow-up

1. Patients and their families will be knowledgeable about AS and its treatment.
2. Patients will not experience any complications from this health problem or its treatment.
3. Patients will follow-up as indicated with their health providers after noninvasive and invasive therapies.

Aortic Regurgitation (AR)

Description

AR may be caused by disease of the valve leaflet and/or aortic root so that the orifice does not close completely during diastole.

Etiology

1. Rheumatic heart disease is the most common cause.
2. Trauma
3. Degeneration
4. Infective endocarditis
5. Ankylosing spondylitis
6. Systemic HTN
7. Marfan syndrome
8. Rheumatoid arthritis

Incidence and Demographics

Chronic AR more frequent with advancing age

Risk Factors

1. Infectious processes such as GAS
2. Injury to the heart
3. Advancing age
4. Systemic diseases

Assessment

1. History
   a. Most patients are asymptomatic until the forth or fifth decade.
   b. Symptoms associated with chronic AR include exertional dyspnea, orthopnea, and paroxysmal nocturnal dyspnea.
2. Physical Findings
   a. De Musset sign (perceptible head shake with each heartbeat) in chronic severe AR

   b. Bisferiens (twice striking) pulse
   c. Widened pulse pressure
   d. Decrescendo diastolic murmur
   e. Inspiratory crackles, productive cough from pulmonary congestion
3. Diagnostic Tests
   a. ECG may demonstrate LVH and nonspecific ST segment and T-wave changes.
   b. Chest x-ray cardiac enlargement and left ventricular enlargement
   c. Echocardiography to evaluate valve function
   d. Angiography

Management

1. Invasive Management
   a. Aortic valve replacement with acute AR
2. Pharmacologic Management
   a. Cardiac glycosides such as digoxin (Lanoxin)
   b. Afterload reducers such as vasodilators
   c. Antidysrythmic medications to treat dysrhythmia
   d. Antihypertensives to treat systolic HTN
      1) Avoid using beta-adrenergic blockers
3. Patient/Family Education
   a. Teach patients and their families about the etiology, risk factors, and course of their disease.
   b. Educate them about pharmacological interventions such as actions, dosages, and side effects.
   c. Discuss with them the symptoms associated with acute aortic valve dysfunction. Family members of people with cardiac disease should learn CPR and how to activate the EMS in the event of cardiac arrest.
   d. If surgery is indicated, teach patients about preoperative preparation along with postoperative and discharge care before leaving the hospital.

Outcomes and Follow-up

1. Patients and their families will be knowledgeable about AR and its treatment.
2. Patients will not experience any complications from this health problem or its treatment.
3. Patients will follow-up as indicated with their health providers after noninvasive and invasive therapies.

Acute Pericarditis

Description

Acute pericarditis is an inflammation of the visceral and parietal pericardium.

Etiology

1. Acute pericarditis may be idiopathic, or caused by viral or bacterial infections, neoplastic disease, autoimmune disorders (eg, rheumatoid arthritis, systemic lupus erythematosus, rheumatoid arthritis, polyarteritis nodosa), inflammatory disorders (eg, amyloidosis, sarcoidsis), medications (eg, hydralazine, procainamide, phenytoin, isoniazid), or trauma (thoracic surgery, pacemaker insertion, cardiovascular diagnostic procedures).
2. Postmyocardial infarction (Dressler) syndrome or postpericardiotomy syndrome are forms of acute pericarditis.

Incidence and Demographics

1. More frequent in men than women
2. Associated with advancing age

Risk Factors

1. Infectious processes
2. Systemic diseases
3. CHD
4. Noninvasive and invasive cardiac therapies

Assessment

1. History
   a. The most frequent symptom is retrosternal chest pain that radiates to the neck. The pain is aggravated by lying down or coughing and is relieved by leaning forward.
   b. Associated symptoms include dyspnea, cough, and weight loss.
2. Physical Findings
   a. Pericardial friction rub
   b. Pericardial effusion muffles heart sounds
   c. Rales from pulmonary compression
   d. Cardiac tamponade results in pulsus paradoxus, hypotension, tachypnea, tachycardia or bradycardia, rales, and jugular venous distention from cardiac compression.

3. Diagnostic Tests
    a. ECG to detect diffuse ST segment elevations and PR segment depression
    b. Chest x-ray to detect enlargement of the cardiac silhouette
    c. Echocardiogram to detect the presence and quantity of pericardial fluid.

Management

1. Invasive Management
    a. Pericardiocentesis if there is evidence of cardiac compression
2. Pharmacologic Management
    a. Nonsteroidal antiinflammatory drugs such as aspirin or indomethicin (Indocin).
    b. Corticosteroids, such as prednisone, are used for severe pain.
    c. Antibiotics are used for the treatment of purulent pericarditis.
3. Patient/Family Education
    a. Teach patients and their families about the etiology, risk factors, and course of their disease.
    b. Educate them about pharmacological interventions such as actions, dosages, and side effects.
    c. Discuss with them the symptoms associated with acute cardiac tamponade and resources for activating emergency care.

Outcomes and Follow-up

1. Patients and their families will be knowledgeable about acute pericarditis and its treatment.
2. Patients will not experience any complications from this health problem or its treatment.
3. Patients will follow-up with their health providers after noninvasive and invasive therapies.

Dilated Congestive Cardiomyopathy (DCCM)

Description

DCCM is a syndrome that results in cardiac enlargement and systolic dysfunction of one or both ventricles.

Incidence and Demographics

1. 4.9 million patients in the US per year are treated for heart failure.
2. 26–35% of heart failure is a result of nonischemic heart disease such as cardiomyopathy.

Etiology

1. Primary, also known as idiopathic, cardiomyopathy is often without a known cause.
2. Secondary cardiomyopathy is an end result of a known cause or disease process such as alcohol abuse, viral infection, chemotherapy, or pregnancy.

Risk Factors

1. Infectious process
2. Genetic predisposition
3. Toxic substances such as alcohol or chemotherapeutic agents

Assessment

1. History
   a. As cardiac workload increases and exceeds capacity the patient becomes symptomatic.
   b. Cardinal congestive symptoms include fatigue, from the low cardiac output, and dyspnea (in 75% of patients). Weight gain is a cardinal sign.
   c. Non-congestive symptoms include chest pain, palpitations, light-headedness, and syncope.
   d. Other symptoms may include paroxysmal nocturnal dyspnea, chronic cough, orthopnea, right upper quadrant pain (secondary to hepatic engorgement), and nausea.
   e. Rarely the first presentation may be an embolic event.
2. Physical Findings
   a. Tachypnea and tachycardia
   b. Cardiac rhythm is usually sinus early in the disease process, but atrial fibrillation is also seen. Rhythm disturbances have been attributed to the enlarged myocardium interfering with the normal conduction pathways.
   c. Diminished stroke volume results in a narrowed pulse pressure.
   d. Apical impulse (formerly known as the PMI) is displaced inferiorly and laterally secondary to increased cardiac size.
   e. S_3 heart sound, if ventricular failure is present
   f. S_4 heart sound may be heard and may precede signs of heart failure
   g. If valvular disease is also present, systolic murmurs of mitral or tricuspid regurgitation will be heard.
   h. Jugular vein distention
   i. Hepatomegaly and liver pulsatility
   j. Ascites from hepatic congestion is often seen.
   k. Peripheral edema

3. Diagnostic Tests
   a. ECG may demonstrate low voltage; dysrhythmia such as atrial fibrillation and ventricular ectopy (atrial ectopy is seen less frequently); and nonspecific ST-T wave changes.
   b. Chest x-ray signs include enlarged heart and evidence of pulmonary venous congestion. Acute interstitial edema may be evident by Kerley's B lines and peribronchial cuffing.
   c. Echocardiogram may be difficult to distinguish DCCM from ischemic left ventricular failure. Characteristic findings include:
      1) Biventricular dilation in early disease that may include all four cardiac chambers in later disease
      2) Decreased EF as a result of the decreased cardiac muscle function
      3) Decreased mitral valve opening if the mitral annular opening or papillary muscles have been affected
      4) Other findings may include mural thrombus in any chamber, pericardial effusion, and mitral or tricuspid regurgitation.

Clinical Course

1. Progressive downhill course over a 3 to 5 year period.
2. Most patients, especially those over 55 years of age, die within five years of the onset of symptoms.
3. Most powerful prognostic factor is the ejection fraction (EF). Those with an EF of less than twenty percent have a 1-year mortality rate of 50%.
4. As symptoms worsen the patient experiences progressive exercise intolerance, symptoms refractory to treatment, and increasing cardiac size.
5. Initially only systolic dysfunction will be present, but as the disease process progresses diastolic dysfunction may develop also.
6. Most patients develop some form of mitral valvular heart disease. As the ventricle enlarges it dilates the anterior annular ring and displaces the papillary muscles, pulling the leaflets apart and causing functional MR.
7. Heart failure (HF) results from various mechanisms, which include neurohormonal changes leading to ventricular remodeling, and changes in pumping capacity.13 HF is classified by impact on function. Different levels of treatment are indicated for each class. The classification scale used currently is the New York Heart Association Functional Classification Scale.
8. Sudden death in severe DCCM is most often a result of dysrhythmia.

Management

1. Invasive Management
   a. Cardiac valve repair or replacement
   b. Implantable defibrillators and permanent pacemakers are useful for patients with malignant or symptomatic dysrhythmias.
   c. Cardiac transplantation is used for patients who are refractory to medical therapy.
   d. Studies of implantable ventricular assist devices in end-stage DCCM are on-going.
   e. The use of left ventricular volume reduction for pharmacologically refractory DCCM is increasing. The surgical techniques have been refined and with the shortage of cardiac donors health care providers are seeking other treatment option.
   f. Left ventriculectomy (Batista operation) is a treatment option for a select few candidates.
2. Pharmacologic Management
   The goals of therapy are to control symptoms, slow the disease progression, and prevent the complications of thromboembolism and sudden death. Treatment is based on presenting symptoms, the type of ventricular dysfunction, and co-morbid conditions. The initial health history and physical examination establish the baseline data. Treatment is based on careful monitoring for any changes from baseline and daily body weight.
   a. Systolic dysfunction treatment to reduce cardiac workload
      1) Diuretics reduce volume overload, which decreases both preload and afterload.
      2) Vasodilators reduce afterload.
      3) Inotropes increase cardiac contractility.
   b. ACE inhibitors decrease ventricular remodeling as well as decreasing cardiac workload through vasodilation.
   c. Antidysrythmics treat dysrhythmia.
   d. Recent studies have shown that beta-blockers decrease mortality in DCCM. Current recommendation is for all patients with severe HF to take a beta-blocker.
3. Noninvasive Management
   a. Eliminate exacerbating factors. Stressors, both emotional and physical, worsen the HF symptoms. Infections increase the metabolic processes, cardiac workload, and symptoms.
   b. Other conditions that increase the cardiac workload and worsen symptoms include dysrhythmia, volume overload (non-adherence to low sodium diets), pulmonary embolism, and coexisting cardiac diseases.

c. Life style modifications that will help the patient control symptoms include:
   1) Reduced physical activity and spacing of energy intense activities.
   2) Eating small frequent meals to decrease the gastric distention if hepatomegaly is present.
   3) Elimination of alcohol, which may increase the cardiomyopathy.

4. Prognosis
   a. Overall prognosis is dependent upon the underlying pathology of the DCCM and the severity of associated HF.
5. Patient/Family Education
   a. Teach patients and their families about the etiology, course, and prognosis of their disease.
   b. Educate them about pharmacologic interventions such as actions, dosages, and side effects.
   c. Discuss the symptoms associated with acute HF and pulmonary edema. Family members of people with cardiac disease should learn CPR and how to activate the EMS in the event of cardiac arrest.
   d. If surgery is indicated, teach patients about preoperative preparation along with postoperative and discharge care before leaving the hospital.

Outcomes and Follow-up

1. Patients and their families will be knowledgeable about DCCM and its treatment.
2. Patients will follow-up as indicated with their health providers after noninvasive and invasive therapies.
3. Patients will adapt to changes in their functional status as their disease progresses.

Hypertrophic Cardiomyopathy (HCM)

Description

1. HCM is a familial Mendelian-linked autosomal dominant disorder that is characterized by idiopathic myocardial hypertrophy and myocyte disarray at the cellular level.
2. Obstructive HCM is the presence of idiopathic LVH without dilation of the ventricle causing abnormal diastolic function and a dynamic subaortic pressure gradient.

3. Obstructive HCM most often involves hypertrophy of the ventricular septum, which results in narrowing of the left ventricle (LV) outflow tract. The mitral valve leaflet is pulled into contact with the ventricular septum and creates a subaortic pressure gradient. The degree of gradient varies according to the patient's activity level or after pharmacologic therapy.
4. Both forms of HCM have diastolic dysfunction.
   a. There is decreased ventricular compliance and incomplete relaxation of the thickened ventricular wall.
   b. These factors impede diastolic filling and increase the left ventricular end-diastolic pressure.
   c. MR may occur secondary to the anterior motion of the mitral valve during systole.

Etiology

1. Idiopathic
2. Genetic predisposition

Incidence and Demographics

1. Obstructive HCMs are estimated to have a prevalence of 1 in 500 (0.2%) of the general population.
2. 50% of HCM is due to an autosomal dominant familial disease.
3. Patients without a family history of the disease may have a sporadic gene mutation.

Risk Factors

1. Abnormalities of myocardial calcium kinetics
2. Diastolic dysfunction

Assessment

1. History
   a. Asymptomatic patients may be identified during screening after a relative has been diagnosed.
   b. Symptom severity does not always correlate with the functional severity of the cardiomyopathy.
   c. Most frequently seen symptoms are those of congestive HF and are not related to the presence or severity of outflow obstruction.
      1) Dyspnea due to increased LV stiffness and diastolic dysfunction
      2) Orthopnea and lethargy due to pulmonary congestion and decreased cardiac output

d. Angina and palpitations may be due to impaired coronary flow reserve and myocardial ischemia. Luminal obstruction (stenosis) of the coronary arteries may cause angina.
e. Atrial fibrillation may result from increased left atrial size and MR.
f. Patients often present with sudden death secondary to dysrhythmia that may be ventricular, atrial, or bradycardia in origin. Exercise with it's associated peripheral vasodilation and induced myocardial ischemia has also been proposed as a possible cause of sudden death.

2. Physical Findings
   a. The apical impulse (also known as PMI) is displaced inferiorly and laterally due to increased cardiac size.
   b. A third (S_3), if diastolic failure is present, and fourth (S_4) heart sound may be heard.
   c. A harsh systolic murmur is heard in those patients with significant outflow gradients.
      1) Palpable systolic thrill my be present
   d. Tachypnea, inspiratory crackles, and productive cough
   e. Jugular venous distention
   f. Hepatosplenomegaly may be present
3. Diagnostic Tests
   a. ECG characterized by nonspecific ST-T wave abnormalities, which have been attributed to the thickened ventricle wall. Pseudo-Q waves (no actual infarct has occurred) may be seen in the anterolateral and inferior leads. Large inverted T-waves in the precordial leads in those with apical hypertrophy. As a consequence of MR, atrial fibrillation is seen in 25% of those with HCM.
   b. Chest x-ray will be normal unless pulmonary congestion and HF are present.
   c. Echocardiogram findings may include LVH, small left ventricular cavity, vigorous posterior wall motion, reduced septal wall movement with or without asymmetrical septal hypertrophy, abnormal systolic anterior motion of the mitral valve leaflets; varying degrees of MR may be seen, and increased left atrial size.
   d. Angiography is not routinely done nor is it needed for diagnosis. Two findings often seen are elevated left ventricular diastolic pressure secondary to the decreased ventricular wall compliance and systolic pressure gradient if an obstruction is present.

Management

1. Invasive Management
   a. Treatments are based on the risk for sudden death. Risk stratification is based on the criteria of survival of cardiac arrest with documented ventricular fibrillation, non-sustained ventricular tachycardia, family history of sudden death, or high-risk genetic mutation.
      1) If high risk, long-term amiodarone (Cordarone), an implantable cardioverter-defibrillator (ICD), or permanent dual chamber pacing are the treatments of choice.
      2) If not high risk, prognosis is good and no restrictions on work or recreational activities are needed. Pharmacologic agents are used for symptom management.
   b. Patients with left ventricular outflow pressure gradients greater than 50 mm Hg that are refractory to medications have three treatment options.
      1) Ventricular septal myotomy-myectomy, known as the Marrow procedure, resects a small amount of the hypertrophic ventricular septum. A resultant reduction if not resolution of the outflow obstruction normalizes the left ventricular pressure and provides symptomatic relief. This procedure is not widely used secondary to the limited number of HCM patients who are suitable candidates.
      2) Transcoronary ablation of the septal hypertrophy is accomplished through the use of an ethanol injection into the left anterior descending artery that precipitates a MI to the hypertrophic area. This procedure is associated with a 17% risk of complete atrioventricular block requiring a pacemaker implantation.
      3) Dual chamber pacing has been used as an alternative to the septal ablation or the Marrow procedure. A 40–50% reduction in the outflow gradient was noted, though the mechanism of this reduction was unclear.
   c. Cardiac transplantation is indicated for patients in the dilated phase of cardiomyopathy with HF not responsive to therapy.
2. Pharmacologic Management
   a. Beta-blockers reduce the obstructive gradient seen in obstructive HCM. By slowing the heart rate, beta-blockers lengthen diastolic filling time, reduce the myocardial oxygen consumption, and reduce the outflow gradient. Beta-blockers are used by patients with atrial fibrillation to control ventricular rate and by some patients with paroxysmal atrial fibrillation.

b. Calcium channel blockers have both a negative inotropic and chronotropic effect that lessens the outflow tract pressure gradient, increases ventricular filling, and increases coronary sinus profusion thus decreasing myocardial ischemia. Care must be taken in observing for adverse effects of peripheral vasodilation of the calcium channel blockers. Patients with high outflow gradients need higher filling pressures to overcome the gradient.
c. Antidysrhythmics are used to treat dysrhythmia. Disopyramide, a class 1A antidysrhythmic, decreases the outflow tract gradient through its actions of negative inotropy and peripheral vasoconstriction. It is the drug of choice in symptomatic obstructive HCM.
d. The risk benefit ratio of anticoagulation must be evaluated individually. Patients with atrial fibrillation and those with severely depressed ventricular function would most benefit from anticoagulation26 as their risk for an embolic event is high.

3. Prognosis
   a. There is wide variability in both the presentation and prognosis of HCM.
   b. Sudden death is the major cause of death in both symptomatic and asymptomatic patients.
   c. No correlation has been found between the severity of the HCM and the risk for sudden death.
4. Patient/Family Education
   a. Teach patients and their families about the etiology, course, and prognosis for their disease.
   b. Educate them about pharmacological interventions such as actions, dosages, and side effects.
   c. Discuss the symptoms associated with acute HF and pulmonary edema along with ways to activate resources for emergency care.
   d. If surgery is indicated, teach patients about preoperative preparation along with postoperative and discharge care before leaving the hospital.

Outcomes and Follow-up

1. Patients and their families will be knowledgeable about HCM and its treatment.
2. Patients will follow-up as indicated with their health providers after noninvasive and invasive therapies.
3. Patients will adapt to changes in their functional status as their disease progresses.

Restrictive Cardiomyopathy (RCM)

Description

RCM is characterized by ventricular stiffness classically associated with abnormal diastolic filling. The ventricles become stiff as a result of fibrosis, hypertrophy, or secondary infiltration. The ventricular cavity may become partially obliterated by fibrous tissue and thrombus. Though primarily associated with diastolic dysfunction, systolic dysfunction may develop as the disease progresses.

Etiology

1. RCM may be idiopathic or have a primary cause such as endomyocardial fibrosis or eosinophilic endomyocardial disease.
   a. Endomyocardial fibrosis is most common in the African and tropical regions.
   b. Hypereosinophilic syndrome may be a result of an idiopathic process, a parasitic infection, hypersensitivity to various allergens, connective tissue disease, or autoimmune disorder.
2. Secondary causes of RCM include amyloidosis, sarcoidosis, Fabry disease (glycogen storage disease process), carcinoid, and hemochromatosis. Less common secondary causes are fibroelastosis, tumors, and collagen-vascular diseases.

Incidence and Demographics

1. Least common form of the cardiomyopathies

Risk Factors

1. Predisposition for endomyocardial fibrosis
2. Hypersensitivity to allergens
3. Systemic inflammatory disease

Assessment

1. History
   a. Patients may remain asymptomatic or present with symptoms of increasing exercise intolerance and HF. Exercise intolerance results from limited ventricular filling and inability to increase cardiac output (also known as "fixed cardiac output").
   b. The underlying cause of the disease determines the patient's presentation.
      1) Patients with endomyocardial fibrosis may present initially with pulmonary and venous congestion.

2) Patients with amyloidosis may present with venous congestion, HF, dysrhythmia, or orthostatic hypotension.
   c. RCM presentation may mimic constrictive pericarditis.
2. Physical Findings
   a. S_3 and/or S_4 heart sounds
   b. Cardiac murmurs
   c. Pulmonary rales, hypotension, narrowed pulse pressure
   d. Jugular venous distention is persistent as preload and impedance to ventricular filling increases.
   e. Dependent edema, ascites, and hepatomeg-aly result from the persistently elevated venous pressure associated with right ventricular failure.
3. Diagnostic Tests
   a. ECG demonstrates low voltage as a result of the replacement of normal myocardium with fibrotic tissue; left axis deviation as the impulse vector is displaced secondary to the myocardial fibrosis; and pseudo-Q waves are often seen. Atrial dysrhythmia is frequently present.
   b. Chest x-ray may show pulmonary vascular redistribution if pulmonary congestion is present. There should be no pericardial calcification unless constrictive pericarditis is present. Cardiomegaly with or without atrial enlargement may be seen.
   c. Echocardiogram demonstrates symmetrical thickening of the ventricular walls. Ventricles are normal in size thus excluding HCM and valvular heart disease. Ventricular volumes and systolic function may be normal or slightly reduced. Early diastolic filling is evident. Diastolic mitral or tricuspid regurgitation is observed in RCM as a physiologic indicator of marked elevation of the ventricular diastolic pressure.
   d. Cardiac catheterization results will show decreased cardiac output and elevated right and left ventricular end diastolic filling pressures. Systolic function is well preserved. Pulmonary artery pressures are elevated.
   e. Endomyocardial biopsy is a definitive method of diagnosis. Myocyte hypertrophy and interstitial fibrosis are seen in RCM without the evidence of myocardial disarray that would be seen with HCM.

Management

1. Invasive Management
   a. Cardiac transplantation is used in those patients with intractable HF.

2. Pharmacologic Management
   A general goal of therapy for all types of RCM is to relieve symptoms of right and left ventricular failure. Specific interventions depend upon the underlying pathology. Each patient has a critical level needed for preload and afterload to maintain adequate ventricular filling and cardiac output.
   a. Diuretics are used to relieve fluid overload that is seen in the form of peripheral edema, ascites, and pulmonary congestion.
   b. Vasodilators, such as calcium channel blockers, are used cautiously. Aggressive reduction of the preload or afterload will affect adversely the patient's status.
   c. ACE inhibitors are used cautiously, because they may decrease ventricular filling and cardiac output.
   d. Digitalis is not used, because it may predispose the patient to dysrhythmia. In amyloidosis, digoxin binds to the amyloid fiber in the heart.
3. Prognosis
   a. Primary RCM has a 9-year survival from time of early diagnosis and treatment. Once HF occurs mean survival rate drops to less than five years.
   b. Prognosis of secondary RCM depends on the etiology of the cardiomyopathy.
4. Patient/Family Education
   a. Teach patients and their families about the etiology, course, and prognosis for their disease.
   b. Educate them about pharmacological interventions such as actions, dosages, and side effects.
   c. Discuss the symptoms associated with acute HF and pulmonary edema along with ways to activate resources for emergency care.
   d. If surgery is indicated, teach patients about preoperative preparation along with postoperative and discharge care before leaving the hospital.

Outcomes and Follow-up

1. Patients and their families will be knowledgeable about RCM and its treatment.
2. Patients will follow-up as indicated with their health providers after noninvasive and invasive therapies.
3. Patients will adapt to changes in their functional status as their disease progresses.

Heart Failure (HF)

Description

HF is "a clinical syndrome or condition characterized by (1) signs and symptoms of intravascular and interstitial volume overload, including shortness of breath, rales, and edema or (2) manifestations of inadequate tissue perfusion, such as fatigue or poor exercise tolerance."

Etiology

1. HF has many causes. The left ventricle (LV), right ventricle (RV), or both may be affected with symptoms reflecting the respective areas of damage.
   a. Systolic failure decreases EF (≤40%). It results from ventricular damage, most often due to ischemia or infarction. The heart is dilated and the cardiac silhouette is enlarged on x-ray.
   b. Diastolic failure restricts ventricular filling. It results from concentric LVH, most often due to HTN or AS. The cardiac silhouette appears normal in size. The EF remains normal but cardiac output is reduced. Diastolic failure is responsible for approximately 40% of all cases of HF; however, guidelines have not been established for management of diastolic HF.
2. HF may be acute or chronic. Acute HF may occur in persons with a previously normal cardiovascular system as a result of an acute stressor (eg, thyrotoxicosis, acute MI, acute hemorrhage) or a reversible valvular dysfunction. Chronic HF results from chronic disorders (eg, HTN or AS) or myocardial damage after MI.

Incidence and Demographics

1. HF affects 4.7 million people (2.3 million males and 2.4 million females) in the US.
2. There are 550,000 new cases of HF each year.
3. HF is a major cause of morbidity, with 438,000 hospital discharges among males and 540,000 among females attributed to HF.
4. HF results in 46,980 deaths annually; 17,694 among males (37.7% of total HF deaths); 29,286 among females (62.3% of total HF deaths). About 50% of patients with HF will die within 5 years.

Risk Factors

1. HF results from ischemic and nonischemic causes. CHD causes HF in two thirds of those with systolic HF.28 Within 6 years after MI, 22% of males and 46% of females will be disabled as a result of HF.

2. Nonischemic causes of HF include HTN, valvular heart disease, cardiomyopathy, congenital heart disease, endocarditis, myocarditis, thyroid disease, and alcohol excess. Three of four HF patients have history of HTN.

Assessment

1. History
   a. LV failure may present with dyspnea, orthopnea, paroxysmal nocturnal dyspnea, or cough. Other symptoms include activity intolerance, fatigue, weakness, palpitations, diaphoresis, and alteration in sleep or confusion.
   b. RV failure may present with weight gain, peripheral edema, abdominal distension, and gastrointestinal complaints.
   c. Chest pain may indicate an ischemic cause of HF; however, ischemia may be present without chest pain.
   d. History of HTN, MI, valvular or congenital disease, rheumatic heart disease, atrial fibrillation, recent viral illness, thyroid disease, lung disease, treatment with cardiotoxic drugs, or alcohol abuse
   e. History of CABG, angioplasty, valvular repair or replacement, or thyroid surgery
2. Physical Findings
   a. Tachycardia may be seen in response to decreased cardiac output.
   b. Apical impulse may be displaced laterally as a result of cardiac enlargement.
   c. S_3 reflects left HF.
   d. S_4 indicates cardiac ischemia, HTN, or hypertrophy.
   e. Cardiac murmurs occur with valvular dysfunction.
   f. Elevated JVP may be seen with RV failure.
   g. Rales (crackles) indicate pulmonary congestion.
   h. Pale, cool, diaphoretic skin, with dependent edema
   i. Hepatomegaly and/or splenomegaly because of venous congestion
3. Diagnostic Tests
   a. Chest x-ray may reveal cardiomegaly, pulmonary edema, or pleural effusions.
   b. ECG with acute ST or T-wave changes indicates myocardial ischemia or infarction. Q-waves or bundle branch block may reflect cardiac dysfunction from previous MI. Tachycardia or atrial fibrillation may reflect thyrotoxicosis or increased heart rate to compensate for decreased cardiac output or anemia. Bradycardia secondary to heart block or medications may

result in HF. A low voltage ECG or electrical alternans may reveal pericardial effusion. Left ventricular hypertrophy may reflect diastolic dysfunction.

c. Echocardiogram is used to assess ventricular EF and to differentiate systolic from diastolic failure, detect ventricular enlargement or hypertrophy, valvular dysfunction or congenital heart disorder, and hypokinesis or akinesis secondary to ischemia or infarction.

d. Radionuclide ventriculogram permits more precise measurement of EF than echocardiogram, particularly of RVEF.

e. Laboratory tests include CBC to detect anemia or infection, electrolytes, serum creatinine and BUN to identify electrolyte imbalances secondary to volume overload or diuretic treatment and renal impairment, serum albumin (increased extravascular volume due to hypoalbuminemia), T_4 and TSH for patients over age 65 or with evidence of thyroid disease or atrial fibrillation, and urinalysis to detect renal dysfunction.

f. Right heart catheterization can measure cardiac output, as well as right and left ventricular filling pressures, permitting assessment and treatment of hemodynamically unstable patients.

Management

1. Invasive Management
   a. Cardiac surgery may be indicated to repair AS or other valvular dysfunction.
   b. After MI, there may be viable stunned or hibernating myocardial tissue surrounding infarcted tissue, which can be salvaged by revascularization, preventing HF.
   c. Patients with acutely decompensated HF may require a left ventricular assist device (LVAD). These devices are used for patients with profound hemodynamic instability resulting from MI and to support the circulation while awaiting cardiac transplant.
   d. Continuous arteriovenous hemofiltration (CAVH) is used to reduce fluid overload in acutely decompensated HF.
   e. Patients with symptomatic dysrhythmia may need a pacemaker or an implanted cardioverter-defibrillator. Sudden death secondary to dysrhythmia is a major cause of death in patients with HF.
   f. Cardiac transplantation should be considered for patients with HF who have severe limitations or require frequent hospitalizations secondary to HF, in whom aggressive medical therapy fails and surgical revascularization is not appropriate.

2. Pharmacologic Management
   a. ACE inhibitors are recommended for all patients with systolic dysfunction. They have been shown to improve symptoms and prolong life. Angiotensin II receptor blockers (ARBs) are an alternative to ACE inhibitors, and may be used for patients intolerant of ACE inhibitors due to angioedema or intractable cough, but they have not been proven to be equal to or better than ACE inhibitors.
   b. Combined therapy with hydralazine and isosorbide dinitrate may be used for patients unable to tolerate ACE inhibitors or ARBs due to angioedema, intractable cough, hypotension, or renal insufficiency. Neither drug taken alone is recommended for HF.
   c. Beta-blockers are recommended for patients in NYHA class II or III, but are not recommended for patients in NYHA class IV (symptomatic at rest). Beta-blockers are indicated for long-term management of HF, but should not be used in acutely decompensated HF requiring hospitalization for aggressive diuresis or intravenous therapy, nor should be used for patients with symptomatic bradycardia, hypotension or advanced heart block.
   d. Spironolactone reduces morbidity and mortality in patients with recurrent dyspnea at rest (NYHA class IV).
   e. Diuretics are recommended for all symptomatic patients, with dosage as needed to control symptoms. Loop diuretics (furosemide, bumetanide, torsemide) are the most potent diuretics. A thiazide diuretic such as metolazone may be added to potentiate diuresis.
   f. Digoxin is a positive inotrope and negative chronotrope recommended to improve the clinical status of patients who remain symptomatic despite treatment with ACE inhibitors, beta-blockers, diuretics, and spironolactone.
   g. Most calcium channel blockers (CCBs) are not recommended for treatment of HF. Amlodipine and felodipine have been shown to not affect survival adversely in HF, however clinical evidence is lacking in support of CCBs in treatment of HF.
   h. Dysrhythmia is a frequent cause of death for patients with HF. Class I antidysrhythmic agents (quinidine, procainamide, flecainide, encainide) should not be used in HF, except in treatment of refractory life-threatening dysrhythmia. Class II antidysrhythmics (beta-blockers) are recommended for patients with HF, as previously discussed. Class III antidysrhythmics (sotalol, amiodarone) are not recommended for general use in patients already receiving beta-blockers and ACEIs, but are

preferred over Class I antidysrhythmics in the treatment of atrial dysrhythmias in patients with HF. Amiodarone is also recommended for treatment of ventricular tachycardia and ventricular fibrillation.

i. IV medications used for inpatient management of acutely decompensated HF include positive inotropes such as dopamine, dobutamine, and phosphodiesterase inhibitors (milrinone, amrinone), which enhance cardiac contractility and increase renal blood flow (promoting diuresis). These drugs provide short-term improvement in symptoms, but long-term use is associated with increased mortality.

3. Patient/Family Education: The AHCPR (now AHRQ) lists the following topics for patient, family, and caregiver education.
   a. Information should be provided about HF, its causes, symptoms, self-monitoring with daily weights, and what to do if symptoms worsen. Smoking cessation should be emphasized. Patients should be encouraged to obtain influenza and pneumococcal vaccinations.
   b. Patients and family should be informed about their prognosis (life expectancy), and advance directives should be discussed.
   c. Work, recreation, sex, and other exercise recommendations should be based upon the patient's age, comorbidities, and exercise stress test results. Cardiac rehabilitation improves symptoms and functional capacity, and reduces morbidity and mortality related to HF.
   d. A low-sodium diet (less than 2g Na+) is generally recommended for HF patients. Fluid restrictions may be required. Moderation or abstinence in intake of alcohol is recommended (≤2 drinks per day).
   e. Patients should be instructed about their medications, their benefits, possible side effects and what to do if they occur, dosages, and timing of medications.
   f. Patients should be advised about the importance of compliance with the treatment plan, and should receive counseling about qualified support groups and HF management programs.

Outcomes and Follow-up

1. Patients and their families will be knowledgeable about HF and its treatment.
2. Patients will follow-up as indicated with their health providers after noninvasive and invasive therapies.
3. Patients will adapt to changes in their functional status as their disease progresses.

Atrial Fibrillation (A fib)

Description

1. A fib is a cardiac dysrhythmia characterized by absent P waves, irregularly irregular R-R intervals, and baseline undulations of variable shape and amplitude (f waves). A fib can occur in chronic or paroxysmal forms. Chronic A fib is often well-tolerated, however it carries the risk of developing mural thrombi within the atria, thromboembolism, and the need for long-term anticoagulation therapy. Acute presentations of a fib are often not well tolerated, as the body has not had time to adjust to the loss of atrial kick, which decreases the cardiac output by 1015%. ECG manifestations of a fib are:
   a. PR interval: unable to measure, no P waves
   b. QRS duration: 0.04–0.12 seconds
   c. Rate: Atrial rate estimated to be 400–600 impulses per minute, ventricular rate ranges from normal to a rapid ventricular response.
   d. Regularity: Irregularly irregular R-R intervals

Etiology

1. A fib is caused by multiple ectopic foci and reentry circuits that lead to chaotic depolarization of the atria. Many conditions that lead to stretching or inflammation of the atrial tissue, decreased velocity of conduction through the atria, or ischemia can trigger the dysrhythmia.

Incidence and Demographics

1. A fib is the most frequently occurring dysrhythmia; incidence increases with age.
2. A fib occurs in 9% of people over 70 years of age and in 20% to 30% of patients undergoing coronary artery bypass graft surgery.

Risk Factors

1. Pulmonary diseases
2. Valvular disease
3. Congenital heart disease
4. Coronary artery bypass surgery
5. Congestive heart disease
6. Atherosclerosis

7. MI
8. Rheumatic heart disease
9. Thyrotoxicosis

Assessment

A fib causes loss of atrial kick, which is responsible for 10–15% of cardiac output. It is important to determine when the symptoms started to estimate the length of time in a fib, and whether it is chronic or intermittent.

1. History
   a. Fatigue, dizziness, activity intolerance, inability to perform activities of daily living, palpitations, shortness of breath
2. Physical Findings
   a. Rapid or irregular heart rate
   b. Varying intensity of S_1
   c. Hypotension
3. Diagnostic Tests
   a. ECG to confirm rhythm and differentiate from atrial flutter
   b. Echocardiogram to evaluate cardiac structure and function, and assess for presence of mural thrombi that would impact treatment.
   c. Thyroid function studies to correct hyperthyroidism, as it interferes with treatment success.

Management

Treatment is aimed at restoring sinus rhythm, controlling ventricular response and preventing thromboembolism by identifying and treating the cause of the dysrhythmia.

1. Electrical Management
   a. Synchronized electrical cardioversion is indicated for hemodynamic instability, to restore sinus rhythm in acute onset, and for conversion to sinus rhythm after anticoagulation in chronic cases.
      1) Length of time in a fib should be less than 48 hours for acute onset and
      2) Confirmation of the absence of mural thrombus by echocardiogram prior to cardioversion to prevent thromboembolism
   b. Permanent atrial pacemaker can be implanted to pace the atria at a set rate.

2. Pharmacologic Management
   a. Medications are used to slow the ventricular rate if it is >100 beats per minute.
      1) Calcium channel blockers
      2) Beta blockers
      3) Digitalis
   b. Antidysrhythmic agents are used to convert to sinus rhythm.
      1) Type 1A agents (quinidine, procainamide)
         a) May speed conduction at the atrioventricular node
         b) An agent to slow ventricular response is used before attempting to convert.
      2) Type IC agents: Flecainide, propafenone
      3) Type III agents: Amiodarone, sotolol, ibutilide
   c. Anticoagulants are used to reduce thromboembolism
      1) Heparin is used acutely in the inpatient setting until the INR is therapeutic on coumadin.
      2) Coumadin is used for 4 weeks before cardioversion is performed. If cardioversion is unsuccessful, then long-term coumadin therapy is indicated.
3. Patient/Family Education
   a. Patients and their families should learn the signs and symptoms of a fib and to report them to their healthcare provider. They should also be instructed on the signs and symptoms of stroke.
   b. Patients on coumadin should learn to self-monitor for signs of bleeding and to avoid situations that will put them at risk for bleeding (eg, falls, vigorous activities, and shaving with a straight razor). Medications that interact with coumadin should be identified and avoided.
   c. Family members of people with cardiac disease should learn CPR and how to activate the EMS in the event of cardiac arrest.

Outcomes and Follow-up Care

1. Approximately, 50% of patients treated for a fib with antidysrhythmic agents remain free from further recurrence at 12 months
2. Patients receiving antidysrhythmic drugs should be monitored carefully on a regular basis with blood levels and physical examination.
3. Health care providers should treat the underlying disease or condition that caused the a fib.

Atrial Flutter (AF)

Description

1. AF is a regular reentry dysrhythmia characterized by identical saw tooth "F" waves at rapid rates and varying ventricular responses. Conduction ratios between the atria and ventricles usually occur at even intervals (ie, 2:1, 4:1, 6:1) but can also vary. Like A fib, AF can occur acutely or chronically. The acute presentation may cause the patient to be unstable due to loss of atrial kick, and chronic manifestations may include mural thrombus that could lead to thromboembolism. AF can occur in combination with A fib.
2. ECG manifestations of AF
   a. PR interval: Unable to measure
   b. QRS duration: Normal
   c. Rate: Atrial rate between 250–450, ventricular rate varies as the AV node blocks most of the impulses. It usually presents with an atrial rate of 300 and a ventricular rate of 150 beats per minute. Ventricular rates <100 are considered controlled, and rates >100 are considered a rapid ventricular response.
   d. Regularity: Regular "F" waves with varying ventricular response, can be regular or irregular depending on the AV node.

Etiology

1. AF arises from a reentry circuit in the right atrium which achieves depolarization rates between 250–450 times per minute in rapid identical waves. There are 2 types of AF, type 1 results in an atrial rate of 300 and type 2 is responsible for much faster rates, averaging 400–450 per minute. Underlying cardiac and pulmonary conditions predispose patients to AF.

Incidence and Demographics

1. AF is less common than a fib and the two often occur concomitantly. AF can be intermittent or sustained, and is more common in adults than in children. AF used to be considered a transient rhythm, it is now understood to be chronic in some patients.

Risk Factors

1. Pulmonary diseases
2. Valvular heart disease
3. Congenital heart disease

4. Coronary artery bypass surgery
5. Congestive heart disease
6. Atherosclerosis
7. MI
8. Rheumatic heart disease
9. Thyrotoxicosis

Assessment

AF causes loss of atrial kick, which is responsible for 10–15% of cardiac output. It is important to determine when the symptoms started to estimate the length of time in AF, and whether it is chronic or intermittent.

1. History
   a. Fatigue, dizziness, activity intolerance
   b. Inability to perform activities of daily living
   c. Palpitations, shortness of breath
2. Physical Findings
   a. Rapid or irregular heart rate, depending on the conduction ratio through the AV node
   b. Varying intensity of S_1 with irregular conduction ratios
   c. Hypotension
3. Diagnostic Tests
   a. ECG to confirm rhythm and differentiate from A fib
   b. Echocardiogram to evaluate cardiac structure and function, and assess for formation of mural thrombi, which would impact treatment
   c. Thyroid function studies to correct hyperthyroidism as it interferes with treatment success
   d. Electrophysiology studies (EPS) to identify reentry circuits

Management

The choice of treatment for the patient will depend on hemodynamic stability and how long they have been in AF.

1. Invasive Management
   a. Radiofrequency ablation of reentry circuits can be done in an electrophysiology lab to prevent recurrence.
   b. Rapid atrial pacing is used to overdrive the reentry circuit with the sinus node.
   c. Electrical cardioversion may convert AF to sinus rhythm. The amount of time the patient has been in AF should be assessed,

and if greater than 48 hours, an echocardiogram should be done to assess for a thrombus prior to converting the rhythm.

2. Pharmacologic Management
   a. Medications are used to slow the ventricular rate if it is >100 beats per minute.
      1) Calcium channel blockers
      2) Beta blockers
      3) Digitalis
   b. Antidysrhythmic agents are used to convert to sinus rhythm.
      1) Type 1A agents-quinidine, procainamide
      2) Type IC agents-flecainide, propafenone
      3) Type III agents-amiodarone, sotolol, ibutilide
   c. Anticoagulants to reduce thromboembolism
      1) Heparin is used acutely in the inpatient setting until the INR is therapeutic on coumadin.
      2) Coumadin is used for 4 weeks before cardioversion is done. If cardioversion is unsuccessful, then long-term coumadin therapy is indicated.
3. Patient/Family Education
   a. Patients and their families should learn the signs and symptoms of AF and report them to their healthcare provider. They should be instructed on the signs and symptoms of stroke also.
   b. Patients on coumadin should learn to self-monitor for signs of bleeding and to avoid situations that will put them at risk for bleeding (eg, falls, vigorous activities, and shaving with a straight razor). Medications that interact with coumadin should be identified and avoided.
   c. Family members of people with cardiac disease should learn CPR and how to activate the EMS in the event of cardiac arrest.

Outcomes and Follow-up Care

1. The goal of treatment is to restore sinus rhythm.
2. Patients receiving antidysrhythmic drugs should be monitored carefully on a regular basis with blood levels and physical examination
3. Health care providers should treat the underlying disease or condition that caused the AF.

First Degree Atrio-Ventricular Block (1°AVB)

Description

1. A delay in the conduction of impulses from the SA node to the AV node, seen on ECG as a prolonged PR interval. It is usually asymptomatic.
2. ECG manifestations of 1°AVB
   a. PR Interval: Prolonged >0.20 seconds
   b. QRS Duration: Normal
   c. Rate: Normal or often bradycardic
   d. Regularity: Regular P-P and R-R intervals

Etiology

1. Normal impulse from the SA node with prolonged relative refractory period in the AV node leads to a delay in ventricular response.
2. Causes for this delay include:
   a. Ischemia, MI, CHD
   b. Scarring of atrial tissue in the area of the internodal pathways
   c. Infiltration by amyloid, sarcoid, Lyme carditis, endocarditis
   d. Degenerative diseases
   e. Rheumatic heart disease
   f. Electrolyte imbalances
   g. Atrial stretch
   h. Increased vagal tone.
   i. Inflammatory diseases
   j. Cardiac medications such as digoxin, calcium channel blockers, beta blockers
3. Prolonged PR interval can occur as a normal variant in some people.

Incidence and Demographics

1°AVB can occur in individuals of all ages and may go undiagnosed due to its benign nature and multitude of common etiologic factors.

Risk Factors

1. Individuals with known cardiac disease or any of the condition listed above are at higher risk for developing 1°AVB.
2. Cardiac medications are often the cause of intermittent 1°AVB, requiring dose adjustments with telemetry monitoring.

Assessment

1. History
   a. 1°AVB is often asymptomatic and discovered during ECG monitoring as an incidental finding.
   b. Activity intolerance or shortness of breath is often associated with higher degrees of AV block.
2. Physical Findings
   a. There may be no findings on physical examination to indicate 1°AVB, unless the patient is bradycardic (heart rate <60).
   b. There may be findings consistent with an underlying disease state such as a murmur from rheumatic heart disease.
3. Diagnostic Tests
   a. ECG to diagnose 1°AVB.
   b. Laboratory studies including cardiac markers, electrolytes, blood gases, and drug levels may identify underlying conditions that cause 1°AVB.

Management

1. Invasive Management
   a. There are no recommended invasive procedures for 1°AVB. Cardiac pacing may be implemented for higher degrees of AV block.
2. Pharmacologic Management
   a. Atropine may be used if the patient is bradycardic and symptomatic due to increased vagal tone.
   b. More commonly, current cardiac medications are held or doses reduced during episodes of 1°AVB until it resolves.
3. Patient/Family Education
   a. Medication education is extremely important for patients and their families when cardiac medications are prescribed. Schedules, food-drug, and drug-drug interactions should be discussed.
   b. Instruct patients to report signs and symptoms of drug overdose and adverse reactions to their healthcare providers.

Outcomes and Follow-up Care

1. Patients will keep scheduled appointments with their healthcare providers to monitor response to medications and for diagnostic testing, if indicated.
2. Patients will adhere to medication schedules.

Second Degree Atrio-Ventricular Block (2°AVB) Type I (Wenckebach, Mobitz I)

Description

1. Progressively lengthening PR intervals until a P-wave occurs that is not followed by a QRS complex, then the pattern begins again. This dysrhythmia is usually asymptomatic.
2. ECG manifestations of 2°AVB type I
   a. PR interval: Gradually increasing until a QRS is dropped
   b. QRS duration: Usually normal
   c. Rate: Normal, with atrial rate faster than ventricular rate due to dropped QRS complexes
   d. Regularity: Regularly irregular pattern with grouped beating and progressively lengthening PR intervals. Cycles range from 2 to 8 beats.

Etiology

1. Excessive parasympathetic tone or medications that slow conduction through the AV node.
2. Conditions that lead to increased parasympathetic tone include:
   a. Inferior MI
   b. CHD
   c. Aortic and mitral valve disease
   d. Atrial septal defects
   e. Medications (eg, digitalis, beta blockers, calcium channel blockers)

Incidence and Demographics

2°AVB type I occurs primarily in adults, and may be asymptomatic if the ventricular rate is fast enough to support cardiac output. It occurs most often with inferior wall ischemia or MI. It can be a normal variant in some people.

Risk Factors

1. CHD, medications that slow conduction through the AV node, and the conditions listed above predispose patients to this type of heart block.
2. Conditions that impair cardiac perfusion and stimulate parasympathetic tone.

Assessment

1. History
   a. Symptoms of decreased cardiac output: light-headedness, activity intolerance, shortness of breath, chest pain, and syncope
2. Physical Findings
   a. There may be detectable pauses in pulse if the delay is long enough.
   b. Hypotension
3. Diagnostic Tests
   a. ECG is diagnostic for 2°AVB type I
   b. Holter monitor may capture the dysrhythmia during normal activity if it occurs intermittently
   c. Electrolytes and drug levels should be measured to identify contributing factors

Management

1. Invasive Management
   a. In symptomatic patients with impaired cardiac output, a pacemaker may be indicated. Usually no invasive treatment is necessary.
2. Pharmacologic Management
   a. Atropine can be used to decrease vagal tone and increase heart rate in symptomatic patients.
   b. Cardiac medications including digoxin and antidysrhythmic agents may need to be held and doses readjusted.
3. Patient/Family Education
   a. Patients and their families should be instructed to identify symptoms of impaired cardiac output such as syncope, activity intolerance, shortness of breath, and report them to their healthcare provider right away, or seek treatment in an emergency room.
   b. Patients should be instructed on the medications that are prescribed, side effects, and monitoring tests.
   c. Family members of people with cardiac disease should learn CPR and how to activate the EMS in the event of cardiac arrest.

Outcomes and Follow-up Care

1. 2°AVB type I is often benign and requires no immediate treatment. If it is the result of medications, by holding them and readjusting doses the block resolves. Resolution of the underlying cause is the best way to achieve the goal of returning to sinus rhythm.

2. Patients will keep scheduled appointments with their healthcare providers to monitor response to medications and for diagnostic testing, if indicated.
3. Adherence to medication schedules should be emphasized

Second Degree Atrio Ventricular Block (2°AVB) Type II, Mobitz II

Description

1. 2°AVB type II is an intermittent failure of conduction of impulses below the AV node, resulting in dropped QRS complexes with consistent PR intervals. Location of the block within the AV node effects QRS duration.
2. ECG manifestations 2°AVB type II
   a. PR interval: Normal, consistent when beats are conducted, may be >0.20
   b. QRS duration: If the block is in the bundle of His the QRS duration can be <0.12 seconds. If the block is lower in the bundle branches, the QRS duration can be >0.12 seconds.
   c. Rate: Normal, atrial rate greater than ventricular rate due to dropped QRS complexes. May be bradycardic with high degree of block.
   d. Regularity: Atrial rhythm is regular, ventricular is irregular, can occur in varying conduction ratios

Etiology

1. 2°AVB type II is often associated with HIS-Purkinje system cardiac disease, which can progress to complete heart block or ventricular asystole from bilateral bundle branch blocks.
2. Conditions that cause this type of block include:
   a. Anterior wall MI
   b. Rheumatic heart disease
   c. Congestive heart disease
   d. Coronary artery disease
   e. Primary diseases of the conduction system

Incidence

1. 2°AVB type II occurs most often in adults and is associated with a high mortality rate when it occurs in the setting of an anterior wall MI.

Risk Factors

1. The most common risk factor for 2°AVB type II is anterior wall MI.
2. Conditions that impair the conduction system will also put a patient at risk for developing this type of block, such as those mentioned above.

Assessment

1. History
   a. Symptoms of activity intolerance, syncope, shortness of breath, chest pain, and nausea
2. Physical Findings
   a. Hypotension
   b. Diaphoresis
   c. Pauses in pulse may indicate heart block of this degree, which causes decreased cardiac output
3. Diagnostic Tests
   a. ECG is diagnostic for 2°AVB type II.
   b. Electrolyte and medication levels should be monitored to identify contributing factors.
   c. Electrophysiology studies may be helpful in identifying high degree blocks.

Management

1. Invasive Management
   a. Cardiac pacing may be indicated because this type of block is often permanent and can progress to complete heart block.
   b. Transcutaneous pacing can be used in the acute setting, until a transvenous or permanent pacemaker is placed.
2. Pharmacologic Management
   a. Atropine in not indicated for high degree AV blocks because it can further challenge the impaired conduction system, enhancing the progression to complete heart block.
   b. Isoproterenol and dopamine can be used to achieve hemodynamic stability in an acutely symptomatic patient if a pacemaker is not readily available.
3. Patient/Family Education
   a. Patients and their families should be instructed to activate EMS (call 911) and seek immediate care for signs of MI, shortness of breath and syncope related to 2°AVB type II. Because this is a higher degree of block, patients will be much more symptomatic than with previously mentioned blocks.

b. Pacemaker education, routine checks, and battery changes should be discussed with patients and their families.
c. Family members of people with cardiac disease should learn CPR and how to activate the EMS in the event of cardiac arrest.

Outcomes and Follow-up Care

1. Goal of treatment is to restore sinus rhythm or maintain cardiac output using a pacemaker.
2. Patients will keep scheduled appointments with their healthcare providers to monitor response to medications and for diagnostic testing, if indicated.
3. Patients' will adhere to medication schedules.

Third Degree Atrio-Ventricular Block (3°AVB), Complete Heart Block

Description

1. 3°AVB is the complete dissociation of impulses between the atria and ventricles. The sinus node controls the atria and either a junctional or a ventricular escape pacemaker controls the ventricles. The result is a series of P-waves and QRS complexes that do not relate to each other. This dysrhythmia is not well tolerated related to the loss of atrial kick and bradycardia, and patients usually seek treatment.
2. ECG manifestations of 3°AVB
   a. PR interval: No consistent PR interval, no relationship between P and QRS complexes
   b. QRS duration: <0.12 if controlled by a junctional pacemaker; >0.12 if controlled by a ventricular pacemaker
   c. Rate: Atrial rate is normal, ventricular rate is slow, that of either junctional or ventricular escape pacemaker
   d. Regularity: Both atrial and ventricular activity are regular, but independent of each other.

Etiology

1. 3°AVB can be caused by rate reducing cardiac medications. It can also arise from advanced structural heart disease that completely prevents impulses from traveling from the atria to the ventricles. Cardiac ischemia and infarction can result in 3°AVB. It can also be congenital, diagnosed as an incidental finding.

2. 3°AVB can occur secondary to the following conditions:
    a. CHD
    b. MI
    c. Cardiac surgery
    d. Lev and Lenegre disease
    e. Congenital heart disease

Incidence and Demographics

3°AVB is more common in adults than children, however it can occur in congenital heart disease. It can occur intermittently or persistently, depending on the etiology.

Risk Factors

1. A history of cardiac disease such as those mentioned above
2. Patients with 2°AVB type II have a great risk of progressing to complete heart block, as do patients who are hyperkalemic or have digitalis toxicity.

Assessment

1. History
    a. Symptoms of activity intolerance, syncope, shortness of breath, chest pain, diaphoresis, and nausea
2. Physical Findings
    a. Bradycardia
    b. Hypotension and poor perfusion
3. Diagnostic Tests
    a. ECG is diagnostic for complete heart block.
    b. Digitalis level and electrolytes should be measured to identify contributing factors.
    c. Echocardiogram may be indicated to assess cardiac function.
    d. Electrophysiology studies may be used also to assess conduction.

Management

1. Invasive Management
    a. A cardiac pacemaker should be inserted for complete heart block if the patient is symptomatic. Transcutaneous and transvenous pacemakers can be used in the acute management, until a permanent pacemaker is inserted.
2. Pharmacologic Management
    a. Atropine is not indicated for 3°AVB because it is often unresponsive to it.

b. Medications used to maintain hemodynamic stability and cardiac output such as dopamine and isoproterenol can be used for acute management.
c. Medications that slow conduction through the AV node such as digoxin and antidysrhythmic agents should be held, and often the heart block will resolve.

3. Patient/Family Education
   a. Patients and their families should be instructed to activate EMS and seek immediate care for signs of an MI, shortness of breath and syncope related to 3°AVB. Because this is a higher degree of block, patients will be much more symptomatic than with previously mentioned blocks.
   b. Pacemaker education, routine checks, and battery changes should be discussed with patients and their families.

Outcomes and Follow-up Care

1. Goal of treatment is to restore sinus rhythm or maintain cardiac output using a pacemaker.
2. Patients will keep scheduled appointments with their healthcare providers to monitor response to medications and for diagnostic testing, if indicated.
3. Patients will adhere to medication schedules.

Ventricular Tachycardia (VT)

Description

1. VT is a rapid, regular, wide QRS complex tachycardia with dissociation between atria and ventricles. QRS complexes in VT are often in the opposite direction of the QRS complexes of the sinus rhythm. VT that originates in the right ventricular outflow track will have the same QRS deflection as the sinus rhythm. VT that lasts longer than 30 seconds is called sustained, and VT that lasts less than 30 seconds is called non-sustained. QRS complexes that look identical come from the same ectopic focus, and are called monomorphic VT. QRS complexes that come from different ectopic foci have different shapes and are called polymorphic. Polymorphic VT has a worse prognosis than monomorphic VT.
2. ECG manifestations of VT
   a. PR interval: Unable to measure, often no evidence of atrial activity, or a sporadic dissociated P wave
   b. QRS duration: >0.12 seconds
   c. Rate: Fast, ranging from 120 to 300 beats per minute
   d. Regularity: Usually regular, often paroxysmal in short runs

Etiology

1. VT can be caused by a reentry circuit in the ventricles, and irritable ectopic foci that propagate impulses from cell to cell instead of through the conduction system.
2. Causes ofVT
   a. Hypoxia
   b. Myocardial ischemia, MI, cardiac surgery
   c. Hypokalemia, hypomagnesemia, acidosis
   d. Increased catecholamines
   e. Exercise
   f. Digitalis toxicity
   g. Caffeine, nicotine, cocaine and other sympathomimetic agents

Incidence

1. VT occurs often in asymptomatic, non-sustained runs.
2. Conditions that cause VT occur equally in men and women, young and old, and across all races.
3. The majority of adult cardiac arrests are due to lethal dysrhythmia, which include VT and ventricular fibrillation (VF). VT often precedes VF in cardiac arrest.

Risk Factors

Untreated premature ventricular complexes (PVC) can be a risk factor for developing VT

Assessment

1. History
   a. Syncope, fainting, palpitations, chest pain or pressure, shortness of breath
   b. History of MI, cardiac surgery, structural heart disease, HF, or cardiomyopathy
   c. Social history including alcohol abuse and drug use
   d. History of renal failure could cause electrolyte imbalances and metabolic disturbances.
2. Physical Findings
   a. May have a pulse or be pulseless and in full cardiac arrest
   b. Rapid heart rate, either sustained or intermittent
   c. Hypotension
   d. S_3 with concurrent HF
   e. Inspiratory crackles and productive cough from pulmonary edema

3. Diagnostic Tests
   a. ECG to diagnose and distinguish from supraventricular tachycardia with aberrant conduction
   b. Laboratory studies of electrolytes, arterial blood gases (ABG), magnesium, and drug levels to identify contributing factors

Management

1. Invasive Management
   a. Synchronized electrical cardioversion for sustained VT with a pulse; electrical defibrillation for pulseless VT
   b. Overdrive pacing may be indicated.
   c. Radiofrequency ablation can be done to obliterate a reentry circuit or excitable ectopic foci.
   d. Implantable cardioverter defibrillators (ICD) are indicated for patients with recurrent episodes of VT, inducible clinically significant VT, or hypotensive VT.
2. Pharmacologic Management (ACLS Protcols)
   a. Pulseless VT is treated with epinephrine or vasopressin as a choice of catecholamines, followed by either lidocaine or amiodarone as an antidysrhythmic agent. Procainamide can also be used.
   b. VT with a pulse is treated with lidocaine, amiodarone, procainamide, or sotalol.
3. Patient/Family Education
   a. Teach the signs and symptoms of cardiac arrest and the procedure for activating the EMS.
   b. Medication indications, doses, schedules, interactions, and side effects should also be taught.
   c. Family members should learn basic life support skills in the event of cardiac arrest.
   d. ICD education, routine checks, and battery changes should be discussed with patients and their families.

Outcomes and Follow-up Care

1. The goal of treatment is to restore and maintain sinus rhythm. This may be accomplished by correcting reversible causes of VT or by long-term antidysrhythmic therapy and ICD.
2. Patients will keep scheduled appointments with their healthcare providers to monitor response to medications and for diagnostic testing, if indicated.
3. Patients will adhere to medication schedules.

Ventricular Fibrillation (VF)

Description

1. A rapid, chaotic dysrhythmia with no organized atrial or ventricular activity. VF can be classified as coarse or fine, depending on the amplitude of the electrical activity. Coarse VF is more responsive to treatment. This is a life threatening dysrhythmia that does not support circulation.
2. ECG manifestations of VF
   a. PR interval: None
   b. QRS duration: No measurable QRS complex
   c. Rate: Rapid, >300 fibrillations per minute, uncoordinated
   d. Regularity: Irregular, chaotic

Etiology

1. VF is caused by an interruption of the normal electrical activity at a point during depolarization when the cells are half polarized and half depolarized. The positive and negative ions are in a state of chaos and lose the ability to either complete depolarization or complete repolarization. The result is ineffective quivering of the ventricles. Another cause of VF is multiple ectopic foci firing at the same time.
2. Causes of VF
   a. CHD
   b. MI
   c. Electrolyte imbalance, hypomagnesemia
   d. Blunt trauma to the chest
   e. Hypoxemia
   f. Structural heart disease
   g. Prolonged QT syndromes
   h. Acidosis
   i. Drug toxicity: poisons, tricyclic antidepressants
   j. Electrocution

Incidence

1. Sudden cardiac death is often attributed to a VF arrest in individuals with CHD.
2. VF can occur at any age, equally in men and women as a result of the causes listed above. VF is rare in children.

Risk Factors

The major risk factor for a VF arrest is CHD. All of the conditions listed above can predispose to VF.

Assessment

1. History
   a. A history may be obtained from bystanders who were present when the patient arrested, as the patient will not be able to give a history. The victim's condition prior to the arrest including illnesses, complaints of chest pain, discomfort, trauma and activity. A complete health history should be obtained from those who know the victim well, and from the victim if he or she survives the arrest.
   b. Risk factors associated with VF
2. Physical Findings
   a. Apnea
   b. Pulselessness
   c. Unresponsive
3. Diagnostic Tests
   a. Immediate cardiac monitoring to analyze the patient's rhythm.
   b. Laboratory tests that include ABG, electrolytes, magnesium, cardiac markers, drug levels, and toxicity screening to identify contributing factors

Management

1. Invasive Management
   a. Immediate CPR and defibrillation within 4–6 minutes for the best chance of survival.
   b. EPS
   c. An ICD may be indicated after EPS.
2. Pharmacologic Management (ACLS Protcols)
   a. Epinephrine or vasopressin should be given initially, followed by an antidysrhythmic agent such as: lidocaine, amiodarone or procainamide.
   b. Magnesium, sodium bicarbonate and calcium chloride may also be given.
3. Patient/Family Teaching
   a. Patients and their families should be taught to call 911 with complaints of chest pain or unresponsiveness.
   b. Family members should learn basic life support skills.

Outcomes and Follow up Care

1. Mortality rate is high for VF arrests unless defibrillation takes place within minutes, and reversible causes are identified and treated.
2. Evaluation in an electrophysiology lab for ICD placement may be indicated for patients surviving a VF arrest.
3. Patients will keep scheduled appointments with their healthcare providers to monitor response to medications and for diagnostic testing, if indicated.
4. Adherence to medication schedules should be emphasized.
5. ICD education, routine checks, and battery changes should be discussed with patients and their families.

Sudden Cardiac Death (SCD)

Description

SCD is the syndrome of death from cardiac causes within 60 minutes of the onset of acute symptoms. The time and form of death are unexpected and the preexisting heart condition may or may not have been known.

Etiology

1. There are multiple causes of SCD. This syndrome results in lethal dysrhythmia (VT, VF, bradydysrhythmia, or asystole) or circulatory failure.
2. Causes of SCD
   a. Coronary atherosclerosis
   b. Abnormalities of the coronary arteries
   c. HF
   d. Myocarditis
   e. Valvular heart disease
   f. Congenital heart disease
   g. VT
   h. VF
   i. Prolonged QT syndrome
   j. Dissecting aortic aneurysm
   k. Cardiac tamponade
   l. Acute pulmonary embolism
   m. Systemic diseases such as sarcoidosis, progressive systemic sclerosis, amyloidosis, hemochromatosis
   n. Electrolyte disturbance

Incidence and Demographics

1. Average age for SCD is 60 years
2. In 90% of the adult victims, two or more coronary arteries were narrowed from atherosclerosis.
3. Two-thirds of the people who experienced SCD had previous MIs.

Risk Factors

The risk factors associated with SCD are the causes of this syndrome

Assessment

1. History
   a. History of conditions associated with SCD.
   b. Symptoms prior to the terminal event such as chest pain, dyspnea, or palpitations.
   c. Before SCD, many people have an acute change in their condition such as dysrhythmia, hypotension, chest pain, or dyspnea.
2. Physical Findings
   a. Loss of cardiac function
   b. Loss of consciousness
3. Diagnostic Tests
   a. ECG to detect cardiac rhythm if present.

Management

1. Invasive Management
   a. Immediate assessment that the collapse is due to cardiac arrest
   b. Once confirmed, start CPR
   c. Initiate ACLS protocol based on the cardiac rhythm or cause of the arrest
2. Pharmacologic Management
   a. ACLS protocol for medications
3. Patient/Family Teaching
   a. Teach the signs and symptoms of cardiac arrest and the procedure for activating the emergency medical services
   b. Patients with conditions contributing to SCD should be taught about the medications and treatments for these health problems.
   c. Family members should learn CPR and how to access EMS in the event of SCD.

Outcomes and Follow-up

1. There are high mortality rates associated with SCD unless prompt treatment is initiated.
2. Patients should adhere to their medication regime especially if antidysrhythmics are indicated.
3. Patients may need further diagnostic testing to determine the contributing cause of this syndrome.

Pulmonary Hypertension

Description

Pulmonary hypertension is present if the pulmonary artery systolic and mean pressures are >30 mm Hg and 20 mm Hg respectively.

Etiology

1. The etiology of primary pulmonary hypertension (PPP) is unknown.
2. Causes of secondary pulmonary hypertension
   a. Cardiac disease: AS, CHD, cardiomyopathy, MS, MR
   b. Lung disease: Chronic obstructive pulmonary disease, restrictive lung disease, interstitial lung disease, chest wall abnormalities
   c. Pulmonary vascular disease: Congenital heart disease, atrial septal defect, PPP
   d. Pulmonary vascular obstruction: Thromboembolic pulmonary hypertension, tumor embolization, mediastinal fibrosis

Risk Factors

1. Portal hypertension
2. HIV infection
3. Systemic infection
4. Pulmonary veno-occlusive disease
5. Pulmonary capillary hemangiomatosis
6. Family history of PPP

Assessment

1. History
   a. Symptoms of dyspnea, fatigue, or syncope
2. Physical Findings
   a. Right ventricular heave
   b. Split S_2 with a pulmonic component

   c. S_4 heart sound
   d. Midsystolic ejection murmur
   e. Hepatomegaly
   f. Ascites
   g. Peripheral edema
3. Diagnostic Tests
   a. ECG to identify right atrial and ventricular enlargement
   b. Chest x-ray to detect enlargement of the pulmonary arteries
   c. Echocardiography to evaluate right atrial and ventricular enlargement and dimensions
   d. Lung scintigraphy to identify perfusion abnormalities
   e. Pulmonary angiography

Management

1. Invasive Management
   a. Heart-lung and lung transplant
2. Pharmacologic Management
   a. Cardiac glycosides to improve myocardial contractility
   b. Diuretic therapy to decrease venous congestion
   c. Vasodilators to decrease pulmonary artery pressure
   d. Prostacyclin infusion therapy for pulmonary artery vasodilation
3. Patient/Family Teaching
   a. Teach patients and their families about the etiology, risk factors, and course of their disease.
   b. Educate them about pharmacological interventions such as actions, dosages, and side effects.
   c. Discuss with them the symptoms associated with acute HF and resources for activating emergency care.

Outcomes and Follow-up

1. Patients and their families will be knowledgeable about pulmonary hypertension and its treatment.
2. Patients will not experience any complications from this health problem or its treatment.
3. Patients will follow-up with their health providers after noninvasive and invasive therapies.

Carotid Artery Occlusive Disease (CAOD)

Description

CAOD, caused by atherosclerosis, may be either asymptomatic or symptomatic. In asymptomatic carotid stenosis, atherosclerotic disease develops slowly and the course is unpredictable. In symptomatic carotid stenosis, patients experience symptoms as the vascular flow through the affected carotid artery becomes increasingly diminished.

Etiology

Most atherosclerotic lesions develop at branch points or in areas where the artery is curved. The most frequently occurring site is the common carotid bifurcation that includes the internal and external carotid arteries.

Incidence and Demographics

1. CAOD is associated with advancing age.
2. Major risk factor for the development of stroke

Risk Factors

1. Risk factors for the development of CAOD are similar to those of other vascular problems associated with atherosclerosis such as hypercholesterolemia, cigarette smoking, and HTN.
2. Concomitant conditions that increase risk are diabetes mellitus, obesity, hypertriglyceridemia, and a family history of cardiovascular disease.

Assessment

1. History
   a. Symptomatic patients may manifest either focal, global, or vertebrobasilar symptoms.
   b. Focal symptoms
      1) Transient ischemia attack (TIA): Symptoms last <24 hours and result in complete recovery. Left carotid TIAs may present as motor dysfunction (dysarthria, weakness or paralysis of face and/or right extremities), loss of vision in the left eye (amaurosis fugax), sensory disturbances (numbness or paraesthesia of the face and/or right extremities), and aphasia. Right carotid TIAs may present with similar symptoms

on the opposite side except that the aphasia occurs only when the right hemisphere is dominant for speech.

2) Reversible ischemic neurologic deficit (RIND): Hemiparesis, monoparesis, and aphasia that last >24 but <72 hours and results in complete recovery.
3) Cerebrovascular accident (CVA): Hemiparesis, monoparesis, and aphasia that results in a permanent deficit.

c. Global symptoms
   1) CVA: Neurological symptoms are related to the area of injury resulting in a permanent deficit that may demonstrate some improvement.
d. Vertebrobasilar symptoms
   1) Dysarthria, aphasia, vertigo, syncope, cognitive deficits and diplopia. The symptoms last for less than 24 hours and there is complete recovery.

2. Physical Findings
   a. Vascular
      1) Carotid bruits although the absence does not exclude CAOD.
      2) Diminished or absent carotid pulses
      3) Blood pressure difference between arms of >10 mm Hg
   b. Neurologic deficits according to the area of injury
3. Diagnostic Tests
   a. Doppler ultrasonography for physiological information of flow velocities
   b. Carotid duplex scan to detect morphologic and hemodynamic abnormalities
   c. CT scan or MRI study to identify abnormalities of the carotid artery
   d. Arteriography to diagnose CAOD and evaluate carotid artery anatomy

Management

1. Invasive Management
   a. Indications for carotid endarterectomy (CEA)
      1) Proven benefit for symptomatic patients (TIA or mild stroke) with ≥70% stenosis
      2) Acceptable benefit for symptomatic patients with 50–69% stenosis
      3) Proven benefit for asymptomatic patients with ≥60% stenosis

2. Pharmacologic Management
   a. Antiplatelet therapy: Aspirin has resulted in a decrease in the percentages of strokes but does not change the progression of COAD.
   b. Coumadin is used to prevent clot formation in selected conditions.
3. Patient/Family Education
   a. Education of patients and their families should be focused on medications and related laboratory testing depending on the type of pharmacologic management.
   b. Teach them about risk factor modification including diet, exercise, weight reduction, smoking cessation, and stress reduction.
   c. Patients and families should be taught the symptoms associated with TIA, RIND, and CVA with resources for activating emergency care.
   d. Patients electing to undergo CEA should have preoperative teaching before the procedure and postoperative and discharge education before leaving the hospital.

Outcomes and Follow-up Care

1. Patients will be knowledgeable about CAOD and its treatment.
2. Patients will not experience any neurological sequelae as a result of CAOD and related invasive and pharmacological interventions.
3. Follow-up care should include monitoring asymptomatic patients for evidence of disease progression and monitoring of all patients for adverse outcomes such as TIA, RIND, or CVA.

Abdominal Aortic Aneurysm (AAA)

Description

1. Aneurysms are areas in the arterial wall that have dilated as a result of weakening and defects.
2. True aneurysms involve the intima, media, and adventitia arterial layers.
   a. Fusiform aneurysm is dilation of the entire circumference of a segment of the aorta.
   b. Saccular aneurysm is an outpouching of one side of the aorta.
3. Dissecting aneurysm occurs when the intima opens and blood separates the intima and some of the media from the adventitia. This process results in a false and true lumen for the vessel.

Etiology

1. Degenerative atherosclerotic lesions weaken the arterial wall
2. Inflammation secondary to infectious arteritis from bacterial or fungal infections or from autoimmune diseases
3. Mechanical trauma that disrupts the integrity of the aortic wall
4. Congenital weakness at the bifurcations due to connective tissue disorders such as Marfan or Ehlers-Danlos syndromes

Incidence and Demographics

1. Aortic aneurysms affect approximately 1% to 5% of the US population.
2. AAA is associated with advancing age and male gender.
3. An aneurysm enlarges approximately 10% a year.
4. Risk for rupture increases with the diameter of the aneurysm.

Risk Factors

1. Risk factors for the development of AAA are similar to those for other vascular problems associated with atherosclerosis such as hypercholesterolemia, cigarette smoking, and HTN.
2. Concomitant conditions that increase risk are diabetes mellitus, peripheral vascular disease, presence of other aneurysms, and a family history of cardiovascular or genetic diseases.

Assessment

1. History
   a. May be asymptomatic
   b. Symptomatic
      1) Abdominal pain either persistent or intermittent
      2) Back pain that is dull or aching
      3) Patients report pulsations especially when recumbent
      4) Weight loss and nausea from abdominal involvement
2. Physical Findings
   a. Palpable, pulsatile mass in the upper abdomen
   b. Bruit heard over the aneurysm
   c. HTN
3. Diagnostic Tests
   a. Abdominal x-ray to detect calcifications of the aorta
   b. Ultrasound to identify and monitor the size of the aneurysm
   c. Abdominal CT or MRI study to identify and monitor the size of the aneurysm
   d. Aortography to visualize the aneurysm and the aorta

Management

1. Invasive Management
   a. AAA repair with a graft for symptomatic aneurysms, rapidly enlarging aneurysms, and infrarenal aneurysm ≥5 cm.
   b. Aneurysms <4 cm and with asymptomatic patients are monitored every 6 months for the size of the aneurysm.
2. Pharmacologic Management
   a. Agents for risk factor management such as antihypertensives, lipid lowering drugs, and glucose lowering drugs.
3. Patient/Family Education
   a. Teach patients and their families about the etiology of the disease, risk factors, and course of the disease.
   b. Teach them about risk factor modification including diet, exercise, weight reduction, smoking cessation and stress reduction.
   c. Discuss symptoms associated with leaking or rupture of the aneurysm and resources for activating emergency care.
   d. If surgery is indicated, teach the patient about preoperative preparation along with postoperative and discharge care before leaving the hospital.

Outcomes and Follow-up

1. Patients and their families will be knowledgeable about aortic aneurysms and its treatment.
2. Patients will not experience any complications from the aortic aneurysm or its related treatment.
3. Patients with aneurysms <4 cm will follow-up with their health care providers for routine monitoring.

Upper Extremity Arterial Occlusive Disease (AOD)

Description

Stenosis of the arteries of the upper extremities from atherosclerosis and other conditions that results in diminished blood flow to the arms and hands.

Etiology

1. Upper extremity AOD may be the result of multiple factors including atherosclerosis, particularly of the proximal left and right subclavian arteries.

2. Embolization from thrombi (A fib, MI), atherosclerotic plaques, or other substances (platelet products, particulate matter) may lodge in the subclavian, axillary, and brachial arteries. Other arteries that may be affected include the ulnar and radial arteries.
3. Trauma from penetrating and blunt injuries. Other factors include radial artery cannulation and hemodialysis cannulation sites in the arm that can contribute to hand ischemia.
4. Immune arteritis, an inflammatory process, results in damage to the intima of the affected arteries leading to stenosis and occlusion. Numerous conditions are associated with this pathology including polyarteritis nodosa and Raynaud's phenomenon.
5. Thoracic outlet syndrome as a congenital abnormality or due to trauma results in atherosclerotic changes and plaque formation. This process results in aneurysm formation, thrombosis, and distal embolization.

Incidence and Demographics

1. Approximately 10% of all embolic events involve the upper extremities.
2. Upper extremity AOD increases with advancing age.
3. Women are affected more often than men by thoracic outlet syndrome and Raynaud phenomenon.

Risk Factors

1. Risk factors for the development of upper extremity AOD are similar to those of other vascular problems associated with atherosclerosis such as hypercholesterolemia, cigarette smoking, and HTN.
2. Concomitant conditions that increase risk are diabetes mellitus, obesity, hypertriglyceridemia, and a family history of cardiovascular disease.

Assessment

1. History
   a. Presence of atherosclerosis risk factors
   b. Coexisting health problems that may precipitate embolic events (eg, A fib, MI, and ventricular aneurysm)
   c. Recent invasive procedures (such as arterial cannulation) or presence of hemodialysis access site
   d. Acute injury to the artery from trauma
   e. Chronic injury from repetitive occupational stress

2. Physical Findings
    a. Diminished or absent pulses in the affected artery
    b. Color changes in the upper extremity such as erythema, pallor, purplish rubor, and cyanosis. Other changes may include muscle atrophy, edema, and gangrene.
    c. Bruits in area of arterial stenosis
    d. Adson maneuver is used to detect compression of the subclavian artery at the thoracic outlet
    e. Allen test to evaluate radial and ulnar artery patency
3. Diagnostic Tests
    a. Doppler ultrasound to detect decreased blood flow
    b. CT or MRI study to detect upper extremity abnormalities
    c. Arteriography to diagnose upper extremity occlusive disease

Management

1. Invasive Management
    a. Embolectomy for acute occlusions due to emboli
    b. Repair of lacerations or intimal injuries from trauma
    c. Arterial bypass procedures with either autologous (eg, saphenous vein) or prosthetic graft material for proximal arterial lesions.
    d. Endarterectomy to remove atherosclerotic plaque
    e. Percutaneous angioplasty with or without a stent for arterial stenosis
2. Pharmacologic Management
    a. Fibrinolytic therapy
    b. Anticoagulation with heparin or coumadin to prevent emboli
    c. Treatment of vasospasm using calcium channel blockers
3. Patient/Family Education
    a. Teach patients and their families about the etiology, risk factors, and course of their disease.
    b. Discuss symptoms associated with acute occlusion of the artery and resources for activating emergency care.
    c. If surgery is indicated, teach the patient about preoperative preparation along with postoperative and discharge care before leaving the hospital.

Outcomes and Follow-up

1. Patients and their families will be knowledgeable about upper extremity occlusive disease and its treatment.
2. Patients will protect the upper extremity from further injury by keeping it warm, stopping occupational trauma, and avoiding undue pressure or constriction of the affected limb.

3. Patients will follow-up as indicated with their health providers after noninvasive and invasive therapies.

Lower Extremity AOD

Description

1. Lower extremity AOD is due to stenosis of the iliac arteries or the infrainquinal vessels (femoral, popliteal, tibial, and pedal arteries) that results in diminished blood flow.
2. Lower extremity AOD may be acute or chronic.

Etiology

1. Acute lower extremity AOD is caused by embolization, thrombosis, or trauma.
2. Chronic lower extremity AOD is usually due to atherosclerosis.

Incidence and Demographics

Lower extremity AOD occurs more frequently than upper extremity AOD.

Risk Factors

1. Embolism, thrombosis, and trauma are the most frequent causes of acute AOD. Other causes include compartment syndrome and low flow states such as circulatory shock or HF.
2. Atherosclerosis is the most common cause of chronic lower extremity AOD.
3. Risk factors for atherosclerosis include advancing age, male gender, diabetes mellitus, cigarette smoking, HTN, increased lipid levels, and family history of cardiovascular disease.

Assessment

1. History
   a. Acute lower extremity AOD
      1) Sudden onset of symptoms with loss of circulation from embolism or trauma
         a) Symptoms occur distal to the site of the blockage and include pain, color changes, and coolness.
         b) There is evidence for the source of the embolism such as a fib, valvular heart disease, or MI.
      2) Gradual onset of changes with thrombosis with some symptoms similar to chronic lower extremity AOD

b. Chronic lower extremity AOD
   1) Progressive decrease in arterial flow resulting in pain with activity and color changes in the affected extremity.

2. Physical Findings
   a. Acute lower extremity AOD
      1) Pain at rest
      2) Absent or diminished pulses
      3) Paresthesia
      4) Tissue necrosis and gangrene
      5) Paralysis is an indicator of irreversible ischemia.
   b. Chronic lower extremity AOD
      1) Intermittent claudication is cramping pain of the lower extremity muscles that occurs with activity or exercise and resolves with rest. The affected arterial segment is proximal to the muscle groups experiencing the symptoms (ie, the superficial femoral artery causes calf pain; external iliac artery causes thigh pain, and aortic disease causes buttock pain).
      2) Rest pain is pain that results from progressive AOD, increases with elevating the foot, and is relieved by placing the extremity in a dependent position.
      3) Color changes from dependent rubor (dusky, purple color) to pallor on elevation.
      4) Diminished or absent pulses
      5) Cooler temperature in the affected extremity
      6) Tissue necrosis from ischemia
      7) Arterial ulcers (toe, heel, or dorsum of foot; ulcer is pale with eschar and perhaps gangrene; associated with moderate to severe pain)
      8) Gangrene from tissue death

3. Diagnostic Tests
   a. Ankle-brachial index to detect arterial stenosis
   b. Doppler ultrasound to detect changes in vascular flow
   c. Arteriography to diagnose lower extremity AOD

Management

1. Invasive Management
   a. Acute AOD
      1) Embolectomy to remove the embolus
      2) Arterial bypass procedures if the cause is thrombosis
      3) Arterial reconstructive procedures for conditions related to trauma
      4) Amputation for gangrene, failed revascularization, or muscle necrosis

b. Chronic AOD
   1) Percutaneous transluminal balloon angioplasty and stenting are acceptable therapies for iliac artery stenosis and other more distant sites.
   2) Surgical procedures may be indicated to either remove the obstruction (endarterectomy) or bypass the obstruction to open the artery. Examples of bypass procedures include the axillopopliteal bypass, infrapopliteal bypass, femoropopliteal bypass, and obdurator foramen bypass. Graft materials for these surgical interventions include autologous (eg, saphenous vein, cephalic vein, or basilic vein) and prosthetic grafts.
   3) Amputation for gangrene, failed revascularization, or muscle necrosis

2. Pharmacologic Management
   a. Thombolytic therapy
   b. Antiplatelet therapy
   c. Drugs for risk factor management such as antihypertensives, lipid, and glucose lower agents.
3. Patient/Family Education
   a. Teach patients and their family about the etiology, contributing conditions, and risk factor modification.
   b. Educate them about risk factor modification including diet, exercise, weight reduction, smoking cessation and stress reduction.
   c. Discuss with them the symptoms associated with acute occlusion of the artery and resources for activating emergency care.
   d. If surgery is indicated, teach patients about preoperative preparation along with postoperative and discharge care before leaving the hospital.

Outcomes and Follow-up

1. Patients and their families will be knowledgeable about lower extremity occlusive disease and its treatment.
2. Patients will adhere to strategies for risk factor reduction such as exercise therapy to develop collateral circulation.
3. Patients will follow-up as indicated with their health providers after noninvasive and invasive therapies.

Deep Vein Thrombosis (DVT)

Description

DVT is caused by thrombosis of the deep veins. This syndrome may affect veins of the upper and lower extremities.

Etiology

The risk factors for DVT are stasis, hypercoagulability, and endothelial injury (Virchow triad).

Incidence and Demographics

Venous thrombosis is more common in the lower than the upper extremities.

Risk Factors

1. Endothelial injury to the intima of the veins from trauma, intravenous catheters, or parenteral medications
2. Stasis of blood flow from immobility, age, and HF
3. Hypercoagulability due to coagulation disorders, pregnancy, oral contraceptives, and certain malignancies

Assessment

1. History
   a. Presence of risk factors for the development of DVT
   b. Recent symptoms such as pain, swelling, and increased temperature of the affected extremity
2. Physical Findings
   a. Color changes from pallor to red to deep purple
   b. Edema of the affected leg
   c. Asymmetry of the legs
   d. Positive Homan sign (Not very sensitive finding; DVT may be present with a negative result)
3. Diagnostic Tests
   a. Venous duplex scan to visualize thrombosis
   b. Plethysmography to identify venous obstruction (rarely used)
   c. Venography to visualize obstructions in the venous circulation
   d. Serum coagulation tests such as partial thromboplastin time, prothombin time, INR, fibrin, and antithrombin III levels

Management

1. Invasive Management
   a. Thrombectomy
   b. Insertion of an inferior vena cava filter
2. Pharmacologic Management
   a. Anticoagulation with heparin or low molecular weight heparin and warfarin (Coumadin)
   b. Fibrinolytic therapy
3. Patient/Family Education
   a. Educate patients and their families about the etiology, risk factors, and course of their disease.
   b. Teach them about pharmacologic and therapeutic interventions such as compression devices (stockings and pneumatic boots), heat, and elevation of affected extremity.
   c. Discuss with patients and their families the symptoms associated with pulmonary embolism and emergency care.

Outcomes and Follow-up

1. Patients and their families will be knowledgeable about DVT and its treatment.
2. Patient will not experience any complications from this health problem and its related treatment.
3. Patient will follow-up as indicated with their health providers after noninvasive and invasive therapies.

Chronic Venous Insufficiency (CVI)

Description

CVI results from the disruption of the venous system that may be congenital or acquired. It usually affects the iliac and femoral veins and less commonly the saphenous veins.

Etiology

1. Venous obstruction from compression of veins by tumor, retroperitoneal fibrosis, or infection
2. Venous valvular insufficiency from congenital or acquired valve incompetence from venous valve prolapse and varicose veins
3. Calf muscle pump malfunction from muscle wasting disease (paraplegia, trauma, disuse syndromes) and muscular fibrosis (multiple sclerosis)

Incidence and Demographics

CVI is more common than acute venous thrombosis.

Risk Factors

1. Family history of CVI
2. Advancing age
3. Female gender
4. Occupation
5. Obesity
6. History of DVT

Assessment

1. History
   a. Presence of risk factors for CVI
   b. Symptoms such as pain or changes in superficial and deeper veins
2. Physical Findings
   a. Telangiectasias or spider veins are often associated with varicose veins.
   b. Distended, tortuous, palpable vessels or varicose veins
   c. Hyperpigmentation of feet and ankles
   d. Lipodermatosclerosis
   e. Venous stasis ulcers (medial distal leg, mild pain, ulcer is pink, and surrounding tissue with stasis dermatitis)
3. Diagnostic Tests
   a. Ambulatory venous pressure measurements to identify venous insufficiency
   b. Duplex scan to detect venous abnormalities
   c. Plethysmography to detect valve incompetency, or calf muscle pump dysfunction
   d. Venography

Management

1. Invasive Management
   a. Stripping of superficial varicosities associated with varicose veins. This usually involves ligation of the greater saphenous vein and vein avulsion.
   b. Venous bypass (eg, cross femoral venous bypass, saphenofemoral venous bypass, saphenopopliteal bypass) has been used to go around obstructed segments of the targeted vein using either autologous vessels or prosthetic grafts.

   c. Sclerotherapy involves injecting caustic substances into veins to promote scar tissue formation and eliminate the venous lesions.
2. Noninvasive Management
   a. Compression stockings
   b. Activity restrictions such as avoiding prolonged standing, elevating legs when seated or recumbent, and wearing loose nonconstricting clothes.
   c. Treatment of venous stasis ulcers such as Unna boot and dressing changes
3. Patient/Family Education
   a. Educate patients and their families about the etiology, risk factors, and course of their disease.
   b. Discuss with them the symptoms associated with infection of venous stasis ulcers.
   c. If surgery is indicated, teach the patient about preoperative preparation along with postoperative and discharge care before leaving the hospital.

Outcomes and Follow-up

1. Patients and their families will be knowledgeable about the disease and its treatment.
2. Patient will not experience any complications as a result of this health problem.
3. Patients will follow-up as indicated with their health providers during noninvasive and invasive therapies.

CHAPTER 14

Invasive Management of Cardiac and Vascular Disease

Percutaneous Transluminal Coronary Angioplasty (PTCA)

Description

1. PTCA is a mechanical procedure in which the narrowed portion of an artery can be enlarged selectively.
2. Balloon pressure is applied to an area of atherosclerotic stenosis and causes plaque rupture, endothelial disruption, and stretching and thinning of the medial wall. The desired outcome is increased blood flow.
3. PTCA can be performed at the time of a diagnostic coronary catheterization, electively some time after catheterization, or urgently in the setting of unstable angina or an acute myocardial infarction (MI).
4. Conscious sedation and local anesthetic are used.

Procedure

1. A guide catheter is introduced through a femoral, brachial, or radial artery sheath into the ostium of the diseased coronary artery.
2. The guide wire is advanced through the central lumen of the balloon catheter into the diseased artery and across the stenosis.
3. The balloon is positioned across the lesion and inflated to variable pressure and for variable duration to achieve optimal results, which are assessed angiographically.

Indications

1. Angina refractory to medical therapy
2. Unstable angina
3. Objective evidence of ischemia such as an abnormal stress test (exercise echocardiogram, dipyridamole sestamibi, exercise thallium)

4. Acute MI with an obstructed or severely stenosed infarct-related coronary artery
5. Angina pectoris after coronary artery bypass surgery (CABG)
6. Unsuitable coronary anatomy for CABG
7. Restenosis after successful PTCA and in-stent restenosis

Contraindications

1. High-risk coronary anatomy that could lead to hemodynamic compromise such as unprotected left main disease.
2. Severe, extensive, diffuse coronary artery disease (CAD) better treated surgically
3. Bleeding disorder
4. Multiple PTCA restenosis

Complications

1. Abrupt closure of the coronary artery
   a. Risk factors for abrupt closure include female gender, unstable angina, diffuse (>10 mm), eccentric, calcified or branched lesions, intracoronary thrombus before intervention, and extensive procedural dissection.
2. Periprocedural MI (3% to 5%)
3. Emergency CABG (<5%)
4. Coronary restenosis
   a. Usually occurs in the first 6 months from a combination of elastic recoil and neointimal hyperplasia causing lumen compromise.
5. Bleeding or hematoma at the vascular access site
6. Arterial embolus (1% to 2%)
7. Pseudoaneurysm of the vessel
8. Retroperitoneal bleeding
9. Death (<1%)

Nursing Implications

1. Pre-procedure
   a. Obtain base line vital signs, including 12-lead electrocardiogram (ECG)
   b. Complete nursing history and physical assessment
   c. Screen the patient for potential problems including:
      1) History of contrast allergy or bleeding disorder
      2) Medications taken day of procedure including insulin, hypoglycemic and antihypertensive agents, coumadin, clopidogrel, and ticlopidine.

3) Prothrombin time >16 seconds or International Normalized Ratio >1.5
4) Potassium <3.0 or >6.0 mEq
5) Hematocrit <30 %
6) Creatinine >1.4 mg/dl

d. Verify that informed consent is obtained and documented. Provisional consent for CABG is usually obtained at the same time.
e. Insert a saline lock in a vein of the patient's arm.
f. Have the patient void on call to the catheterization laboratory.
g. Patient should have nothing by mouth (NPO) except medications as ordered. Aspirin is often given before the procedure.

2. During PTCA (ie, in the cardiac catheterization laboratory)
   a. Anticoagulation with intravenous heparin is usually maintained throughout the procedure and activated clotting time (ACT) is monitored.
   b. Nitroglycerin is frequently administered into the coronary artery to dilate the artery and to prevent coronary artery spasm.
   c. If acute thrombus is present, a glycoprotein (GP) IIb/IIIa receptor inhibitor (eg, abciximab) or intracoronary thrombolytic agent may be given.
3. Post-procedure
   a. Measure and record vital signs and ECG. Connect patient to bedside ECG monitor. Vital signs should be measured every 15 minutes for the first hour or until stable, every 30 minutes twice, hourly four times, and then routinely.
   b. Perform a complete physical assessment, including vascular access. Monitor distal limb perfusion and complications of bleeding or hematoma formation. The patient may return with sheaths in place or the access site may be closed with an arterial closure device.
   c. Evaluate the patient for cardiac ischemic pain.
   d. Review the procedure summary in the clinical record. Note the type of intervention, target lesions, last ACT, and plan for sheath removal.
   e. Sheaths are usually removed 4 hours after the heparin is stopped and can be removed if the ACT is <150 seconds or at ordered value. Most hospitals have specific protocols to follow and these should be used.
   f. Patients are usually discharged the day after the procedure. Laboratory data are obtained in the morning and may include hematocrit, cardiac enzymes, and ECG.

Patient and Family Teaching

1. Pre-procedure
   a. Review planned procedure including conscious sedation, preparation of the vascular access site, and the catheterization environment.
   b. Review informed consent and advance directives.
   c. Explain the estimated length of the procedure.
2. Post-procedure
   a. Instruct patient to report symptoms including chest pain, back pain, or discomfort at arterial access site. Teach patient and family how to access the emergency medical service (EMS) if needed.
   b. Discharge instructions include pictures or diagrams of the lesion or lesions before and after the procedure that are given to the patient and/or family members.
   c. Discuss all medications that the patient is to be taking and give written instructions. All patients are to take aspirin (unless allergic) or other antiplatelet therapy. Additional medications may include a beta blocking agent, antihypertensive agents, anti-lipid therapy and nitrate products.
   d. Assess the patient for atherosclerosis risk factors, including hyperlipidemia, smoking history, hypertension, and activity level. Discuss resources for further interventions, which may include nutritional consultation, use of antilipid agents, smoking cessation programs, and cardiac rehabilitation.
   e. Review prescribed activity level and when patient can return to normal activities or work.

Follow-up Care

1. Follow-up appointment should be made within the first few weeks after intervention.
2. Cardiac stress testing is usually performed 2 to 6 months after PTCA.

Stent

Description

1. Stents are metallic devices, which mechanically support the arterial wall to oppose elastic recoil, prevent vasoconstriction, or treat dissections of the arterial wall.
2. Materials used for stents include stainless steel, tantalum, cobalt alloy and platinum, and nitinol.

3. Balloon-expandable and self-expanding stents are available for clinical use.
4. Intracoronary stenting is the most frequently used percutaneous coronary intervention (PCI).

Procedure

1. Vascular access is similar to PTCA.
2. Balloon-expandable stents are ones in which the stent fits over the balloon. After the lesion is crossed, the balloon is inflated and the stent is deployed.
3. Self-expanding stents are covered by a retaining sheath that, when removed, allows the stent to expand. Dilatation of the stent continues until equilibrium is reached between the circumference of the vessel and the dilating force of the stent. To achieve optimal coronary dilatation, balloon expansion of the device may be performed.
4. Glycoprotein II b/III a receptor inhibitors are a new class of antiplatelet agents that are used often during stent procedures.

Indications

1. Same as for PTCA
2. Patients with focal de novo lesions in native coronary vessels
3. Stenosis of previously placed saphenous vein grafts

Contraindications

1. Similar to those for PTCA.
2. When anticoagulation is used, in particular the GP II b/IIIa receptor inhibitors, additional contraindications include:
   a. Gastrointestinal bleeding that prevents use of antiplatelet therapy
   b. Inability to take antiplatelet drugs
   c. Conditions limiting the use of antiplatelet drugs, which may include intracranial hemorrhage, recent surgery, or bleeding disorder.

Complications

1. Similar to those for PTCA
2. Coronary restenosis is usually related to intimal hyperplasia causing in-stent restenosis.
3. Coronary artery dissection and late coronary aneurysm formation

Nursing Implications

1. Same as for PTCA
2. During stent placement, GP II b/III a receptor inhibitors are usually initiated and are continued for up to 12 hours after procedure.
3. Oral antiplatelet agents (eg, aspirin or clopidogrel) will also be given.
4. Assess carefully for complications of bleeding.

Patient and Family Teaching

1. Same as for PTCA
2. Discuss prescribed medications and give written instructions. Patients take aspirin and clopidogrel for a minimum of 30 days post-procedure. Patients remain on aspirin indefinitely.

Follow-up Care

1. Same as for PTCA

Coronary Atherectomy

Description

1. Atherectomy catheters remove atherosclerotic plaque debulking and smoothing the vessel wall.
2. Atherectomy minimizes the degree of arterial wall stretch and controls vascular injury.
3. Three atherectomy devices are available that have specific applications dependent on the coronary anatomy and lesion morphology.
4. Atherectomy may be done in combination with PTCA and stent placement.

Procedure

1. Vascular access is similar to PTCA.
2. **Directional Coronary Atherectomy (DCA).** This device consists of a catheter-mounted cutterhousing unit, with a flexible nose cone collection chamber, window and cup-shaped cutter, a support balloon, and a battery operated motor drive unit. The catheter is placed at the stenotic lesion and the balloon is inflated at low pressure against one wall of the vessel resulting in the plaque being pushed into the cutter housing. The cutter can be moved manually and the atheroma excised with the cutter rotating at 2,000 rpm by the motor drive unit. The excised atheroma is stored in the nose-cone collection chamber.

3. **Rotational Atherectomy.** This catheter-based device uses a high-speed (140,000 to 180,000 rpm) rotating elliptical metal burr coated with diamond chips that abrade atheromatous plaque into fine micro particles.
4. **Transluminal Extraction Atherectomy (TEA).** The system consists of a conical cutting head with two stainless-steel blades at the distal end of a hollow flexible tube. Attached to the proximal end of the hollow lumen are suction bottles that collect excised material. The TEA increases the luminal dimensions of the coronary artery by cutting plaque and aspirating it.

Indications

1. Directional Coronary Atherectomy
   a. Bifurcation lesions
   b. Ostial lesions, particularly for lesions in the left anterior descending coronary artery
   c. Eccentric lesion
2. Rotational Atherectomy
   a. Calcified lesions
   b. Ostial lesions
   c. Lesion length; rotational atherectomy which shows a 92% success rate for lesions 15 to 25 mm in length.
   d. In-stent restenosis
3. Transluminal Extraction Atherectomy
   a. Lesions in which thrombus or debris has to removed in the artery. This includes patients with acute ischemic syndromes including unstable angina, acute MI, and after failed thrombolytic therapy. TEA has been used in degenerated saphenous vein grafts.

Contraindications

1. Similar to those for PTCA
2. Each device has specific indications, thus contraindicating other uses.

Complications

1. Similar to those for PTCA
2. Vascular spasm at or distal to the treated site
3. Distal embolization in those with acute coronary syndrome and in interventions on saphenous vein grafts
4. Vessel perforation (0.5%)

Nursing Implications

Same as for PTCA and stents

Patient and Family Teaching

Same as for PTCA and stents

Follow-up Care

Same as for PTCA and stents

Percutaneous Transluminal Angioplasty (PTA) of the Lower Extremity

Description

PTA is an alternative to surgical intervention for patients with peripheral artery disease. Similar to coronary balloon angioplasty, the balloon pressure applied to an area of atherosclerotic plaque causes dilation of the artery and increases the arterial lumen diameter and blood flow. Peripheral endovascular therapy includes stents, use of thrombolytic therapy, and atherectomy procedures also.

Procedure

1. Iliac PTA and Stenting
   a. Vascular access is achieved either using a retrograde approach or an iliac crossover approach. If necessary, PTA can be performed from an axillary or brachial artery.
   b. After the lesion is crossed with a guide wire, the balloon is inflated. Balloon size is usually 6 mm to 10 mm.
   c. If the patient has an acute or subacute occlusion of an iliac artery, intraarterial thrombolytic therapy may be needed before PTA or stenting.
   d. Stenting of the iliac artery provides a larger lumen than PTA alone does, preventing and/or treating dissection, inhibiting elastic recoil, and thus decreasing restenosis of the artery.2,6
2. Femoropopliteal PTA
   a. Vascular access is achieved using an antegrade femoral approach or femoral crossover approach.
   b. After the lesion is crossed with a guide wire, the balloon is inflated. Balloon size ranges from 4 mm to 6 mm.
   c. The role of stents in the femoral and popliteal arteries is being studied.

3. Tibioperoneal PTA
   a. PTA below the knee in tibioperoneal vessels is reserved most often for patients who have limb-threatening ischemia.
   b. Vascular access is achieved in an antegrade fashion. Heparin is administered and nitroglycerin is often given intraarterially to prevent vessel spasm. Smaller balloons, 2 to 4 mm, are used.
   c. Rotational atherectomy can be used in heavily calcified lesions of these vessels. There is limited experience with stenting.

Indications

1. Symptoms of claudication that are severe or life-style limiting.
2. Critical limb ischemia in which patient may have rest pain, non-healing ulcer or gangrene.
3. PTA may be performed in conjunction with surgical bypass surgery.

Contraindications

1. Medically unstable
2. Long arterial occlusions, usually >15 mm
3. Poor distal runoff
4. Patients with diabetes, although not absolutely contraindicated to PTA, have shown consistently negative outcomes.

Complications

1. Vasospasm
2. Thrombus formation
3. Arterial dissection
4. Vessel perforation (1%)
5. Compartment syndrome
6. Arterial dissection
7. Restenosis
8. Death (<0.5%)

Nursing Implications

1. Pre-procedure.
   a. Similar to those for PTCA and stents
   b. Assess and document peripheral pulse quality, skin color and temperature of the feet, and severity of rest pain.
2. Post-procedure
   a. Similar to the care of patient undergoing PTCA and stents.
   b. Evaluate the patient for peripheral ischemic pain including

severity of pain, quality of peripheral pulses, sensory and motor function of the extremities, skin color and temperature, and capillary refill.

c. Clinical manifestations of circulatory compromise should be reported immediately.

Patient and Family Teaching

1. Pre-procedure similar to PTCA and stent placement.
2. Post-procedure
   a. Similar to PTCA and stent.
   b. Discuss prescribed medications and give written instructions. Patients will be on long-term aspirin therapy and will receive at least 30 days of the anti-platelet drug clopidogrel. Vasodilators and other antihypertensive agents may be prescribed. Emphasize the importance of blood pressure control.
   c. Atherosclerosis risk factors should be assessed and managed. Refer to self-help clinics such as smoking cessation, weight management, and exercise programs. Tight glycemic control for patients with diabetes and agressive lipid management for those with dyslipidemia.
   d. Foot care is an important aspect of care for the patient with peripheral vascular disease. Daily hygiene, inspection and lubrication of the skin, care of toenails, proper footwear, safety precautions, and activity are topics to be addressed.
   e. Review activity level and when patient can anticipate return to normal activities or work.

Follow-up Care

1. Follow-up appointment should be made within the first few weeks after intervention.
2. Foot-care specialist (eg, podiatrist) may be needed to address the issues of footwear and nail care, particularly in the diabetic patient.

Percutaneous Transluminal Angioplasty (PTA) of the Carotid Artery

Definition

A nonsurgical approach to open a narrowed carotid artery for patients with hemodynamically significant impairment of the cerebral circulation. Stenting is used along with PTA. The type of stent used for carotid placement is self-expandable, flexible, and non-collapsing as the stent needs to adapt to arteries of different endoluminal diameters. The procedure is carried out under conscious sedation and local anesthesia.

Procedure

1. The usual vascular approach to the internal carotid artery (ICA) is via the femoral artery. Alternative approaches are from the brachial or axillary artery.
2. The guide wire is advanced into the distal ICA close to the skull base across the lesion. The stenosis is usually predilated, most often with a 4-mm coronary balloon.
3. A stent is then deployed and post-dilated with a 5 to 6 mm balloon.

Indications

1. Stenosis of the ICA exceeding 70% in a symptomatic patient.
2. High degree of stenosis in patients with recurring transient ischemic attacks (TIA), and if infarcted area is small.
3. Bilateral carotid stenosis and contralateral carotid artery occlusion.
4. Post-operative recurrent carotid artery stenosis.
5. Patients who have had previous neck irradiation or radical neck dissection.
6. Patients with increased operative risk (eg, severe coronary artery disease).
7. Symptomatic restenosis after conventional carotid endarterectomy.

Contraindications

1. Major thrombus formation
2. Thick circular or semicircular stenosis

Complications

1. TIA
2. Stroke (major and minor)
3. Cerebral hemorrhage
4. Amaurosis fugax
5. In-stent restenosis
6. Cranial nerve injury
7. Death (<0.4%)

Nursing Implications

1. Pre-procedure
   a. Similar to the care of the patient undergoing PTCA and stent placement.
   b. Assess and document the base line neurological status.

c. Before the procedure the patient is heparinized and given 5 milligrams (mg) of nifedipine. Patients are premedicated with 0.5 to 1.0 mg of atropine depending on the heart rate. This is done to prevent severe bradycardia as a result of carotid body stimulation during balloon dilatation.

2. Post-procedure
   a. Similar to the care of the patient undergoing PTCA and stent placement.
   b. Assess the patient's neurological function including level of consciousness, reflexes, motor strength, level of sensation, and pupillary size and reaction to light.
   c. Patients usually remain on heparin therapy for 24 to 48 hours and begin clopidogrel along with aspirin immediately after the procedure.

Family and Patient Teaching

1. Similar to the care of the patients undergoing PTCA and stent placement both pre- and post-procedure.
2. Discuss prescribed medications and give written instructions. Patients will be on long-term aspirin therapy and on clopidogrel daily for 4 to 8 weeks post-procedure.
3. Atherosclerosis risk factors should be assessed and managed.
4. Review activity level and when patient can anticipate return to normal activities or work. Also review signs and symptoms to be reported to their provider.

Follow-up Care

1. Follow-up appointment is made within the first week post-procedure. A complete neurological exam is performed.
2. Doppler ultrasound surveillance is performed every 3 to 6 months initially and then on a biannual or annual basis. MRI of the head may be done also 3 months post-procedure.

Percutaneous Transluminal Angioplasty (PTA) of the Renal Artery

Definition

A nonsurgical approach to open a narrowed renal artery, which may alleviate renovascular hypertension or improve renal function. Stenting is usually accomplished along with PTA in patients with atherosclerotic lesions, whereas PTA alone can be used in fibromuscular dysplasia.

Procedure

1. Vascular access is either by the femoral or brachial approach. The patient is pretreated with aspirin and heparin is given. The lesion is crossed with a guide wire and an appropriate size balloon is used (4 to 8 mm).
2. The predominant cause of renal artery stenosis is atherosclerotic plaque. The lesion is usually ostial in location and due to the plaque in the aorta, which encroaches on the lumen of the renal artery. PTA alone may not be successful and renal stenting is used.
3. Renal artery narrowing in the younger patient is fibromuscular dysplasia and responds well to PTA.

Indications

1. Renovascular hypertension caused by atherosclerotic or fibromuscular narrowing of a renal artery after failed medical therapy
2. Renal transplant artery stenosis
3. Renal artery/vein bypass graft stenosis
4. Renal insufficiency with >50 % renal artery stenosis

Contraindications

1. Borderline lesion (<50% or no pressure gradient)
2. Long segment (>2 cm) of total occlusion
3. Aortic plaque extending into the renal artery
4. Unstable medical condition

Complications

1. Complications involving the vascular access site similar to those for PTCA
2. Worsening renal failure
3. Thrombus (1%)
4. Nonocclusive dissection (2–4%)
5. Embolus to peripheral artery (1.5–2.0%) or to distal renal artery (2%)
6. Rupture of artery (1%)
7. Death (1%)

Nursing Implications

1. Similar to the care of patients having PTCA and stent.
2. Careful measurement of urine output, daily serum creatinine levels, and assessment and management of hypotension or hypertension.

3. Discuss prescribed medications and give written instructions. Most patients will be on aspirin, and those with stents will receive at least 30 days of clopidogrel in addition to the aspirin.

Patient and Family Education

1. Similar to PTCA
2. Education regarding hypertension management including antihypertensive medication use, monitoring of blood pressure at home, diet, and activity.
3. Assess for other risk factors including smoking, diabetes, and hyperlipidemia and discuss resources for further intervention.

Follow-up Care

1. Follow-up appointment should be made within the first week following the procedure.
2. Management of hypertension and careful monitoring of renal function is indicated.
3. Renal vascular ultrasound is used to monitor renal blood flow over time.

Percutaneous Balloon Valvuloplasty

Description

Percutaneous technique is an alternative to surgical intervention for the treatment of valvular disease. The procedure is performed in the cardiac catheterization laboratory.

Procedures

1. Percutaneous Balloon Mitral Valvuloplasty (PBMV)
   a. Vascular access is the same as for PTCA.
   b. Transeptal catheterization is performed in which one or two catheters are advanced into the right atrium, through the atrial septum into the left atrium, and across the mitral valve.
   c. A large balloon catheter is placed over the guide wire and positioned with the balloon across the mitral valve. The balloon is inflated increasing the size of the valve orifice. When two balloons are used, they are inflated simultaneously.
2. Percutaneous Balloon Aortic Valvuloplasty (PBAV)
   a. Before PBAV, an evaluation for coronary artery disease and peripheral vascular disease is indicated.
   b. Vascular access is the same for PTCA.

c. A transeptal approach is used as described above. A balloon tipped catheter is advanced in a retrograde fashion across the stenotic valve. After the balloon is positioned it is inflated.

Indications

1. Mitral Valve
   a. Symptomatic mitral valve stenosis, isolated or combined with mixed valvular disease with less than moderate mitral regurgitation.
   b. Patients who are not surgical candidates and are symptomatic with immobile, severely thickened and fused valves or those with severe calcification.
2. Aortic Valve
   a. As a short term palliative procedure, patient selection is limited to:
      1) Symptomatic patients who are not candidates for valve surgery.
      2) Patients with poor left ventricular function as a bridge to surgery.
      3) Symptomatic patients who are scheduled to undergo major noncardiac surgery.

Contraindications

1. Presence of atrial thrombus
2. Severely calcified, thickened or immobile, fused valve leaflets are negative predictors for success.
3. Severe left main coronary artery disease
4. Aortic regurgitation greater than 2+ because the amount of regurgitation may increase after PBAV

Complications

1. Similar to those of PTCA
2. Hemopericardium or tamponade (<2%)
3. Mitral regurgitation (MR) is noted in all patients post-procedure, with increases in 20% to 50% of patients. Significantly increased MR occurs in 8% to 10%; and severe MR that requires valve replacement occurs in 0.9% to 3%.
4. Atrial septal defects, which are usually not of hemodynamic significance
5. Restenosis is a major problem in PBAV, which occurs in approximately half of the patients within 6 months.

6. Precipitation of severe aortic regurgitation (<2%)
7. Mortality (0 to 2%)

Nursing Implications

1. Pre- and post-procedure care is similar to that for PTCA.
2. Carefully assess and document heart sounds, and evaluate for any evidence of heart failure.

Patient and Family Teaching

1. Similar to those for PTCA both pre- and post-procedure.
2. Discuss prescribed medications and give written instructions. Patients are instructed to take an aspirin daily, and to use of antibiotics prophylactically before all dental or surgical interventions.

Follow-up Care

1. Follow-up appointment should be made within the first week after intervention.
2. Transthoracic or transesophageal echocardiogram is usually performed in the 3 to 6 months after, and may be repeated annually or biannually.
3. If symptoms or signs of progressive dyspnea, chest pain, palpitations, or syncope occur, these should be reported to the provider.

Pacemakers

Description

Cardiac pacemakers provide an artificial electrical stimulus to the heart muscle when the intrinsic heart rate (HR) fails to provide a cardiac output adequate to meet physiologic demands, or to stimulate the heart in an effort to terminate tachyarrhythmias. The pacing system consists of a pulse generator and a unipolar or bipolar lead, which is placed in the right atrium or right ventricle in contact with the enocardium.

1. Permanent Pacemaker (PPM)
   a. Implanted under local anesthesia in the cardiac catheterization laboratory or operating room
   b. The pulse generator is placed in a subcutaneous pocket in the pectoral area. The cephalic vein is located and cannulated. Less commonly, the internal or external jugular vein is used. Under

fluoroscopy, the pacing lead is placed into the right ventricular apex (single lead). If a dual-chamber pacemaker is used, a second lead is placed in the right atrial appendage.

2. Temporary Pacemaker
   a. Transvenous Pacing
      1) A temporary, transvenous pacemaker can be placed under fluoroscopy in a cardiac catheterization laboratory or at the bedside. Venous access is established by percutaneous puncture of the internal jugular, subclavian, antecubital, or femoral vein, or by venous cutdown in an antecubital vein. A bipolar, transvenous pacing lead is usually placed. The lead is attached to an external pulse generator, which is kept at the bedside.
   b. Transcutaneous Pacing
      1) Noninvasive method of pacing that uses large surface adhesive electrodes, which are attached to the anterior and posterior chest wall and connected to an external pulse generator. This method of pacing is used temporarily in emergency situations until a transvenous or permanent pacing system can be established.
   c. Epicardial Pacing
      1) Pacing leads are loosely sutured on the epicardial surface of the atria or ventricles or both during cardiac surgery. The proximal end of the lead exits through the chest wall and is attached to an external pulse generator.
   d. Transthoracic Pacing
      1) Temporary method of pacing that is used in extreme cardiac emergencies. A long needle is inserted subxyphoid and the pacing lead is threaded through the needle to the right ventricle. The proximal end of the lead is attached to an external pulse generator.
3. Single Chamber Pacing
   a. The pacing system allows either the atria or the ventricles, but not both to be paced.
4. Dual-Chamber Pacing
   a. The pacing system allows the atria, the ventricles, or both to be paced.
5. Rate Modulated Pacing
   a. This mode of pacing uses a physiologic sensor that responds and helps a patient adapt to physiologic stress with an increased HR. The most common sensors used are motion and minute ventilation sensors. Body movement and muscle

motion activate the motion sensor. Minute ventilation sensor is a respiration sensor that measures transthoracic impedance and increases the pacing rate when the respiratory rate is increased as seen in response to exercise.

6. Atrial Overdrive Pacing
   a. In an attempt to terminate atrial tachydysrhythmias such as atrial tachycardia and atrial flutter, atrial pacing rates of 200 to 500 impulses per minute can be used.
7. Anti-tachycardia Pacing
   a. One to several paced impulses are delivered to the heart to interrupt tachycardia. This is done most frequently to terminate ventricular tachycardia and is incorporated into implantable cardioverter defibrillators (ICD).
8. Pacemaker Code

   Pacemakers are classified using a five-letter code, which describes the various types of pacemakers and their function. Position I describes the chamber(s) being paced. Position II describes the chamber(s) being sensed. Position III describes the device's response to sensing. An I indicates an inhibited mode in which a sensed event inhibits pacing. This is the most common form of sensing. T indicates a triggered response in which the pacemaker senses an event and triggers a pacing stimulus. Position IV describes the programmability and rate modulation function. Position V is restricted to anti-tachycardia functions and is rarely used. (Table 14–1 illustrates the pacemaker code.)
   a. The most common pacing modes are VVI and DDD. In the VVI mode, the pacing lead both senses and paces the ventricle.

TABLE 14–1.
The Generic Pacemaker Code

Position	**I**	**II**	**III**	**IV**	**V**
Category	**Chamber(s) Paced**	**Chamber(s) Sensed**	**Response to Sensing**	**Program-mability**	**Antitachy-cardia**
	O = None	O = None	O = None	O = None	O = None
	A = Atrium	A = Atrium	T = Triggered	P = Simple	P = Pacing
	V = Ventricle	V = Ventricle	I = Inhibited	M = Multiprogram	S = Shock
	D = Dual (A+V)	D = Dual (A+V)	D = Dual (T+I)	C = Commu-nicating	D = Dual (P+S)
Manufacturers' Designation		S = Single (A or V)			

The pacemaker inhibits its output when it senses intrinsic ventricular depolarization. In the DDD mode, pacing leads are able to pace and sense in both the atrium and the ventricle. The pacemaker will either trigger or inhibit its output in response to sensed intrinsic activity.

9. Operational Settings
    a. Rate: The number of times per minute that the pacemaker will fire when patient's own rate drops to less than the set rate.
    b. Output: Intensity of the electrical current used to depolarize the myocardium measured in milliampere or mA.
    c. Sensitivity: The ability of the pacemaker to detect patient's own intrinsic HR measured in millivolts or mV. The lower the number, the more sensitive the pacemaker.

Indications

1. Permanent Pacing
    a. Class I indications for pacing are conditions under which implantation of a permanent pacemaker is considered necessary and acceptable. (Table 14–2 lists the Class I indications for permanent pacing.)
2. Temporary Pacing
    a. Symptomatic bradycardia after acute MI or associated hyperkalemia, drug toxicity (eg, digitalis)
    b. A bridge method before permanent pacing in symptomatic patients
    c. Bradycardia not responsive to atropine or isuprel
    d. New bifasicular bundle branch block or alternating bundle branch block in the setting of an acute MI
    e. Transient right bundle branch block occurring during cardiac catheterization
    f. After cardiac surgery to treat or prevent symptomatic bradycardia and to have available the ability to use atrial overdrive pacing.

Contraindications

(Pacing not recommended)

1. First-degree AV block, asymptomatic Mobitz I second-degree block, transient AV block
2. AV block due to inferior wall MI
3. Asymptomatic sinus node dysfunction including athletes with high vagal tone
4. Suppression of ventricular tachycardia

Complications

1. Permanent Pacing
   a. Related to Venous Access
      1) Pneumothorax, hemothorax, inadvertent entry into an artery
   b. Related to Lead Placement
      1) Perforation of heart or vein, damage to heart valve, damage to lead

TABLE 14–2
Indications for Permanent Pacing in Adults

Pacing for Acquired Atrioventricular (AV) Block
- Third-degree AV block
- Second-degree AV block with symptomatic bradycardia

Pacing for Chronic Bifasicular and Trifasicular Block
- Intermittent third-degree block
- Type II second-degree AV block

Pacing in Sinus Node Dysfunction
- Sinus node dysfunction with documented symptomatic bradycardia, including frequent sinus pauses
- Symptomatic chronotropic incompetence

Pacing for AV Block Associated With Acute Myocardial Infarction
- Persistent second-degree AV block with bilateral bundle branch or third degree heart block
- Persistent and symptomatic second-or third-degree AV block
- Transient advanced second-or third-degree infranodal AV block and associated bundle-branch block

Pacing to Prevent Tachycardia
- Sustained, pause-dependent ventricular tachycardia, with or without prolonged QT, for which the efficacy of pacing is documented

Pacing for Hypertrophic Cardiomyopathy or Dilated Cardiomyopathy
- Sinus node dysfunction or AV block as previously described

Pacing in Hypersensitive Carotid Sinus Syndrome and Neurally Mediated Syncope
- Recurrent syncope caused by carotid sinus stimulation

Pacemakers that Automatically Detect and Pace to Terminate Tachycardia
- Symptomatic recurrent supraventricular tachycardia that is reproducibly terminated by pacing after drugs and catheter ablation fail to control the arrhythmia

Adapted from Gregoratos G, Cheitlin MD, Conill A et al (1998). ACC/AHA guidelines for implantation of cardiac pacemakers and antiarrhythmic devices: Executive summary. Circulation 97:1325–1335.

c. Related to Pulse Generator
   1) Inadequate or improper connection of leads
   2) Pain, erosion, infection in pacemaker pocket, migration
d. Related to Lead Function
   1) Intravascular thrombus or constriction (ie, superior vena cava obstruction)
   2) Brady- or tachydysrhythmias
   3) Infection causing endocarditis; perforation causing pericarditis
   4) Lead failure due to insulation failure
e. Patient Related
   1) "Twiddler's syndrome" in which the patient flips the pulse generator in its pocket often twisting pacing wires with possible disruption of pacing.

2. Temporary Pacing
   a. Transvenous Pacing
      1) Malfunction of the pacing system manifested as inconsistent pacing or sensing occurs in 14% to 43% of patients. The causes are multifactorial and include catheter dislodgment or perforation, local myocardial necrosis or fibrosis, hypoxia, acidosis, lead fracture, and electrocautery or cardioversion damaging the lead.
      2) Ventricular tachycardia during catheter manipulation
      3) Thromboembolic events
      4) Clinical infection or phlebitis (3% to 5%)
   b. Transcutaneous Pacing
      1) Failure to capture
      2) Painful transcutaneous pacing
   c. Epicardial Pacing
      1) Failure to capture or sense appropriately
      2) Infection
   d. Transthoracic Pacing
      1) Pneumothorax or hemothorax
      2) Laceration of the right atrium, ventricles, coronary arteries, venae cavae, great vessels, liver, or lung
      3) Hemopericardium and cardiac tamponade

Nursing Implications

1. For all types of pacemakers, the nurse should have a working knowledge of pacemakers that includes:
   a. Understanding how the pacemaker is programmed (eg, VVI, DDD); the minimum rate of the pacemaker, and any other programmable feature of the pacemaker.

   b. Ability to evaluate appropriate pacemaker function by interpreting ECG or rhythm strips.
   c. Ability to intervene appropriately with corrective measures.
2. Permanent Pacemaker
   a. Pre-procedure
      1) Similar to PTCA including base line vital signs, history and physical, screening of the patient for potential problems, informed consent, IV access, and NPO status.
      2) Obtain posteroanterior chest X-ray
      3) Patients on oral anticoagulants are converted to intravenous heparin, which can be stopped 4 to 6 hours before implant. Heparin can be restarted 8 to 12 hours after the procedure and coumadin restarted the day of the procedure
      4) Antibiotic prophylaxis is usually given intravenously before the procedure.
   b. Post-procedure
      1) Obtain base line vital signs, including ECG. A post-procedure chest x-ray should be done.
      2) Perform a complete physical assessment and evaluate the pacemaker site for evidence of hematoma or infection. A sling to immobilize the arm on the side of the pacemaker generator implant may be used until the day of discharge, which is usually the day after the procedure.
3. Temporary Pacemakers
   a. Maintaining a clean insertion site is important to prevent infection. Guidelines for the care of central venous catheters and dressings should be followed.
   b. Epicardial wires exit through the skin and this area should be cleaned with liquid iodine daily and covered with a dressing. The wires should be insulated to prevent dysrhythmia.
   c. Electrical safety is of key importance as the wire provides a direct pathway for stray electrical current to reach the heart. Care includes:
      1) Wear gloves when handling pacing wires.
      2) Insulate the exposed metal ends of pacing wires that are not in use.
      3) Keep the dressing dry.
      4) Be sure electrical equipment in the room is properly grounded.

Patient and Family Teaching

1. Pre-Procedure
   a. Review planned procedure including conscious sedation and estimated length of procedure

b. Review informed consent and advance directives

2. Post-procedure
   a. Instruct patient about symptoms to report including discomfort over chest wall incision site.
   b. Discharge instructions include information about pacemaker function, how to check the pulse, and importance of follow-up visits. The patient should monitor the incision site and body temperature for signs of infection.
   c. Medications usually include a broad-spectrum antibiotic to be taken orally for 3 to 5 days.
   d. Patients should be instructed to carry the pacemaker identification card with them at all times. They should advise all their health care providers of their pacemaker. They do not need antibiotics for dental work, and can safely use cellular phones and microwaves. They should not be exposed to high fields of radiation such as magnetic resonance imaging (MRI). If they are to undergo surgery where electrocautery is to be used, the physician familiar with the patient and patient's pacemaker should be consulted.
   e. Review activity level and when patient can anticipate return to normal activities or work.

Follow-up Care

1. Follow-up appointments are usually made one week after permanent pacemaker implantation for wound care check up and then in 2 to 3 months for checking threshold(s) and programming chronic output setting(s). Further programming can also be performed. The patient then should be followed on a biannual basis.
2. Trans-telephonic monitoring is a telephone transmission of a rhythm strip that allows the pacemaker battery status to be measured. This method is used by some pacemaker clinics.

Implantable Cardioverter Defibrillator (ICD)

Description

The ICD is an electronic device that is used to automatically treat life-threatening dysrhythmia. The device consists of a pulse generator and a lead system similar to those of a pacemaker. Leads are available for sensing, pacing, and shocking.

1. Implanted under local anesthesia in the cardiac catheterization laboratory, electrophysiology (EP) laboratory or operating room.

2. The pulse generator is implanted subcutaneously in the patient's subclavian area or abdomen.
3. Similar to pacemaker implantation, the transvenous lead system is inserted into the right ventricle and then tunneled and connected to the pulse generator. One ventricular patch is also connected to the pulse generator. Some systems have two leads and two ventricular patches.
4. Programmability includes defibrillation, cardioversion, anti-tachycardia pacing and anti-bradycardia pacing.

Indications

1. Candidates for an ICD are evaluated by a cardiac electrophysiologist.
2. Types of patients include:
   a. Victims of cardiac arrest due to ventricular fibrillation (VF) or ventricular tachycardia (VT) not due to a transient cause.
   b. Individuals with sustained VT
   c. Individuals with a history of undetermined syncope and a positive EP study for inducible VT or VF
   d. Those with non-sustained, inducible VT that is not suppressed by drug therapy and coronary heart disease, left ventricular dysfunction, or prior MI.
   e. Individuals with an inherited or familial condition including prolonged QT syndrome or hypertrophic cardiomyopathy with high risk for sudden cardiac death.

Contraindications

1. Reversible cause of the cardiac arrest such as acute myocardial ischemia or electrolyte abnormalities
2. Terminal illness with a life expectancy <6 months
3. VF or VT resulting from dysrhythmia that is amenable to ablation therapy (eg, Wolff-Parkinson-White syndrome, right ventricular outflow tract and fasicular tachycardia).

Complications

1. Similar to permanent pacemakers
2. Acceleration of the dysrhythmia

Nursing Implications

1. Similar to pre-and post-procedures for permanent pacemaker implantation in regards to pain management and site assessment and care.

2. Consideration of the patient and family's emotional response is an important aspect of nursing care, and counseling either pre- or post-procedure may be indicated.

Patient and Family Teaching

1. Pre-and post-procedure care is similar to the permanet pacemaker (PPM) care.
2. Discharge instructions include what to do if the device discharges, when to notify the provider, and the importance of carrying proper identification that allows medical personnel to quickly check the ICD.
3. Provide information about support groups and encourage attendance of cardiopulmonary resuscitation (CPR) courses by family members.
4. For the patient and family members who have ongoing emotional concerns, professional counseling may be indicated.
5. Review activity level and when the patient can anticipate return to normal activities or work. Driving may be restricted 6 months, and the provider should give approval.

Follow-up Care

1. Initial follow-up appointment is usually within one week. Patients are then seen every 3 to 6 months to review stored data that provide information for any treated episodes of dysrhythmia. Chest x-ray may be done annually to evaluate the ICD.
2. If the ICD discharges, the patient should notify the provider. If the device discharges, and the patient does not feel well, or the device discharges two or more times, EMS should be activated.

Coronary Artery Bypass Graft Surgery (CABG)

Description

Surgical revascularization of ischemic areas of the heart using a graft from the aortic root to a point distal to the ischemic lesion. The internal mammary artery (IMA) and the saphenous vein graft are the most commonly used conduits. The gastroepiploic artery (infrequent) and radial artery (increasingly frequent) can also be used. CABG is performed with the patient under general anesthesia.

Procedure

1. In standard cardiac surgery, a median sternotomy incision is made, the heart is arrested and circulation is maintained by placing the patient on cardiopulmonary bypass (CPB). Cardioplegia is infused to arrest the heart and provide a motionless, bloodless field as well as to protect the ischemic heart during surgery. During the procedure, hypothermia is maintained, usually 82.4°F to 89.6°F (28°C to 32°C). Deep hypothermia at 18°C with CPB stopped is done if circulatory arrest with interruption of circulation through the ascending aorta is needed in surgery involving the ascending aorta and aortic arch.
2. Minimally invasive direct coronary artery bypass (MIDCAB) is done through a small left anterior thoracotomy, a short parasternal incision, or other small incision using port access and video-assisted technology. Because of the small incisions, this approach is usually limited to proximal disease of the right coronary artery or the left anterior descending coronary artery with IMA grafts to these sites. Surgery is performed on the beating heart. Pharmacological agents (eg, adenosine or beta blockers) are used to slow or temporarily stop the heart. CPB is on standby during the procedure to facilitate emergent conversion to standard median sternotomy if necessary.
3. Off-pump CABG is done through median sternotomy, but without the use of CPB. Like MIDCAB, grafts are done on the beating heart. Avoidance of CPB and aortic cross clamping may be necessary for patients with severe aortic arteriosclerosis or poor left ventricular function.

Indications

1. Angina refractory to drugs and PCI
2. Significant left main disease (>50%)
3. Triple vessel coronary artery disease
4. Acute MI (emergent or delayed)
5. Left ventricular failure related to cardiogenic shock or congestive heart failure
6. Complications from or unsuccessful PCI

Contraindications

Relative contraindications include:

1. Lack of adequate conduit
2. Small (≤1 to 1.5 mm) coronary arteries distal to the stenosis
3. Severe aortic sclerosis

4. Severe left ventricular failure and coexisting peripheral vascular, renal and pulmonary disease increase the risk of surgery.

Complications

1. Postoperative bleeding and hematologic conditions which may include:
   a. Heparin induced thrombocytopenia
   b. Disseminated intravascular coagulopathy
   c. Dilutional anemia
2. Myocardial depression
3. Cardiac tamponade
4. Perioperative MI
5. Dysrhythmia including atrial tachydysrhythmia (eg, atrial fibrillation), which can occur in 20% to 40% of patients. Ventricular dysrhythmia requiring medical treatment occurs in 9% to 24% of patients.
6. Pulmonary complications including pulmonary edema, atelectasis, or pneumothorax
7. Renal impairment ranging from mild renal impairment to acute renal failure (0.1% to 0.7%)
8. Gastrointestinal problems such as abdominal distention, ileus, hepatic dysfunction, and mesenteric ischemia
9. Neuropsychological problems may include the following:
   a. Cerebral ischemia, infarction, or emboli
   b. Postcardiotomy delirium, which usually occurs within the first few days postoperatively
   c. Peripheral neurological deficits, which include brachial plexus injury and ulnar nerve injury
10. Postpericardiotomy syndrome occurs when traumatized tissue in the pericardial cavity stimulates an autoimmune response, resulting in inflammation of the pleura and pericardium causing pericardial and pleural pain.
11. Wound infection includes superficial infection, sternal dehiscence, and mediastinitis. **All sternal wound drainage must be reported.**
12. Death

Nursing Implications

1. Preoperative
   a. Obtain base line vital signs, including 12 lead ECG, and labs including blood type and cross-match
   b. Complete nursing history and physical examination

c. Screen patient for potential problems and co-morbid medical conditions including bleeding disorder, diabetes mellitus, lung disease, peripheral vascular disease, liver disease and underlying neurological conditions. A carotid duplex Doppler may be done to evaluate carotid stenosis before surgery. Pulmonary function tests may be done to assess pulmonary status.
d. Assess patient and family learning needs as well as the patient's functional level, coping mechanisms and support systems. Fear and anxiety surrounding anticipated CABG are common and many issues need to be addressed, including knowledge and understanding of the procedure, postoperative course, and long-term rehabilitation.

2. Postoperative: Immediate postoperative care is provided in the intensive care or recovery unit. Patients are transferred to step-down units after extubation for subsequent care. The following parameters should be assessed:
   a. Cardiac status including HR and rhythm, heart sounds, peripheral pulses, BP, and pacemaker status and function. Desirable parameters include the following:
      1) Resting HR >60 and <120 per minute without pacing
      2) Systolic BP >90 and <160 mm Hg
      3) Guidelines for management of atrial fibrillation are often part of post-CABG protocol and may include beta-blockers and amiodarone. Calcium channel blockers (eg, diltiazem) may be used for rate control if beta-blockers are ineffective or contraindicated. Electrical cardioversion is an alternative. Patients who remain in atrial fibrillation for ≥48 hours or have multiple sustained episodes should be started on coumadin.
      4) Nitrates or diltiazem may be used to prevent vasospasm for patients in whom the radial artery was used as a conduit.
   b. Respiratory status including respiratory rate, breath sounds, effective cough and airway clearance, and arterial oxygen saturation (SaO_2)
      1) Desirable parameters include respiratory rate 10 to 20/minute and SaO_2 >92%
   c. Neurological status including level of consciousness, reflexes, motor strength, sensation, and pupil size and reaction to light
   d. Renal function with urine output and daily serum blood urea nitrogen and creatinine levels
      1) Desirable parameter is urine output ≥30 cc per hour
   e. Fluid and electrolyte status including intake and output, potassium, magnesium and calcium levels
   f. Peripheral vascular status including peripheral pulses, skin color and temperature, capillary refill, edema, and condition of inva-

sive lines and dressings. Paresthesia may be experienced by patients who have had an IMA graft due to ulnar nerve compression on the same side of the body as the graft.

g. Gastrointestinal status including bowel sounds, fluid and nutritional intake. Patients who had the gastroepiploic artery used as a conduit may experience abdominal incisional pain and prolonged paralytic ileus.
h. Pain status including the nature, type, location, duration, radiation, and associated symptoms. It is important to differentiate between incisional pain, cardiac ischemic pain, and pericarditis.
i. Complications as described above should be identified and action taken to reverse their progression.
j. Psychosocial status including anxiety, fear, and knowledge deficits

Patient and Family Teaching

1. Provide verbal and written instructions including the following:
   a. Activity progression and exercise (may include enrollment in a cardiac rehabilitation program)
      1) Phase II cardiac rehabilitation occurs after hospital discharge and consists of supervised, individualized exercise training, along with teaching and counseling about lifestyle modification and risk factor reduction.
      2) Phase III focuses on maintaining long-term conditioning and cardiovascular stability and is usually self-directed although supervised programs are available.
   b. Diet, which includes low-sodium, low-cholesterol
   c. Medication regimen
   d. CPR, if appropriate and access to EMS
   e. Deep breathing and lung expansion, wound care
2. Instruct the patient to report the following to their provider:
   a. Symptoms of infection
   b. Palpitations, tachycardia, or irregular pulse
   c. Dizziness or increased fatigue
   d. Sudden weight gain and increase in peripheral edema
   e. Increase in shortness of breath or paroxysmal nocturnal dyspnea

Follow-up Care

1. Follow-up appointments with the cardiovascular surgeon and cardiologist are scheduled in the early post-hospital recovery phase.
2. Provide information regarding follow-up phone calls to surgeons, cardiologist, or nurse.
3. Make appropriate referrals to home care agency, cardiac rehabilitation, and community support groups.

Valvular Repair and Valvular Replacement

Description

1. Valvular repair is a surgical procedure to correct a stenotic or incompetent valve. Acquired valve disease most commonly affects the aortic and mitral valves and this section will focus on these two valves.
   a. Commissurotomy is a procedure in which fused valve leaflets are split apart and then reconstructed.
   b. Annuloplasty is the repair of the valve annulus, which is the junction of the valve leaflets with the muscular heart wall. Two different techniques are used.
      1) The orifice of an incompetent valve is made smaller by remodeling using a ring prosthesis attached to the valve leaflets and annulus.
      2) The other involves tacking the valve leaflets to the atrium with sutures or taking tucks to tighten the annulus.
   c. Chordoplasty is a procedure in which the elongated or ruptured chordae tendinae are repaired.
2. Valvular replacement is used when a dysfunctional valve is not suitable for repair. Two types of prosthetic valves are used, mechanical or biologic (tissue) valves.
   a. Mechanical valves have excellent durability but are usually thrombogenic and require lifelong anticoagulation therapy. Types of mechanical valves include bileaflet, tiltingdisk, and caged-ball valves. Mechanical valves may be preferred over a biologic valve for patients who meet the following criteria.
      1) Age <65 years
      2) History of atrial fibrillation
      3) History of embolic cerebral vascular accident
      4) Already on anticoagulant therapy
   b. Biologic (tissue) valves are less thrombogenic and less durable than mechanical valves. Types of biologic valves include xenografts (porcine or bovine) and homografts or allografts (human valves). Biologic valves may be preferred over mechanical valves for patients who meet the following criteria.
      1) Age >65 years
      2) Unable or unwilling to take coumadin
         a) Desire to become pregnant
         b) Desire to maintain active, athletic life-style
      3) History of bleeding

Procedure

Valvular heart surgery can be accomplished by standard median sternotomy, MIDCAB, or through port access using small incisions and endoscopic techniques. Valve surgery requires an arrested heart, therefore CPB must be used.

1. Types of surgery for valve disease.
   a. Mitral stenosis (MS)
      1) A stenotic mitral valve may be repaired by open chest commissurotomy and reconstruction.
      2) The mitral valve is replaced when repair is not possible. Usually there is severe mitral regurgitation along with the stenosis due to rheumatic heart disease.
      3) PBMV is an alternate, less invasive approach.

   b. Mitral Insufficiency (MI)
      1) Mitral valve repair uses reconstructive techniques that may include direct suture of the valve cusps, repair of the valve annulus (annuloplasty) and remodeling with a rigid ring prosthesis, or repair of the ruptured or elongated chordae tendinae (chordoplasty). The most common mitral valve repair is surgical reconstruction of the posterior leaflet with ring placement.
      2) With chronic MI, valve replacement should occur before the patient experiences irreversible left ventricular dysfunction.

   c. Aortic stenosis (AS)
      1) Aortic valve replacement is the only effective treatment for advanced AS and is recommended for patients with severe, symptomatic AS.
      2) PBAV may be used in symptomatic patients that are not candidates for surgery or as a temporary bridge to surgery.

   d. Aortic insufficiency (AI)
      1) Aortic valve replacement is the only effective treatment for acute and chronic AI.
         a) Patients with acute AI due to infective endocarditis are treated with an appropriate course of intravenous antibiotics before valve replacement.
         b) Patients with ascending aortic dissection or dilation contributing to AI require replacement of the ascending aorta.
         c) With chronic AI, valve replacement should occur before left ventricular function deteriorates.

Indications

1. Acquired valvular disease of the aortic or mitral valve

Contraindications

1. Among patients with high surgical risk as evaluated by cardiac surgeons.

Complications

1. Similar to those patients undergoing CABG
2. Specific complications related to prosthetic valves include:
   a. Thromboembolism
   b. Prosthetic valvular thrombosis
   c. Bacterial endocarditis
   d. Prosthesis malfunction, which has occurred with mechanical valves
   e. Paravalvular leaks
   f. Valve degeneration, which is a primary complication with tissue valves
   g. Hemolytic anemia

Nursing Implications

1. Pre- and post-operative care is the same for the patient undergoing CABG.
2. Assessment and appropriate intervention should also be taken for complications associated with prosthetic valves.
3. Anticoagulation therapy may be started 48 hours after surgery.
   a. Patients with mechanical valves require lifelong anticoagulation.
   b. Patients with biologic valves, except homografts, may require anticoagulation for 6 to 12 weeks after surgery, after which time the patient is converted to aspirin therapy.
   c. Clinical guidelines and protocols for post-operative anticoagulation differ among centers.

Patient and Family Teaching

1. Similar to the care of the CABG patient
2. Medication regimen including duration of anticoagulation therapy and the need for lab work with continuous follow-up of prothrombin time (PT) and international normalized ratio (INR)
3. Teach the patient about the use of coumadin, side effects, and symptoms to report.
4. Antibiotic prophylaxis is prescribed before dental and surgical interventions.

Follow-up Care

1. Follow-up clinic appointments are similar to those for patients undergoing CABG.
2. Anticoagulation guidelines differ among centers and according to valve type (mechanical versus biologic) and position (mitral versus aortic).
   a. For patients with mechanical valves, INR is maintained between 2.5 and 3.5.
   b. Laboratory testing may occur weekly until the effective coumadin dose is established and then every 4 to 6 weeks long-term.
3. The function of the valve can be evaluated at anytime by transthoracic echocardiogram.

Arterial Bypass Surgery

Description

Bypass grafts are performed to reroute blood flow around the peripheral stenosis or occlusion. The distal vessel must be at least 50% patent for the grafts to remain patent. Various locations along the arterial system can be reconstructed using either femoral artery bypass grafting or axillofemoral reconstruction. Bypass grafts may be either synthetic or autologous vein. Selection for surgery is based on careful history and physical and diagnostic assessments, including arteriography.

Procedure

1. Lower abdominal aorta and iliac arteries are the most common areas of atherosclerotic disease. The most frequent operative procedure for aortoiliac occlusive disease is aortobifemoral bypass. Most surgeons place a bifurcated aortic graft using a transabdominal midline approach. Synthetic graft material includes expanded polytetrafluorethylene (ePTFE, such as Gore-Tex), and woven or knitted Dacron. An aortoiliac endarterectomy can also be performed in which atheromatous plaque is removed. The surgeon identifies the area, clamps off the blood supply to the vessel, an incision is made into the artery, plaque is removed and the vessel is sutured to restore vascular integrity.
2. If the occlusion is below the inguinal ligament in the superficial femoral artery, the surgical procedure of choice is the femoral-to-popliteal graft. The grafts can be anastomosed into any of the three lower leg arteries, including the anterior tibial, posterior tibial, or peroneal artery. If the distal anastomosis is above the knee,

prosthetic material may be used for the graft. If the distal anastomosis is below the knee, one of the patient's own veins (autologous) can be used.

a. **In situ graft** is when the saphenous vein is used but left in its anatomic position. A part of the proximal and distal vein is dissected and brought to the artery for anastomosis.
b. In **reversed vein graft,** the vein is harvested, removed from the extremity, reversed and tunneled back into the extremity at the site of the occlusion to form a bypass.

3. Extra-anatomic bypass such as axillofemoral bypass, or femorofemoral bypass are reserved for patients who have increased operative risk, such as those patients with marginal cardiopulmonary status, or those unable to tolerate an abdominal surgery. In the axillofemoral bypass, the graft begins at the axillary artery and is tunneled subcutaneously along the lateral chest wall to the femoral artery.

Indications

1. Severe unilateral or bilateral aortoiliac disease
2. Distal aortic occlusion
3. Critical limb ischemia with diffuse disease and long total occlusions

Contraindications

1. Medically unstable
2. Poor distal runoff

Complications

1. Thrombosis and embolization
2. Bleeding
3. Arterial dissection
4. Infection
5. Restenosis
6. Compartment syndrome
7. Mesenteric ischemia or infarction
8. Death

Nursing Implications

1. Preoperative
   a. Obtain base line vital signs with careful documentation of the character of the peripheral pulses, particularly those that can be palpated and those that can only be assessed by Doppler.

b. Complete nursing history and physical assessment
c. Screen the patient for potential problems including bleeding disorders and co-morbid medical conditions.
d. Verify that informed consent is obtained and documented.
e. Antibiotic therapy is usually prescribed preoperatively.
f. Assess the patient and family's learning needs and the patient's functional level, coping mechanisms, and support systems.

2. Postoperative
   a. Hemodynamic stability and maintenance of adequate circulation through the arterial repair as evidenced by normal tissue perfusion and skin integrity is key.
      1) Observe for signs and symptoms of hemorrhagic shock (eg, increased pulse, decreased BP, pallor, cool clammy skin, and decreasing level of consciousness).
      2) Check hematocrit and hemoglobin levels
      3) Assess pedal pulses every hour for 24 hours, and compare the extremities.
         a) Doppler evaluation of the vessels is usually done.
         b) Measurement of ankle-brachial systolic pressure index may be ordered every 2 hours for 24 hours and then routinely.
         c) Color, temperature, capillary refill, sensory and motor functions are monitored hourly for 24 hours. Then these parameters are assessed every shift unless otherwise ordered.
      4) Leg swelling is common after revascularization. Vascular boots are used for patients who had a loss of sensation before surgery or who are at risk for pressure ulcers. If edema worsens with the legs dependent, elastic wraps may be prescribed.
   b. Assess for complications including infection and compartment syndrome.
      1) Compartment syndrome develops from swelling around the fascial compartments of the leg. In addition to compromise of the circulation, the muscle cells die and release myoglobin, which can cause acute tubular necrosis (rhabdomyolysis).
         a) Manifested by pain out of proportion to the surgery, a tense and swollen leg, and decreased sensation of the extremity. The urine color changes to rusty brown.
         b) Urinalysis that is positive for hemoglobin but negative for red blood cells indicates myoglobin.
   c. Assess the patient's level of pain as to type, severity, duration, and location and provide comfort measures and medication.

d. Medication management may include the following:
   1) Anticoagulants such as heparin or low-molecular-weight heparin (eg, enoxaparin)
   2) Antiplatelet medication (eg, clopidogrel) is recommended by some to preserve graft patency.
   3) Long term use of anticoagulants such as coumadin may be prescribed for patients with poor outflow, complicated procedures, or a small-caliber graft.
   4) Aspirin is prescribed for most patients.
   5) Broad spectrum antibiotics are continued post-surgically.

Patient and Family Teaching

1. Discuss prescribed medications and give written instructions. Patients will be on long term aspirin therapy and may also be on clopidogrel for 4 to 6 weeks or longer. If the patient has had problems with poor out flow or had a complicated procedure, coumadin is prescribed.
2. Management of hypertension is critical, and discussion of antihypertensive medications, diet and weight management, and the importance of keeping a record of BP readings should be reviewed.
3. Atherosclerosis risk factors should be assessed. Refer the patient to self-help clinics such as smoking cessation, weight management, and exercise programs.
4. Foot care is an important aspect of care of the patient with peripheral vascular disease. Daily hygiene, inspection and lubrication of the skin, care of toenails, proper footwear, safety precautions, and activity are topics to be discussed.
5. Review activity level and when the patient can anticipate return to normal activities or work.

Follow-up Care

1. Follow-up appointment with the vascular surgeon is made within one week of hospital discharge.
2. Follow-up graft surveillance can be performed with duplex ultrasound.
3. A foot care specialist (eg, podiatrist) may be needed to address the issues of footwear and nail care.

Aneurysm Repair

Description

Aneurysm resection and bypass grafting are the usual surgical repair procedures. An aneurysm is a localized sac or dilation that formed at a weak point of the vessel wall. The most common type of aneurysm is abdominal, and has been attributed to atherosclerotic changes in the aorta. Other areas include the thoracic aorta, subclavian artery, femoral artery or popliteal artery. Surgical treatment of an aneurysm may be either an emergency surgery or an elective procedure.

Procedure

1. Abdominal aortic aneurysm
   a. The surgical technique involves an incision from the xiphoid process to the symphysis pubis. The aneurysm is exposed and aortic clamps are applied above and below the aneurysm. The aneurysm is opened and a polyester (Dacron) graft is placed within the aneurysm. The aneurysm sac is then wrapped around the graft to protect it.
   b. Elective aneurysm repair occurs when the benefits of the operation to prevent aneurysm rupture are greater than the risk of surgical complications.
   c. Endovascular grafting is an alternative approach for treating infrarenal abdominal aortic aneurysm. This procedure involves the transluminal placement of a sutureless graft across the aneurysm. The procedure may be done under local or regional anesthesia. It cannot be used for a ruptured aneurysm.
2. Ascending thoracic aneurysm
   a. Repair of this type of aneurysm involves exposure of the aneurysm, clamp above the aneurysm, incision into the aneurysm, aortic valve replacement with aortic graft implant to repair the ascending aortic aneurysm. The aortic aneurysm is then trimmed and closed over the graft.

Indications

1. Abdominal aortic aneurysm or thoracic aneurysm as described above. In the event of a dissection, the procedure becomes emergent with increased mortality.

Contraindications

1. Medically unstable, although emergent surgery may be attempted.

Complications

1. Postoperative bleeding
2. Cardiac tamponade
3. Myocardial infarction
4. Pulmonary complications including atelectasis, pulmonary edema, or pulmonary emboli
5. Renal impairment
6. Gastrointestinal problems (eg, abdominal distention, ileus, hepatic dysfunction, and mesenteric ischemia)
7. Hematoma or wound infection
8. Distal ischemia or embolization, dissection or perforation of the aorta, graft thrombosis or graft infection
9. Spinal cord ischemia resulting in paraplegia, rectal and urinary incontinence, or loss of pain and temperature sensation
10. Death

Nursing Implications

1. Preoperative
   a. Obtain baseline vital signs and ECG. Complete nursing history and physical assessment.
   b. Screen the patient for potential problems including bleeding disorder and co-morbid medical conditions.
   c. Verify that informed consent is obtained and documented.
   d. Assess the patient and family's learning needs and the patient's functional level.
   e. Assess for signs of impending rupture which include:
      1) Abdominal aneurysm: Severe back or abdominal pain, whichmay be persistent or intermittent.
         a) Low back pain may also be present due to pressure of the aneurysm on the lumbar nerves.
      2) Thoracic aneuryms: Intense chest, back, shoulder or abdominal pain often described as a "ripping pain'.
      3) Impending rupture of either thoracic or abdominal aneurysm may present with hypotension, symptoms of heart failure, and falling hematocrit.
   f. BP management is critical preoperatively, and the systolic BP should be maintained at about 100 to 120 mm Hg with anti-hypertensive agents.
      1) ß-blockers, especially labetalol α–and ß-blocker), are the drugs of choice as they reduce shear force on the aortic wall, as well as reducing HR and BP.

2. Postoperative
   The following areas should be assessed. (See desirable parameters under CABG.)
   a. Cardiac status
   b. Respiratory status
   c. Neurological status
   d. Peripheral vascular status
   e. Gastrointestinal status particularly as ileus can occur as well as mesenteric ischemia causing ischemic colitis.
   f. Pain status
   g. Psychosocial status
   h. Complications as described above should be identified and measures instituted to reverse their progression.

Patient and Family Teaching

1. Similar to the care of the patient undergoing CABG
2. Provide verbal and written instructions to include activity, diet, and medication regimen.
3. Assess the patient for atherosclerosis risk factors, including hyperlipidemia, smoking history, hypertension, diabetes, and obesity. Discuss resources for further interventions.

Follow-up Care

1. Follow-up appointment is usually made one week after surgery.
2. Ultrasound or CT scanning are used to monitor graft patency.

Carotid Endarterectomy

Description

Carotid endarterectomy (CEA) is a surgical procedure with the opening of the carotid artery to remove obstructing and embolizing plaque. After CABG, it is the second most common vascular surgery.

Procedure

1. An incision is made on the anterior border of the sternocleidomastoid muscle, the vessel is clamped, and the plaque or atheroma is removed.
2. Intraoperative electroencephalogram (EEG) and transcranial doppler monitoring may be used to monitor cerebral blood flow.

Indications

1. Severe carotid stenosis (>70% by duplex doppler ultrasound) in symptomatic or asymptomatic patients.
2. Ulcerated or intermediate degrees of stenosis (>50% by duplex ultrasound) if they remain or become symptomatic despite use of antiplatelet therapy.
3. Greater than 50% stenosis (by duplex ultra sound) if it is in conjunction with contralateral internal carotid occlusion.

Contraindications

1. Thick circular calcifications may increase operative risk
2. Totally occluded arteries
3. Patient with co-morbid conditions, particularly cardiovascular disease may have increased operative risk and may be better treated by PTA and stent.

Complications

1. Thrombus formation and embolization
2. Transient ischemic attack or stroke
3. Cranial nerve injury
4. Infection or hematoma of the surgical incision
5. Intracerebral hemorrhage
6. Restenosis
7. Death

Nursing Implications

1. Preoperative
   a. Baseline vital signs, 12 lead ECG, complete nursing history and physical examination, and screen for co-morbid conditions.
   b. Assess and document base line neurological status.
   c. Assess patient and family learning needs.
2. Postoperative
   a. Neurological assessment is made every 1 to 2 hours including level of consciousness, reflexes, motor strength, level of sensation, and pupil size and reaction to light.
   b. Cranial nerve assessment for nerve damage is also important.
      1) Facial nerve (VII)
      2) Vagus nerve (X)
      3) Spinal accessory (XI)
      4) Hypoglossal (XII)
      5) The most common cranial nerve damage causes vocal cord paralysis, difficulty in managing saliva, or tongue deviation.

c. Cardiopulmonary assessment including HR and BP monitoring and lung status.
    1) BP should be maintained within 20 mm Hg of the preoperative baseline.
    2) Labile blood pressure is common.
    3) Hypertension may precipitate cerebral hemorrhage, edema, or hemorrhage at the incision site.
    4) Hypotension may cause cerebral ischemia and thrombosis.
d. Assess incision for evidence of excessive swelling or hematoma.
e. If neurologic deficits are identified, appropriate referral to speech, occupational, or physical therapy.

Patient and Family Teaching

1. Discuss prescribed medications and give written instructions. Patients are instructed to take an aspirin daily, and may also be on clopidogrel for 4 to 6 weeks or longer.
2. Management of hypertension is critical, and discussion of use of antihypertensive medications, diet and weight management, and the importance of keeping a record of BP readings should be reviewed.
3. Review signs and symptoms to report to the provider which may include:
    a. Numbness or weakness of the face, arm, or leg especially if one-sided
    b. Trouble speaking or understanding speech
    c. Sudden severe headache
    d. Visual disturbances
    e. Difficulty walking
    f. Confusion or memory loss
4. Assess the patient for atherosclerosis risk factors such as smoking, diabetes, and hyperlipidemia and discuss resources for further intervention.
5. Review activity level and when the patient can anticipate return to normal activities or work.

Follow-up Care

1. Follow-up appointment is usually made in the first week postoperatively.
2. Follow-up doppler studies are performed 3 months postoperatively to assess for artery patency and again at 6 months to a year and then annually to detect restenosis on the operated side and disease on the non-operated side.

Peripheral Thromboembolectomy

Description

A balloon catheter technique, which removes arterial emboli and restores peripheral circulation. Systemic arterial emboli may originate from a variety of sites, but 80% to 85% arise in the heart, usually due to atherosclerotic heart disease. The left ventricle in the setting of MI accounts for 60% to 65% of systemic emboli, which tend to travel to the lower extremities, with 75% to 79% lodging in the iliac, femoral or popliteal arteries.

1. Aortic and Iliac Occlusions
   a. The initial approach to an aortic occlusion is via bilateral vertical groin incisions. The superficial, common and deep femoral arteries are isolated and looped with silastic tapes. The arteriotomy is made in the common femoral artery proximal to the bifurcation. The vessel is carefully palpated for location of the plaque.
   b. The embolectomy catheter is passed through the affected artery and distal to the occlusion. The balloon is inflated with sterile saline solution and the thrombus is extracted as the catheter is extracted. Repeated passes are made to ensure all obstructing emboli are removed.
   c. Heparinized solution is injected into the distal artery through an irrigating catheter.
   d. A similar procedure is performed on the opposite leg after extraction of the clot from one side.
2. Femoral and Popliteal Occlusions
   a. The most current approach for occlusion at the level of the adductor tendon and popliteal areas is through an incision in the distal common femoral artery. This is a more satisfactory approach than making an incision over the site of the occlusion. The balloon technique is the same as described above.
3. Adjunctive endovascular procedures such as balloon dilatation and atherectomy may be used if thromboembolectomy alone fails.
4. Immediate anticoagulation and early operative embolectomy is the recommended treatment.

Indications

1. Acute arterial occlusion with symptoms including loss of sensation and proprioception of the affected limb, loss of motor function and rigor.
2. A surgeon may elect to proceed with embolectomy even in the presence of gangrene to achieve a lower level amputation.

Contraindications

Advanced ischemia of 24 to 48 hours usually has increased risk of poor outcome, and ischemia >48 hours increases the risk of amputation.

Complications

1. Thrombus formation
2. Vessel vasospasm
3. Hemorrhage
4. Bleeding or hematoma formation along incision site
5. Artery dissection
6. Compartment syndrome
7. In advanced ischemia with motor loss and rigor, significant complications and death can occur if not recognized or handled appropriately. These include:
   a. Venous thrombosis and development of edema
   b. Hyperkalemia and acidosis secondary to pooled blood in ischemic limbs, which may lead to hypotension and cardiac arrhythmia
   c. Rhabdomyolysis and renal failure

Nursing Implications

1. Pre-procedure
   a. Obtain base line vital signs with careful documentation of the character of the peripheral pulses, particularly those that can be palpated and those that can only be assessed by doppler. Keep the extremity level or slightly (15°) dependent.
   b. Complete nursing history and physical assessment
   c. Screen the patient for potential problems including bleeding disorder and co-morbid medical conditions.
   d. Verify that informed consent is obtained and documented.
   e. Administered heparin intravenously, as prescribed.
   f. Assess the patient and family's learning needs and the patient's functional level, coping mechanisms, and support systems.
2. Post-procedure
   a. Similar to the care of patient undergoing peripheral bypass surgery including:
      1) Hemodynamic stability and maintaining adequate circulation through the arterial repair as evidenced by normal tissue perfusion and skin integrity is key, with assessment of patient's pedal pulses (doppler, ankle-brachial indices), leg swelling and signs of hemorrhage.

b. Assess for complications including infection, and compartment syndrome.
c. Assess the patient's level of pain as to type, duration and location and provide comfort measures and appropriate medication.
d. Medication management may also include use of anticoagulants such as heparin or low-molecular-weight heparin (eg, enoxaparin) post-procedure. Some recommend antiplatelet medication such as clopidogrel along with aspirin while others recommend long-term use of anticoagulants.

Patient and Family Teaching

1. Similar to the care of the patient undergoing peripheral bypass surgery including diet, activity level and management of hypertension. Other risk factors should be assessed including smoking and weight management and appropriate referral should be made. Tight glycemic control is recommended for patients with diabetes.
2. Discuss prescribed medications and give written instructions. If the patient is taking coumadin, careful instructions are given including use, side effects and need for monitoring of the PT and INR.
3. Discussion with the vascular surgeon to explore further interventions that may be required.
   a. Approximately 60% of patient sustaining an acute arterial occlusion require an additional operative procedure within one month of the original procedure.

Follow-up Care

1. Follow-up appointment is made within one week of discharge.
2. Follow-up surveillance can be performed with duplex ultrasound
3. A foot care specialist (eg, podiatrist) may be needed to address the issues of footwear and nail care.

Overview of Cardiac Transplantation

Description

Cardiac transplantation is a surgical procedure for patients with end stage heart disease.

Procedure

1. A bicaval heart transplant is the most common procedure in which the recipient's heart is removed and the donor heart

implanted with direct anastomosis to the aorta, pulmonary artery, inferior and superior vena cava. The procedure involves a median sternotomy and the use of CPB.
2. The heterotopic heart transplant is performed rarely in which the donor heart is placed parallel to the recipient's heart. The right side of the patient's heart can continue to function, while the dysfunctional left ventricle is bypassed.

Indications

Selection criteria

1. End-stage heart failure, New York Heart Association III or IV
2. Life expectancy <one year
3 Under 65 years of age, non-smoker
4. No drug or alcohol abuse
5. Patient is psychologically stable and able to follow postoperative instructions and long-term medication use.
6. No underlying conditions that would limit survival such as systemic infection, irreversible renal, pulmonary or hepatic insufficiency, active peptic ulcer, or recent pulmonary emboli.

Nursing Implications

1. Preoperative and perioperative care
   a. The care of the cardiac transplant patient is very complex, and the nurse works collaboratively with the multidisciplinary team. The care focuses on immunosuppression, acute renal failure, bradycardia, and right ventricular dysfunction.
2. Postoperative and long-term care
   a. Rejection, infection, and transplant coronary artery disease are the major long-term problems.
   b. Other long-term problems include nephrotoxicity, hypertension, hyperlipidemia, transplant lympho-proliferative disease, and malignancy.
   c. Medication management includes immunosuppressive agents, antibiotic prophylaxis, and may include antihypertensive agents, diuretics, H2 blockers and lipid lowering drugs.

Patent and Family Teaching

1. Importance of rigorous medication regimen and side effects of the various medications.
2. Discuss the signs and symptoms of rejection and infectious complications and when to notify the health care team in order to intervene early.

3. Cardiac rehabilitation provides a benefit of improving exercise tolerance and psychosocial support for the transplant participant and family members.

Follow-up Care

1. Follow-up visits are made with the multidisciplinary team, and the patient should adhere to these follow-up appointments. This may include laboratory surveillance, and enodmyocardial biopsies.

CHAPTER 15

Cardiovascular Pharmacology

The cardiovascular system consists of three anatomical components: the autonomic nervous system, the heart, and the vasculature. These three components interact in a complex manner to control blood flow to organs throughout the body. A clear understanding of the basic principles of cardiovascular physiology is needed to appreciate the complex mechanisms and pharmacological effects of many of the cardiovascular drugs.

In this chapter, a hierarchy is used for the organization of cardiovascular drugs: Groups, Classes, and Drugs. In this hierarchy, groups represent the major headings, classes represent categories of drugs within the groups, and drugs represent individual class members. For example, positive inotropic agents are a group, cardiac glycosides are a class of inotropic agent, and digoxin is a drug that is a cardiac glycoside. It is important to realize that some drugs may belong to two different groups (eg, dobutamine is a sympathomimetic but it is also a positive inotropic agent).

Adrenergic Group

1. Classes within this group include Sympathomimetics, $Alpha_1$-Selective Adrenergic Agonists, $Alpha_2$-Selective (Centrally-Acting) Adrenergic Agonists, Alpha-Adrenergic Antagonists, and Beta-Adrenergic Antagonists.

Sympathomimetics

1. Drugs within Class
   a. Dobutamine (Dobutrex)
   b. Isoproterenol (Isuprel)
   c. Dopamine (Intropin)
   d. Metaraminol (Aramine)
   e. Epinephrine (Adrenalin)
   f. Norepinephrine (Levophed)

2. Mechanism of action
   a. Sympathomimetic drugs mimic the effects of endogenous catecholamines and stimulate (to varying degrees) both alpha and beta-adrenergic receptors.
   b. Epinephrine and norepinephrine are endogenous catecholamines that interact with both alpha and beta-receptors.
   c. Metaraminol is a synthetic agent that is very similar to norepinephrine and has prominent direct effects on alpha-receptors.
   d. Dopamine is another endogenous catecholamine that primarily interacts with dopamine receptors, in addition to alpha- and beta-receptors.
   e. Isoproterenol is a synthetic catecholamine with higher affinity for beta-receptors.
   f. Dobutamine is another synthetic catecholamine with higher affinity for $beta_1$ receptors.
3. Pharmacological effects
   a. Stimulation of alpha-receptors causes vasoconstriction.
   b. Stimulation of cardiac $beta_1$ receptors increases the force and rate of cardiac contraction.
   c. Stimulation of dopamine receptors increases the force of cardiac contraction and dilates renal blood vessels.
4. Therapeutic uses
   a. Hypotension and shock
      1) Epinephrine and norepinephrine are used to treat shock or during cardiac arrest.
      2) Dopamine increases renal blood flow and does not cause the renal shutdown that has been associated with the other sympathomimetics.
      3) Dobutamine is used in the treatment of severe, decompensated heart failure (HF) because it increases myocardial contractility without a marked increase in heart rate or oxygen demand.
5. Adverse effects
   a. GI: Nausea and vomiting
   b. CV: Tachycardia, dysrhythmia, hypertension, palpitations, and angina
   c. CNS: Throbbing headache and cerebral hemorrhage
6. Contraindications
   a. Tachydysrhythmia and ventricular fibrillation
   b. Pheochromocytoma
7. Nursing implications
   a. Use extreme caution in calculating and preparing doses of these drugs.

b. Monitor patient response closely (monitor vital signs) and adjust dosage accordingly to ensure the most benefit with the least amount of toxicity.
c. Maintain phentolamine or another adrenergic antagonist in case extravasation occurs (infiltration of the site with 5 to 10 mg phentolamine dissolved in 10 to 15 ml saline is usually effective in saving the area).
d. Administer via central line, if available.

Alpha₁-Selective Adrenergic Agonists

1. Drugs within class
   a. Methoxamine (Vasoxyl)
   b. Phenylephrine (Neo-Synephrine)
   c. Midodrine (ProAmatine)
2. Mechanism of action
   a. Stimulate alpha-adrenergic receptors in vascular smooth muscle
3. Pharmacological effects
   a. Increase peripheral vascular resistance
   b. Maintaine or increase blood pressure (BP)
4. Therapeutic uses
   a. Limited clinical utility
   b. Midodrine may be useful in the treatment of some patients with persistent hypotension.
5. Adverse effects
   a. Extension of the therapeutic effects (eg, increased BP, sweating).
6. Contraindications: hypertension, tachycardia, vasospasm, and lactation
7. Nursing implications
   a. Do not discontinue drug abruptly as sudden withdrawal can result in rebound hypertension, dysrhythmia, hypertensive encephalopathy, and death. Taper drug over 2 to 4 days.
   b. Do not discontinue prior to surgery; mark the patient's chart and monitor BP carefully during surgery. Sympathetic stimulation may alter the normal response to, and recovery from, anesthesia.
   c. Intravenous administration via central line, if available.

Alpha₂-Selective Adrenergic Agonists (Centrally Acting)

1. Drugs within class
   a. Clonidine (Catapres)
   b. Guanfacine (Tenex)

c. Guanabenz (Wytensin)
d. Methyldopa (Aldomet)

2. Mechanism of action
   a. Activate $alpha_2$ receptors in the cardiovascular control centers of the central nervous system (CNS)
   b. Methyldopa is metabolized to alphamethylnorepinephrine in the brain, and this compound is thought to activate central $alpha_2$ receptors in a manner similar to that of clonidine, guanfacine, and guanabenz.
3. Pharmacological effects
   a. Activation of $alpha_2$ receptors in the CNS suppresses the outflow of sympathetic nervous system activity from the brain, thus decreasing BP and heart rate.
4. Therapeutic uses
   a. $Alpha_2$-selective adrenergic agonists are used primarily in the treatment of systemic hypertension.
   b. Methyldopa is the drug of choice in pregnant women who are hypertensive.
5. Adverse effects
   a. CNS: Depression, nightmares, sedation, drowsiness, fatigue, and headache
   b. CV: Hypotension, HF, and bradycardia
   c. Other: Dry mouth, sexual dysfunction, and decreased urinary output.
6. Contraindications: Severe coronary heart disease, vascular disease, and chronic renal failure
7. Nursing implications
   a. Withdrawal reactions may follow abrupt discontinuation of long-term therapy.
   b. Clonidine can be used in hypertensive urgencies or emergencies because of its rapid onset of action.

Alpha-Adrenergic Antagonists

1. Drugs within class
   a. Doxazosin (Cardura)
   b. Prazosin (Minipress)
   c. Phenoxybenzamine (Dibenzyline)
   d. Terazosin (Hytrin)
   e. Phentolamine (Regitine)
   f. Tolazoline (Priscoline)
2. Mechanism of action
   a. Alpha-adrenergic receptor antagonists

1) $Alpha_1$ receptors are postsynaptic receptors that produce the effects of the sympathetic nervous system.
2) $Alpha_2$ receptors are presynaptic receptors that modulate norepinephrine release.

b. Some of these drugs have markedly different affinities for $alpha_1$ and $alpha_2$ receptors.
   1) Prazosin, terazosin, and doxazosin are more potent in blocking $alpha_1$ than $alpha_2$ receptors (and are termed $alpha_1$-selective).
   2) Phenoxybenzamine and phentolamine have similar affinities for both of these receptor sites.

3. Pharmacological effects
   a. Decrease vascular tone and produce vasodilation, which lowers blood pressure.
   b. Because $alpha_1$-selective antagonists do not block the presynaptic $alpha_2$ receptor sites, the reflex tachycardia that accompanies the reduction in blood pressure is less likely to occur.
4. Therapeutic uses
   a. Hypertension, either alone or as part of combination therapy
   b. Phenoxybenzamine and phentolamine are used in the treatment of pheochromocytoma.
   c. Phentolamine is used also to manage extravasation of tissue toxic agents.
5. Adverse effects
   a. CV: Postural hypotension, dysrhythmia, edema, HF, and angina. Vasodilation from these agents can cause flushing, rhinitis, reddened eyes, nasal congestion, and priapism.
   b. CNS: Dizziness, weakness, fatigue, drowsiness, and depression
   c. First-dose phenomenon: Marked postural hypotension and syncope are sometimes seen 30 to 90 minutes after a patient takes an initial dose.
6. Contraindications: Use cautiously in the presence of HF or renal failure, because drug effects could exacerbate these conditions. Caution also should be used with pregnancy and lactation.
7. Nursing Implications
   a. Monitor BP, pulse, rhythm and cardiac output regularly in order to arrange to adjust dosage or discontinue drug if cardiovascular effects are severe.
   b. Observe the patient for any hypotensive effects for approximately 90 minutes following administration of first dose.
   c. Administer doxazosin, prazosin and terazosin at bedtime

Beta-Adrenergic Antagonists (Beta-Blockers)

1. Drugs within class (See Table 15–1.)
2. Mechanism of action
   a. Beta-receptor antagonists occupy beta-receptors and block receptor action
      1) $Beta_1$ receptors are found in the heart, where they stimulate myocardial contraction and increase heart rate

Table 15–1. Properties and Therapeutic Uses of Beta-Receptor Blocking Drugs

	Trade Name	Selectivity	Partial Agonist Activity	Therapeutic Uses
Acebutalol[A]	Sectral	$Beta_1$	Yes	Hypertension, ventricular dysrhythmias
Atenolol	Tenormin	$Beta_1$	No	Hypertension, chronic angina, status-post myocardial infarction (MI)
Betaxolol[A]	Kerlone	$Beta_1$	No	Hypertension
Bisoprolol	Zebeta	$Beta_1$	No	Hypertension
Carteolol	Cartrol	None	Yes	Hypertension
Carvedilol[B]	Coreg	None	No	Hypertension, heart failure (HF)
Esmolol	Brevibloc	$Beta_1$	No	Supraventricular tachycardia
Labetolol[A,B]	Normodyne Trandate	None	Yes	Hypertension
Metoprolol[A]	Lopressor Toprol	$Beta_1$	No	Hypertension, angina, prevention of reinfarction after MI
Nadolol	Corgard	None	No	Hypertension, angina
Penbutolol	Levatol	None	Yes	Hypertension
Pindolol[A]	Visken	None	Yes	Hypertension
Propranolol[A]	Inderal	None	No	Hypertension, angina, idiopathic hypertrophic subaortic stenosis, dysrhythmias, pheochromocytoma
Sotalol	Betapace	None	No	Ventricular dysrhythmias
Timolol	Blocadren	None	No	Hypertension, prevention of reinfarction after MI

[A]Beta blockers with local anesthetic action. [B]Carvedilol and labetalol also cause $alpha_1$ adrenergic receptor blockade.

2) $Beta_2$ receptors are found predominately in bronchioles (where they cause dilation), smooth muscle of blood vessels (where they cause dilation), and the uterus (where they cause relaxation).
3) Some of these drugs have markedly different affinities for $beta_1$ and $beta_2$ receptors — selectivity.

b. Other mechanisms of action include partial agonist activity at beta-receptors and local anesthetic action, which differ among the beta-blockers.

c. Table 15–1 summarizes the properties of various beta-adrenergic antagonists.

3. Pharmacological effects
   a. Decrease heart rate and BP
   b. Beta-receptor blockade has relatively little effect on the normal heart of an individual at rest but has profound effects when sympathetic control of the heart is dominant, as during exercise, stress, or from an underlying pathophysiology.
4. Therapeutic uses (See Table 15–1)
5. Adverse effects
   a. CV: Bradycardia, heart block, HF, hypotension, and peripheral vascular insufficiency
   b. Pulmonary (with nonselective beta-blockers): Difficulty breathing, coughing, and bronchospasm
   c. CNS: Fatigue, dizziness, depression, paresthesia, sleep disturbances, memory loss, and disorientation
   d. Other: Nausea, vomiting, diarrhea, colitis, decreased libido, sexual dysfunction, slowed recovery from hypoglycemia, and decreased exercise tolerance
6. Contraindications
   a. CV: Bradycardia or heart block; use with caution in HF (eg, Metoprolol)
   b. Pulmonary: Bronchospasm, chronic obstructive pulmonary disease, or acute asthma
   c. Nonselective beta-blockers should be used with great caution in people with diabetes and frequent hypoglycemic reactions.
7. Nursing implications
   a. Do not withdraw these drugs abruptly after chronic therapy; taper gradually over 2 weeks, because long-term use of these drugs can sensitize the myocardium to catecholamines and severe reactions can occur.
   b. Give the oral form of these drugs with food to improve absorption.

c. If beta-blockers are used in people with HF, be aware that HF symptoms may worsen initially. Dosage may need to be adjusted if the person experiences weight gain, significant bradycardia, or dizziness.
d. Selectivity may be lost with high doses of beta$_1$ selective antagonists.

Inotropic Agents

Classes within this group include Cardiac glycosides, Phosphodiesterase inhibitors, and sympathomimetics (Dopamine and Dobutamine) discussed at the beginning of this chapter.

Cardiac Glycosides

1. Drugs within class
   a. Digitalis
   b. Digitoxin (Crystodigin)
   c. Digoxin (Lanoxin)
2. Mechanism of action: Cardiac glycosides act by inhibiting the enzyme Na+/K+ ATPase ("the sodium pump"), which is responsible for maintaining the resting membrane potential of nerve and muscle cells.
3. Pharmacological effects: Inhibition of the sodium pump increases sodium and calcium influx during the cardiac action potential. Thus, the cardiac glycosides allow more calcium to enter myocardial cells during depolarization resulting in the following effects:
   a. Increased force of contraction of the heart (positive inotropic effect), increased cardiac output, and increased renal perfusion;
   b. Decreased heart rate (negative chronotropic effect) due to decreased rate of repolarization (increased duration of the "plateau phase" of the cardiac action potential) and from indirect stimulation of the vagal nerve; and
   c. Decreased conduction velocity through the AV node.
4. Therapeutic uses
   a. Treatment of HF; and
   b. Treatment of atrial flutter, atrial fibrillation, and paroxysmal atrial tachycardia (PAT).
5. Adverse effects
   a. CV: Cardiac effects are the most dangerous and include premature ventricular contractions (PVC), dysrhythmia, and bradycardia.
   b. GI: Nausea, vomiting, and anorexia resulting from the central stimulation of the chemoreceptor trigger zone (CTZ) — an

area of the brainstem responsible for producing nausea and vomiting.

c. CNS: Neurologic effects include the presence of yellow green halos in the visual field, headaches, fatigue, confusion, and depression.

6. Toxicity and drug interactions
   a. Factors influencing toxicity
      1) Electrolyte imbalances (decreased potassium levels potentiate toxicity because potassium competes with cardiac glycosides for binding to Na+/K+ ATPase)
      2) Renal (digoxin) and hepatic (digitoxin) insufficiency.
   b. Treatment of digitalis-related toxicity
      1) Decontamination (emesis)
      2) Continuous monitoring of plasma potassium levels
      3) Administration of anti-dysrhythmics such as phenytoin (Dilantin) or lidocaine if necessary
      4) Administration of digitalis antibodies (digoxin immune fab [Digibind])
   c. Pharmacokinetic drug interactions
      1) Examples of drugs that decrease the effect of digoxin are antacids, cholestyramine, neomycin, and sulfasalazine.
      2) Examples of drugs that increase the effect of digoxin are albuterol, amiodarone, captopril, cyclosporine, diltiazem, erythromycin, nifedipine, omeprazole, tetracycline, and thyroxine.
7. Contraindications: ventricular tachycardia or fibrillation, heart block, idiopathic hypertrophic subaortic stenosis, acute MI, Wolff-Parkinson-White (WPW) syndrome
8. Nursing implications
   a. Digoxin is the drug within this class most often used to treat HF
      1) Rapid onset of action
      2) Available for parenteral and oral use
   b. Digitoxin is only available in the oral form and has a slow onset of action and a long duration, making it less useful than digoxin in managing acute HF.
      1) Metabolized by the liver and can reach toxic levels in patients with diminished liver function.
   c. Cardiac glycosides have a very narrow margin of safety (that is, the therapeutic dose is very close to the toxic dose), so extreme care must be taken when using these drugs. Periodic blood levels should be determined to assure appropriate dosing.

Phosphodiesterase Inhibitors

1. Drugs within class
   a. Amrinone (Inocor)
   b. Milrinone (Primacor)
2. Mechanism of action
   a. Inhibit phosphodiesterase, the enzyme responsible for the inactivation of the second messengers cAMP and cGMP. These second messengers mediate calcium levels within the cell.
   b. By blocking phosphodiesterase metabolism, these agents increase calcium levels within the myocardial cell.
3. Pharmacological effects
   a. Increased intracellular calcium causes a stronger contraction, thus increasing cardiac output with little or no effect on heart rate or blood pressure.
   b. Although the acute effects are beneficial in some patients, the toxicity of these agents prevents their long-term use.
4. Therapeutic uses: Treatment of decompensated HF in patients who do not respond to conventional HF therapy (digoxin, diuretics, and vasodilators).
5. Adverse effects
   a. CV: Dysrhythmia
   b. GI: Nausea and vomiting (high incidence), liver enzyme changes
   c. Heme: Thrombocytopenia (TCP), bone marrow toxicity
6. Contraindications: Aortic or pulmonary valvular disease, acute MI, ventricular dysrhythmia
7. Nursing implications
   a. Use caution with older adults because they are more likely to develop adverse effects.
   b. Life support equipment should be available in case of severe reaction to drug or development of ventricular dysrhythmia.
   c. Assure accurate dosing because these drugs are given IV only.

Anti-dysrhythmics

Classes and drugs within this group are listed in Table 15–2.

Mechanisms of Action

1. Class I anti-dysrhythmic drugs block sodium channels, to varying degrees.
2. Class II drugs are beta-adrenergic receptor antagonists.
3. Class III drugs block potassium efflux during repolarization.

4. Class IV agents are calcium channel blockers.
5. Digitalis and related compounds slow conduction velocity (discussed with cardiac glycosides).
6. Adenosine is an endogenous nucleoside that activates adenosine receptors. The mechanism of action of adenosine involves enhanced potassium conductance and inhibition of cAMP-induced calcium influx.

TABLE 15–2. Anti-Dysrhythmic Drug Classification and Major Therapeutic Uses

Class	Drugs	Therapeutic Uses
IA	Quinidine (Cardioquin, etc.)	Atrial dysrhythmias, ventricular tachycardia
	Procainamide (Pronestyl)	Atrial dysrhythmias, WPW,[A] Life-threatening ventricular dysrhythmias
	Moricizine (Ethmozine)	Life-threatening ventricular dysrhythmias
	Disopyramide (Norpace)	Life-threatening ventricular dysrhythmias
IB	Lidocaine (Xylocaine)	Life-threatening ventricular dysrhythmias, WPW[A]
	Tocainamide[C] (Tonocard)	Life-threatening ventricular dysrhythmias
	Mexiletine[C] (Mexitil)	Life-threatening ventricular dysrhythmias
	Phenytoin (Dilantin)	Digitalis-induced dysrhythmias
IC	Flecainamide (Tambocor)	Ventricular dysrhythmias, prevention of PAT[B]
	Propafenone (Rythmol)	Ventricular dysrhythmias, prevention of PAT[B]
II	Propranolol (Inderal)	Atrial dysrhythmias, sinus tachycardia, AV reentry, WPW[A]
	Acebutolol (Sectral)	Premature ventricular contractions
	Esmolol (Brevibloc)	Short-term or intraoperative management of supraventricular tachycardia
III	Bretylium (Bretylol)	Ventricular tachycardia and as last resort for ventricular fibrillation
	Amiodarone (Cordarone)	Life-threatening ventricular dysrhythmias
	Ibutilide (Corvert)	Atrial fibrillation or flutter
	Sotalol[D] (Betapace)	Ventricular tachycardia, life-threatening ventricular dysrhythmias
	Dofetilide (Tikosyn)	Cardioversion of atrial fibrillation and flutter
IV	Verapamil (Calan, Isoptin)	Atrial tachycardia, atrial flutter
	Diltiazem (Cardizem, etc.)	Atrial tachycardia, atrial flutter
Others	Digoxin (Lanoxin)	Atrial fibrillation, atrial flutter, PAT[B]
	Adenosine (Adenocard)	PAT[B], ventricular tachycardia

[A]WPW: Wolff-Parkinson-White syndrome

[B]PAT: Paroxysmal atrial tachycardia

[C]Mexiletine and tocainide are analogs of lidocaine with structures that have been modified to reduce first-pass hepatic metabolism (associated with lidocaine) to make chronic oral therapy effective.

[D]Sotalol is a nonselective beta-blocker, but acts as a Class III antidysrhythmic that prolongs the action potential.

Pharmacological Effects

1. Class IA anti-dysrhythmic drugs have moderate potency for activated sodium channel blockade and prolonging repolarization, thus lengthening the refractory period between action potentials.
   a. Class IA drugs have little effect on SA node automaticity, while most other antidysrhythmics reduce sinoatrial (SA) node automaticity. (Automaticity occurs when one or more regions of the heart are beating asynchronously with the rest of the heart.)
2. Class IB agents block both activated and inactivated sodium channels and shorten action potential duration.
3. Class IC agents are the most potent sodium channel blockers and have limited effects on repolarization.
4. Class II agents decrease heart rate and SA automaticity.
5. Class III agents block potassium channels, thus prolonging repolarization and slowing the conduction rate of the heart.
6. Class IV agents are calcium channel antagonists, causing a depression of depolarization and prolongation of repolarization, which acts to slow automaticity and conduction.
7. Adenosine can produce a bradycardia that is resistant to atropine, and it depresses SA automaticity, conduction velocity, and atrial-ventricular (AV) nodal conduction.
   a. Administration of adenosine could be considered the pharmacological "shocking" of the heart.

Therapeutic Uses

(See Table 15–2.)

Adverse Effects

1. CV: All anti-dysrhythmic agents include the development of new dysrhythmia ("prodysrhythmia"), heart block, hypotension, vasodilation, and the potential for cardiac arrest.
2. Some of the more notable, non-cardiovascular side effects of individual anti-dysrhythmic agents are listed below:
   a. Quinidine: Nausea and vomiting are common; quinidine syncope, hypersensitivity, hemolytic anemia, anticholinergic effects, "cinchonism" (tinnitus, headache, blurred vision)
   b. Procainamide: Hypersensitivity, systemic Lupus-like syndrome (arthralgia and arthritis)
   c. Moricizine: Orthostatic dizziness, euphoria, perioral numbness
   d. Lidocaine: Agitation, disorientation, paraesthesia, tremor, lightheadedness, slurred speech, seizures

e. Tocainamide: Bone marrow suppression
f. Propranolol: Bronchospasm; see beta-adrenergic receptor antagonists
g. Amiodarone: Photosensitivity, pulmonary fibrosis, liver enzyme dysfunction, thyroid dysfunction
h. Verapamil: Constipation, lassitude, nervousness, peripheral edema
i. Adenosine: Shortness of breath, flushing, headache, nausea, paresthesia

Contraindications

1. Contraindicated with allergy, bradycardia, sick sinus syndrome, AV block, shock, hypotension, and respiratory depression
2. Use with caution in patients with HF

Nursing Implications

1. Continually monitor cardiac rhythm when initiating therapy or changing dose to detect potentially serious adverse effects and to evaluate drug effectiveness.
2. Arrange for periodic monitoring of cardiac rhythm when the patient is on long-term therapy to evaluate the effects on cardiac status.
3. Maintain life support equipment on standby to treat adverse reactions that might occur.
4. Give parenteral forms only if the oral form is not feasible; convert to an oral form as soon as possible to decrease potential for adverse effects.
5. Consult the prescriber to reduce the dosage in patients with renal or hepatic insufficiency.

Vasodilators

The three main classes of drugs used in the treatment of angina are beta-blockers, calcium channel blockers, and direct-acting vasodilators, nitrates/nitrites. Because beta-blockers and calcium channel blockers are discussed elsewhere within this chapter, the emphasis of this section will be on the direct-acting vasodilators used in the treatment of angina, as well as vasodilators used in the treatment of hypertension.

Classes within the vasodilator group are Anti-Anginal Vasodilators (Nitrates/Nitrites) and Anti-Hypertensive Vasodilators

Anti-Anginal Vasodilators (Nitrates/Nitrites)

1. Drugs within class
   a. Amyl nitrite (Aspirols, Vaporole)
   b. Isosorbide dinitrate (Isordil, Sorbitrate)
   c. Isosorbide mononitrate (Imdur, Ismo, Monoket)
   d. Nitroglycerin (Nitrobid, Nitrostat, Nitrong, Nitro-Dur, Nitrol, Nitrogard)
2. Mechanism of action: Nitrates and nitrites directly relax all types of vascular smooth muscle (from large arteries to large veins) by releasing nitric oxide, a potent vasodilator.
3. Pharmacological effects
   a. Vasodilators increase coronary blood flow by relaxing coronary blood vessels, leading to an increase in the supply of oxygen to myocardial cells.
      1) Because coronary heart disease causes stiffening and decreased responsiveness in coronary arteries, nitrates probably have little effect on increasing blood flow through these vessels.
      2) Nitrates do, however, increase blood flow through healthy coronary arteries.
   b. Vasodilators decrease cardiac oxygen demand and workload by decreasing venous return (preload) and peripheral resistance (afterload).
   c. Vasodilators relax all types of smooth muscle, but have practically no direct effect on cardiac or skeletal muscle.
4. Therapeutic uses
   a. Nitroglycerin is the most commonly used anti-anginal agent and is useful in treating all types of angina.
   b. Isosorbide is used for prophylaxis of angina and is not used for acute attacks.
   c. Amyl nitrate is used in the treatment of acute attacks as an inhalant with an onset of action of about 30 seconds.
   d. In addition, the utility of nitrates/nitrites to relieve pulmonary congestion and to increase cardiac output in HF is well established.
5. Adverse effects
   a. CV: Hypotension, rebound tachycardia, bradycardia, flushing, sweating
   b. CNS: Throbbing headache, dizziness
   c. Other: Nausea, vomiting, incontinence, contact dermatitis
6. Contraindications: Head trauma, cerebral hemorrhage, pregnancy, and lactation

7. Nursing implications
   a. Bioavailability of the traditional oral nitrates is very low. The sublingual route, which avoids the first-pass effect, is therefore preferred for achieving a therapeutic blood level rapidly.
   b. Sublingual or buccal preparations produce a fizzle or burning sensation, which indicates potency.
   c. Ensure that translingual spray is used under the tongue and not inhaled.
   d. With continuous exposure to nitrates, smooth muscle may develop complete tolerance (tachyphylaxis), and patients may become more tolerant when long-acting preparations (oral, transdermal) or continuous intravenous infusions are used for more than a few hours without interruption.
      1) Transdermal nitrates should be discontinued during the night (or at another nitrate-free interval of approximately 12 hours) to prevent tolerance development.
      2) Increasing the dose of nitrate can overcome tolerance also.

Anti-Hypertensive Vasodilators

1. Drugs within class
   a. Diazoxide (Hyperstat)
   b. Minoxidil (Loniten)
   c. Fenoldopam (Corlopam)
   d. Nitroprusside (Nipride)
   e. Hydralazine (Apresoline)
   f. Tolazoline (Priscoline)
2. Mechanism of action
   a. These agents directly act on vascular smooth muscle.
   b. All vasodilators used in hypertension produce direct relaxation of the arterioles. Nitroprusside also relaxes the veins.
3. Pharmacological effects
   a. Decreased arteriolar resistance and decreased arterial blood pressure elicit compensatory responses, mediated by baroreceptors and the sympathetic nervous system, as well as the renin-angiotensin-aldosterone system.
      1) These compensatory responses oppose the antihypertensive effect of vasodilators. Because sympathetic reflexes are intact, antihypertensive vasodilator therapy usually does not cause orthostatic hypotension or sexual dysfunction.
   b. Vasodilators work best in combination with other antihypertensive drugs that oppose the compensatory cardiovascular responses.

4. Therapeutic uses: hypertension, hypertensive crisis (nitroprusside, diazoxide, fenoldopam), pulmonary hypertension in the newborn (tolazoline)
5. Adverse effects
   a. CV: Sweating, flushing, edema, dizziness, hypotension, reflex tachycardia
   b. CNS: Throbbing headache
   c. Other:
      1) Systemic Lupus-like syndrome (hydralazine)
      2) Hypertrichosis (increased hair growth; minoxidil)
      3) Nitroprusside can increase thiocyanate levels, and therefore should be used with caution in patients with renal failure.
6. Contraindications
   a. Contraindicated with pregnancy and lactation
   b. Use with caution with peripheral vascular disease, coronary heart disease (CHD), HF, or tachycardia
7. Nursing Implications
   a. Monitor BP closely during administration to evaluate for effectiveness and to ensure quick response if BP falls rapidly or too much.
   b. Monitor carefully in any situation that might lead to reduced fluid volume (eg, excessive sweating, vomiting, diarrhea, dehydration).

Calcium Channel Blockers

Drugs within Class

(See Table 15–3.)

Mechanism of Action

These agents act by antagonizing L-type calcium channels in both smooth and cardiac muscle.

Pharmacological Effects

1. Marked reduction in transmembrane calcium current
   a. Long-lasting relaxation in smooth muscle
   b. Reduced contractility, decreased SA pacemaker rate, and decreased AV conduction velocity in heart.

Therapeutic Uses, Adverse Effects and Contraindications

See Table 15–3.

Nursing Implications

1. Monitor blood pressure very carefully if the patient is also on nitrates or beta-blockers because there is increased risk of hypotensive episodes.
2. Provide comfort measures to help the patient tolerate drug effects, including small, frequent meals, and access to bathroom facilities if GI upset is severe.
3. Monitor for edema resulting from vasodilation.

TABLE 15–3. Therapeutic Uses and Special Considerations of Calcium Channel Blocking Drugs

	Trade Name	Therapeutic Uses	Adverse Effects and Contraindications
Amlodipine	Norvasc	Prinzmetal angina, chronic angina; hypertension; HF	Headache, dysrhythmias, edema, bleeding gums
Bepridil	Vascor	Chronic, stable angina	Serious dysrhythmia, agranulocytosis, dizziness, nausea
Diltiazem	Cardizem	Prinzmetal angina, chronic angina, exercise-flushing, bradycardia associated angina; hypertension; Raynaud phenomenon; atrial tachycardia, atrial flutter	Serious dysrhythmia, dizziness,
Felodipine	Plendil	Hypertension; Raynaud phenomenon; HF	Dizziness, headache
Isradipine	DynaCirc	Hypertension	Headache, fatigue
Nicardipine	Cardene	Chronic, stable angina; hypertension	Dysrhythmia, severe GI upset, edema, headache, constipation
Nifedipine	Adalat, Procardia	Prinzmetal angina, chronic angina; hypertension	Dysrhythmia, tachycardia, GI upset, edema, dizziness, flushing, constipation
Nimodipine	Nimotop	Subarachnoid hemorrhage	Headache, diarrhea
Nisoldipine	Sular	Hypertension	Dysrhythmia, GI upset, edema, dizziness, flushing, constipation
Verapamil	Calan, Isoptin	Prinzmetal angina, chronic angina, unstable preinfarction angina; hypertension; atrial tachycardia, atrial flutter	Hypotension, myocardial depression, constipation, edema; Do not use with any heart block; Has strong negative inotropic effects

Anticoagulant, Anti-Thrombotic (Anti-Platelet), and Thrombolytic (Fibrinolytic) Drugs

Classes within Group: Anticoagulants, Anti-Thrombotics (Anti-Platelets), and Thrombolytic (Fibrinolytic) Drugs

Anticoagulants

1. Drugs within class
   a. Antithrombin III (Thrombate III)
   b. Heparin (Liquaemin)
   c. Lepirudin (Refludan)
   d. Warfarin (Coumadin)
   e. Danaparoid (Orgaran)
   f. Low molecular weight (LMW) Heparins: Ardeparin (Normiflo), Dalteparin (Fragmin), Enoxaparin (Lovenox), Tinzaparin (Innohep)
   g. Argatroban (Acova)
   h. Vivalirudin (Angiomax)
2. Mechanism of action
   a. Antithrombin III is a naturally occurring clotting inhibitor.
   b. Heparin is a naturally occurring protein that inhibits the conversion of prothrombin to thrombin, thus blocking the conversion of fibrinogen to fibrin — the final step in clot formation.
   c. Lepirudin is a recombinant hirudin (leech polypeptide) that directly inhibits thrombin formation.
   d. LMW heparins inhibit thrombus and clot formation by blocking factors Xa and IIa.
   e. Warfarin acts by interfering with the formation of vitamin K-dependent clotting factors in the liver.
3. Pharmacological effects: The eventual effect of all anticoagulants is a depletion of clotting factors (or inhibition of their formation or activity) and a prolongation of clotting times.
4. Therapeutic Uses
   a. Antithrombin III is used in patients with hereditary antithrombin III deficiency who are undergoing surgery or obstetric procedures that might put them at risk for thromboembolism.
   b. Heparin is indicated for acute treatment and prevention of venous thrombosis and pulmonary embolism; treatment of atrial fibrillation with embolization; prevention of clotting in blood samples and dialysis and venous tubing; and diagnosis and treatment of disseminated intravascular coagulation (DIC), as well as an adjunct in the treatment of MI and stroke.

   c. Lepirudin and argatroban are used for anticoagulation in patients with heparin-induced TCP.
   d. LMW heparins are used for the prophylaxis or treatment of deep venous thrombosis and pulmonary emboli.
   e. Warfarin is used to treat patients with atrial fibrillation, artificial heart valves, or valvular damage that makes them susceptible to thrombus or embolus formation.
5. Adverse effects: Bleeding, hemorrhage, nausea, GI upset, TCP, hepatic dysfunction
6. Contraindications
   a. Conditions that could be compromised by increased bleeding tendencies; these include hemorrhagic disorders, recent trauma, spinal puncture, GI ulcers, recent surgery, intrauterine device placement, tuberculosis, the presence of indwelling catheters, and threatened abortion.
   b. Warfarin is contraindicated in pregnancy (use heparin only if an anticoagulant must be used).
   c. Use with caution in HF, thyrotoxicosis, diarrhea (which could alter the normal clotting process by loss of vitamin K from the intestines), and fever (which could activate plasminogen).
7. Nursing implications
   a. Warfarin's onset of action is about 3 days, and its effects last for about 5 days. Because of this time delay, warfarin is not the drug of choice for acute situations, but is convenient and useful for prolonged effects.
   b. Heparin is injected IV or SC and has an almost immediate onset of action.
   c. Warfarin has documented drug-drug interactions with a vast number of drugs. It is wise practice never to add or remove a drug from the drug regimen of a patient receiving warfarin without careful patient monitoring and possible adjustment of the warfarin dosage to prevent serious adverse effects.
   d. Maintain availability of antidotes to anticoagulants in case of overdose.
      1) Protamine sulfate for heparin
      2) Vitamin K for warfarin

Antithrombotic (Anti-Platelet) Drugs

1. Drugs within class: See Table 15–4.
2. Mechanism of action: See Table 15–4.
3. Pharmacological effects: The end result of the various actions of all antithrombotic drugs is the inhibition of platelet aggregation.

4. Therapeutic uses: See Table 15–4.
5. Adverse effects: Bleeding and hemorrhage. Some of the more notable, non-cardiovascular side effects of some of the individual antithrombotic agents are listed below:
    a. Aspirin, clopidogrel, ibuprofen, sulfinpyrazone: GI ulceration

TABLE 15–4.
Mechanism of Action and Therapeutic Uses of Anti-Thrombotic (Anti-Platelet) Drugs

	Trade Name	Mechanism of Action	Therapeutic Uses
Abciximab	Reopro	Glycoprotein IIb/IIIa inhibitor; blocks platelet aggregation	Used to treat ischemia in high risk patients; Adjunct to percutaneous coronary intervention (PCI)
Aspirin Ibuprofen Sulfinpyrazone	Easpirin, etc. Motrin, etc. Anturane	Cycloxygenase inhibitor; inhibits formation of thromboxanes; blocks platelet aggregation	Reduction of risk of recurrent TIAs in males (aspirin only); reduction of risk of death or MI in patients with history of MI or unstable angina (aspirin only); reduction of emboli in rheumatic valve disease, atrial fibrillation
Clopidogrel	Plavix	ADP receptor blockade; block ADP from binding to platelets; blocks platelet aggregation	Treatment of patients with high risk for ischemic events (history of MI, peripheral artery disease, stroke)
Dipyridamole	Persantine	Phosphodiesterase inhibitor; increases cAMP which potentiates prostacyclins (platelet aggregation inhibitor)	With warfarin to prevent thromboembolism; With aspirin to enhance life-span of platelets in patients with thrombotic disease
Eptifibatide	Integrilin	Glycoprotein IIb/IIIa inhibitor; blocks platelet aggregation	Treatment of acute coronary syndrome; prevention of cardiac ischemic complications; often used with heparin
Ticlodipine	Ticlid	ADP receptor blockade; block ADP from binding to platelets; blocks platelet aggregation	Prevention of thrombotic stroke, especially in patients intolerant to aspirin or ibuprofen
Tirofiban	Aggrastat	Glycoprotein IIb/IIIa inhibitor; blocks platelet aggregation	With heparin to treat acute coronary syndrome; prevention of cardiac ischemic complications

b. Dipyridamole: may worsen angina, dizziness, headache, syncope, GI upset, rash
c. Eptifibatide, tirofiban: headache, dizziness, TCP
d. Ticlodipine: neutropenia, rash, nausea, diarrhea, and TCP
e. Abciximab: TCP

6. Contraindications: Caution should be used in the following conditions: the presence of any known bleeding disorder because of the risk of excessive blood loss, recent surgery, and closed head injuries.
7. Nursing implications
   a. Provide comfort measures and analgesia for headache to relieve pain and improve compliance
   b. Suggest safety measures, including the use of an electric razor and avoidance of contact sports

Thrombolytic (Fibrinolytic) Drugs

1. Drugs within class
   a. Alteplase (t-PA, Activase)
   b. Streptokinase (Kabikinase, Streptase)
   c. Anistreplase (Eminase)
   d. Urokinase (Abbokinase)
   e. Reteplase (Retevase)
   f. TNK t-PA (TNKase, Tenecteplase)
2. Mechanism of action
   a. Streptokinase, urokinase and anistreplase activate the conversion of plasminogen to plasmin and inhibit the formation of fibrin.
   b. Alteplase, tenecteplase and reteplase are recombinant forms of tissue plasminogen activator (t-PA) and activate the conversion of fibrin-bound plasminogen to plasmin.
3. Pharmacological effects: The production of plasmin causes the digestion of fibrin. The result is the degradation of fibrin clots to open up blood vessels and restore blood flow to the dependent tissue.
4. Therapeutic uses
   a. Lysis of thrombi in ischemic, but not necrotic, coronary arteries after infarction, acute MI, stroke, pulmonary embolism, deep venous thrombosis, occluded AV cannulas in dialysis patients, and peripheral artery thrombosis.
5. Adverse effects
   a. Bleeding, bruising, anaphylaxis, hematoma
   b. Aminocaproic acid (Amicar) is a fibrinolytic inhibitor that can be administered to antagonize the action of the thrombolytic drugs.

6. Contraindications: These drugs should not be used with any conditions that could be compromised by dissolution of clots; these include recent surgery, hemorrhage, cerebrovascular accident within the past two months, aneurysm, obstetric delivery, organ biopsy, serious GI bleeding, major trauma, or hypertension.
7. Nursing implications
   a. Evaluate the patient regularly for any sign of blood loss.
   b. Initiate treatment within 6 hours of the onset of symptoms of acute MI to achieve optimum therapeutic effectiveness.

Drugs Influencing the Renin-Angiotensin System

Classes within this group: Angiotensin Converting Enzyme (ACE) Inhibitors; Angiotensin II antagonists

ACE Inhibitors

1. Drugs within class
   a. Benazepril (Lotensin)
   b. Moexipril (Univasc)
   c. Captopril (Capoten)
   d. Perindopril (Aceon)
   e. Enalapril (Vasotec)
   f. Quinipril (Accupril)
   g. Fosinopril (Monopril)
   h. Ramipril (Altace)
   i. Lisinopril (Prinivil, Zestril)
   j. Trandolapril (Mavik)
2. Mechanism of Action: These drugs inhibit the converting enzyme that hydrolyzes angiotensin I to angiotensin II and that inactivates bradykinin, a potent vasodilator.
3. Pharmacological effects
   a. Inhibits the renin-angiotensin system
      1) Blocks the formation of angiotensin II, a potent vasoconstrictor
      2) Blocks the release of aldosterone from the adrenal glands, thus decreasing sodium and water reabsorption in the kidneys
   b. Stimulates the kallikrein-kinin system
      1) By inhibiting ACE, increased bradykinin
      2) Bradykinin is a vasodilator
   c. Cumulative effect of ACE inhibition is a decrease in BP

4. Therapeutic uses
   a. Primary therapeutic use is in the treatment of hypertension.
   b. Particularly useful role in treating patients with diabetic nephropathy because they diminish proteinuria and stabilize renal function (even in the absence of lowering of blood pressure).
      1) These benefits probably result from improved intrarenal hemodynamics, with decreased glomerular efferent arteriolar resistance and a resulting reduction of intraglomerular capillary pressure.
   c. Extremely useful in the treatment of HF and after MI. ACE inhibitors result in better preservation of left ventricular function in the years following MI by reducing post-infarction remodeling.
5. Adverse effects: Hypotension, glomerular damage, acute renal failure, hyperkalemia, dry cough (resulting from increased bradykinin and substance P; dry cough is sometimes accompanied by wheezing and angioedema), agranulocytosis, GI upset, skin rash, or other hypersensitivities
6. Contraindications: ACE inhibitors are contraindicated during the second and third trimesters of pregnancy because of the risk of fetal hypotension, anuria, and renal failure, sometimes associated with fetal malformations or death.
7. Nursing Implications
   a. All of the ACE inhibitors, except fosinopril and moexipril, are eliminated primarily by the kidneys; doses of these drugs should be reduced in patients with renal insufficiency.
   b. Monitor the patient carefully in any situation that might lead to decreased fluid volume (eg, excessive sweating, vomiting, diarrhea, dehydration) to detect and treat excessive hypotension that may occur.
   c. Potassium and renal function should be monitored periodically.

Angiotensin II Antagonists

1. Drugs within class
   a. Candesartan (Atacand)
   b. Losartan (Cozaar)
   c. Eprosartan (Teveten)
   d. Telmisartan (Micardis)
   e. Irbesartan (Avapro)
   f. Valsartan (Diovan)

2. Mechanism of action
   a. Block angiotensin II receptors (specifically blocking a subtype of angiotensin II receptor known as AT_1).
   b. No effect on bradykinin metabolism and are therefore more selective than ACE inhibitors.
3. Pharmacological effects
   a. By blocking AT_1 receptors in blood vessels and in the adrenal cortex, angiotensin II antagonists block the pressor and aldosterone-releasing effects of angiotensin II, resulting in decreased blood pressure caused by a decrease in both peripheral resistance and blood volume.
   b. Because the angiotensin II antagonists do not alter the levels of bradykinin, patients may escape the cough and other related side effects of ACE inhibition.
4. Therapeutic uses: Hypertension
5. Adverse effects: GI upset, dry mouth, tooth pain, headaches, dizziness, some cough, dry skin, alopecia
6. Contraindications: Angiotensin II antagonists are contraindicated during the second and third trimesters of pregnancy because of associated fetal malformations or death.
7. Nursing implications
   a. Administer with food to decrease GI distress if necessary.
   b. Monitor the patient carefully in any situation that might lead to decreased fluid volume (eg, excessive sweating, vomiting, diarrhea, or dehydration) to detect and treat excessive hypotension.
   c. Potassium and renal function should be monitored periodically.

Diuretics

Classes and Drugs within this Group: Table 15–5.

Mechanism of Action & Pharmacological Effects

1. Diuretics prevent cells lining the tubules of the nephron from reabsorbing sodium ions from the glomerular filtrate.
   a. As a result, sodium and other ions (and therefore water) are lost in the urine instead of being reabsorbed into the blood.
2. Each class of diuretic drugs works at a slightly different site in the nephron, and therefore produces effects by a slightly different mechanism.
3. The net result of diuresis is a decrease in intravascular volume, resulting in decreased BP and decreased workload of the heart (from decreased stroke volume and cardiac output).

4. The specific mechanisms of each of the diuretic classes are listed below.
   a. Thiazide diuretics inhibit sodium and chloride reabsorption in the distal convoluted tubule of the nephron. The resulting loss of sodium, chloride, and potassium causes an increase in urine output. Sodium loss also decreases the glomerular filtration rate. These agents are associated with a moderate potassium loss.
   b. Loop diuretics inhibit sodium and chloride reabsorption from the thick ascending limb of the loop of Henle. The resulting loss of sodium, chloride, and potassium causes an increase in urine output. These agents are powerful and associated with a high potassium loss.
   c. Potassium-sparing diuretics increase sodium excretion and decrease potassium secretion from the distal convoluted tubule. These agents are associated with less potassium loss ("potassium-sparing") compared to the thiazide and loop diuretics.

TABLE 15–5.
Diuretic Drug Classification and Major Therapeutic Uses

Class	Drugs	Therapeutic Uses
Thiazide Diuretics	Bendroflumethiazide (Naturetin) Benzthiazide (Exna) Chlorothiazide (Diuril) Chlorthalidone (Hygroton) Hydrochlorothiazide (Hydrodiuril, etc.) Hydroflumethiazide (Diucardin) Indapamide (Lozol) Methyclothiazide (Enduron) Metolazone (Mykrox) Polythiazide (Renese) Quinethazone (Hydromox) Trichlormethiazide (Diurese)	HF; hypertension; edema
Loop Diuretics	Bumetanide (Bumex) Ethacrynic Acid (Edecrin) Furosemide (Lasix) Torsemide (Demadex)	HF; pulmonary edema; hypertension;edema from HF, renal, or liver disease
Potassium-Sparing Diuretics	Amiloride (Midamor) Spironolactone (Aldactone) Triamterine (Dyrenium)	Hypertension; edema from HF, renal, or liver disease; replacement diuretic if patient develops hypokalemia
Osmotic Diuretics	Glycerin (Osmoglyn) Mannitol (Osmitrol)	Intracranial pressure; brain edema

d. Osmotic diuretics inhibit sodium and water reabsorption from the proximal convoluted tubule and descending limb of the loop of Henle.

Therapeutic Uses

See Table 15–5.

Adverse Effects

1. The most common adverse effects are imbalances in electrolytes and fluids, hypotension, oliguria, anuria, and dizziness.
2. Specific adverse effects of each of the diuretic classes are listed below.
   a. Thiazide diuretics: Hypokalemia, hyponatremia, hypocalcemia, hyperglycemia, hyperuricemia, GI distress
   b. Loop diuretics: Hypokalemia, hyponatremia, hypocalcemia, hyperglycemia, hyperuricemia, ototoxicity resulting in hearing loss, GI distress
   c. Potassium-sparing diuretics: Hyperkalemia, some hyponatremia, glucose intolerance in diabetics, gynecomastia, GI distress

Contraindications

Thiazides and loop diuretics should be used with caution with renal disease, hypokalemia, dysrhythmia, glucose intolerance, and gout.

Nursing Implications

1. Use of the potassium-sparing diuretic, triamterene, may cause the urine to turn blue.
2. Administer these agents early in the day so that increased urination will not interfere with sleep.
3. Monitor the dose carefully and reduce the dosage of one or both drugs if administered with an antihypertensive drug.
4. Provide a potassium-rich or poor diet as appropriate for the administered drug to maintain electrolyte balance. Electrolyte and renal function should be monitored periodically.

Antihyperlipidemics

Classes within Group: Resins, Niacin, Statins (HMG-CoA Reductase Inhibitors), and Fibric Acid Derivatives

Resins

1. Drugs within class
   a. Cholestyramine (Questran)
   b. Colestipol (Colestid)
   c. Covesevelam (Welchol)
2. Mechanism of action: These agents act as bile acid sequestrants by forming an insoluble complex with bile salts that is excreted in the feces. The resulting low level of bile acids feeding back to the hepatic circulation stimulates the production of more bile acids. The body compensates by increasing liver low-density lipoprotein (LDL) receptors, removing LDL from the circulation, and oxidizing the cholesterol from LDL to form bile acids.
3. Pharmacological effects
   a. Decrease LDL lipoprotein (15% to 30%)
   b. Increase HDL lipoprotein (3% to 5%)
   c. No effect or increase triglyceride
4. Therapeutic uses
   a. Single drug therapy should be evaluated before drug combinations are used.
   b. Treatment of hypercholesterolemia and hyperlipidemia
      1) Provided that diet therapy has failed, these agents are used if LDL is >160, or if LDL is >130 with the presence of 2 or more risk factors (eg, obesity, poor diet, smoking, HDL <40 mg/dL).
      2) The LDL goal for people with CHD or CHD equivalents and those at highest risk for CHD is <100 mg/dL.
   c. Resins are the only antihyperlipidemic currently recommended for children 11–20 years of age, although data now are emerging that document the safety of statin therapy for children in this age range.
5. Adverse effects: GI irritation, bloating, constipation, malabsorption of Vitamins A, D, and K
6. Contraindications: Hypertriglyceridemia, biliary obstruction, abnormal intestinal function, with pregnancy and lactation (to avoid malabsorption of important vitamins)
7. Nursing implications
   a. Do not administer powder in dry form; the drug must be mixed with fluids to be effective.
   b. Tablets must not be cut, chewed, or crushed. Tablets are designed to break down in the GI tract, and if the tablet is crushed the active ingredients will be ineffective.

Niacin

1. Drugs within class: Niacin (Nicotinic acid, Nicobid, Niaspan)
2. Mechanism of action:
   a. Inhibits lipolysis of triglycerides in adipose tissue, which reduces the transport of free fatty acids to the liver and decreases hepatic triglyceride synthesis.
   b. Decreased triglyceride synthesis reduces very low density lipoprotein (VLDL) production by the liver, which results in reduced LDL levels.
3. Pharmacological effects
   a. Best agent available for increasing HDL (increase of 15% to 35%);
   b. Lowers triglyceride (decrease of 20% to 50%) and
   c. Lowers LDL (decrease of 5% to 25%)
4. Therapeutic uses
   a. Single drug therapy should be evaluated before drug combinations are used.
   b. Treatment of hypertriglyceridemia, hypercholesterolemia, and hyperlipidemia
      1) Provided that diet therapy has failed, these agents are used if LDL is >160, or if LDL is >130 with the presence of 2 or more risk factors.
      2) The LDL goal for people with CHD or CHD equivalents and those at highest risk for CHD is <100 mg/dL.
5. Adverse effects: Niacin can cause cutaneous flushing, pruritus or dry skin, hyperpigmentation, GI distress, liver dysfunction (transaminase activity should be monitored), abnormal glucose tolerance, and hyperuricemia. Flushing and dyspepsia are two of the most common adverse effects, limiting patient compliance with this drug.
6. Contraindications: gout or pregnancy
7. Nursing implications
   a. Oral nicotinamide (source of niacin in many vitamin supplements) does not affect lipid levels.
   b. The dose of niacin for antihyperlipidemic therapy is high: 1–2 grams per day or more.
   c. Flushing is worse when therapy is initiated or the dosage is increased, but after 1 or 2 weeks of a stable dose, most patients no longer flush.
   d. Taking an aspirin (one-half hour prior to taking niacin) alleviates the flushing in many patients.
   e. Flushing is more likely to occur when niacin is consumed with hot beverages or alcohol.

3-Hydroxy–3-Methylglutaryl-Coenzyme-A (HMG-CoA) Reductase Inhibitors (Statins)

1. Drugs within class
   a. Atorvastatin (Lipitor)
   b. Pravastatin (Pravachol)
   c. Fluvostatin (Lescol)
   d. Simvastatin (Zocor)
   e. Lovastatin (Mevacor)
2. Mechanism of action
   a. Competitive inhibition of HMG-CoA reductase
   b. HMG CoA reductase catalyzes an early, rate-limiting step in cholesterol biosynthesis
3. Pharmacological effects
   a. The statins are the best-tolerated and most effective agents for treating dyslipidemia
   b. Decrease LDL (18% to 55%)
   c. Increase HDL (5% to 15%)
   d. Higher doses of the more potent statins (atorvastatin, simvastatin) also can reduce triglyceride (7% to 30%)
4. Therapeutic uses
   a. Single drug therapy should be evaluated before drug combinations are used.
   b. Treatment of hypertriglyceridemia, hyper-cholesterolemia, and hyperlipidemia
      1) Provided that diet therapy has failed, these agents are used if LDL is >160, or if LDL is >130 with the presence of 2 or more risk factors.
      2) The LDL goal for people with CHD or CHD equivalents and those at highest risk for CHD is <100 mg/dL.
5. Adverse effects
   a. Statins can cause liver dysfunction and increase liver transaminases. Therefore, a liver function test to measure alanine aminotransferase (ALT) is recommended at base line and 3 to 6 months after initiation of therapy. If the ALT values are normal, it is not necessary to repeat the ALT test more than every 6 to 12 months.
   b. Statins can cause myopathy and rhabdomyolysis, both associated with myalgia and fatigue. These side effects can be severe, prompting the removal of cerevastatin (Baychol) from the market after the drug had been linked to rhabdomyolysis, particularly when used with gemfibrozil.
   c. These agents also can cause cataracts, hypersensitivities, and renal failure.

6. Contraindications: liver disease or pregnancy
7. Nursing implications
   a. Administer the drug at bedtime because the highest rates of cholesterol synthesis occur between midnight and 5 am.
   b. Arrange for periodic ophthalmic exams to monitor for cataract development.
   c. Monitor liver function tests prior to and periodically during therapy.
   d. Ensure that patients attempt a cholesterol-lowering diet for at least 3–6 months before beginning therapy. Patients should continue to limit their fat intake and exercise routinely after drug therapy is initiated.
   e. Instruct patients to report muscle or joint pain.

Fibric Acid Derivatives

1. Drugs within class
   a. Clofibrate (Atromid-S)
   b. Fenofibrate (Tricor)
   c. Gemfibrozil (Lopid)
2. Mechanism of action: Unclear
3. Pharmacological effects
   a. Decrease VLDL synthesis with subsequent decrease in LDL (decrease 5% to 20%)
   b. Reduce triglycerides (20% to 50%) by stimulating lipoprotein lipase activity
   c. Increase HDL levels (10% to 20%)
4. Therapeutic uses
   a. Single drug therapy should be evaluated before drug combinations are used.
   b. Treatment of hypertriglyceridemia, hypercholesterolemia, and hyperlipidemia
      1) Provided that diet therapy has failed, these agents are used if LDL is >160, or if LDL is >130 with the presence of 2 or more risk factors.
      2) The LDL goal for people with CHD or CHD equivalents and those at highest risk for CHD is <100 mg/dL.
   c. Fibric acid derivatives are the drugs of choice for type III hyperlipidemia and hypertriglyceridemia.
5. Adverse effects: GI distress, rash, alopecia, fatigue, headache, impotence, and anemia. A myositis flu-like syndrome also can occur.
6. Contraindications: Renal and liver failure

7. Nursing implications
   a. Fibric acid derivatives have potential antiplatelet effects, so potential drug interactions need to be addressed.
   b. Gemfibrozil should not be combined, or used with extreme caution, with statins because of increased risk of rhabdomyolysis.

Hormone Replacement Therapy and CHD

1. Drugs within class: Estrogen, Estrogen-progesterone, Tamoxifen (Nolvadex), and Raloxifene (Evista)

Role of Hormone Replacement Therapy

1. The role of hormone replacement therapy (HRT) in preventing acute MI or in secondary prevention of acute MI is controversial.
2. The putative benefits of the use of HRT for the prevention of clinical CHD among postmenopausal women have been documented by most, but not all, observational studies.
   a. The Nurses' Health Study research group estimated that there was about a 20% reduction of cardiovascular disease among hormone users and a 30% reduction in risk.
   b. The results of these observational studies have led to widespread use of HRT among postmenopausal women for the prevention of cardiovascular disease.
   c. New studies, however, are providing less than convincing, and even contradictory, results.

HRT and Hypertension

1. Antihypertensive therapy reduces the risk for stroke, MI, and HF in both men and women.
2. Estrogen or estrogen-progesterone therapy has no effect on BP.
3. Estrogen might improve compliance of large blood vessels.
4. Estrogen therapy has no apparent benefit in reducing the risk for stroke.
5. Estrogen is contraindicated in postmenopausal women with a history of thromboembolic disorders.

Estrogen Antagonists and CHD

1. Estrogen antagonists like tamoxifen or selective estrogen receptor modulators (SERMs) like raloxifene, may have equal benefits in reducing CHD as compared with estrogen and estrogen-progesterone.

2. These newer agents may reduce the risk for breast cancers as well as other cancers.
3. No evidence that tamoxifen or SERMs reduce the risk for CHD.
4. Caution should remain in the presence of a history of venous thrombosis or smoking because of an increased risk of blood clot formation when smoking and estrogen or SERMs are combined.

HRT and Osteoporosis

1. Estrogen therapy and estrogen-progesterone therapy is effective in the prevention and treatment of osteoporosis and osteoporotic fractures.
2. The best approach now, absent definitive evidence, is to consider estrogen or estrogen-progesterone therapy as a specific drug therapy for the possible prevention of CHD in the context of other available therapies on a patient by patient basis and evaluate the risk-benefit ratio on each individual.

CHAPTER 16

Special Situations

This chapter addresses some of the special situations encountered in cardiac and vascular nursing practice. It provides a brief overview of cardiac and vascular emergency conditions that are often treated in the emergency department or intensive care unit. Individual differences of race, ethnicity, and culture that influence cardiac and vascular nursing practice are described. Co-morbid and concomitant conditions are discussed.

Emergency Conditions

Cardiac Arrest

Sudden cessation of cardiac function that may be reversible if appropriate actions are taken but will lead to death if no intervention is initiated.

1. Etiology
   a. Ventricular fibrillation
   b. Bradydysrhythmia
   c. Asystole
   d. Sustained ventricular tachycardia
   e. Pulseless electrical activity
   f. Ventricular rupture
   g. Cardiac tamponade
   h. Acute disruption of blood flow
2. Risk factors
   a. Coronary heart disease (CHD)
   b. Myocardial infarction (MI)
   c. Cardiac dysrhythmia
   d. Multiple conditions may be risk factors for cardiac arrest including pericardial effusion, cardiac surgery, pulmonary embolism, and acute respiratory failure.
3. Assessment
   a. History
      1) Symptoms of chest pain, dyspnea, fatigue, and palpitations preceding arrest
      2) Increased cardiac electrical ectopic activity prior to ventricular fibrillation such as tachycardia and ventricular ectopy

3) Symptoms of conditions associated with cardiac arrest before the event

b. Physical findings
   1) Loss of effective cardiac function
   2) Loss of effective circulation (pulseless)
   3) Loss of consciousness

c. Diagnostic tests
   1) ECG to identify cardiac rhythm if present.

4. Management of cardiac arrest
   a. Non Pharmacologic
      1) Assess that the collapse is due to cardiac arrest
      2) Once confirmed start basic life support (BLS) and activate emergency medical system (EMS)
   b. Pharmacologic
      1) Initiate ACLS protocol based on the cause of the cardiac arrest or type of dysrhythmia

5. Predictors of outcomes
   a. Prehospital care and admission to the hospital alive
      1) Increased survival with the initiation of bystander CPR
      2) Increased survival with immediate defibrillation
   b. Predictors of in hospital mortality
      1) Before arrest: Presence of hypotension, pneumonia, renal failure, cancer, or home bound life style
      2) During arrest: Duration of arrest greater than 15 minutes, intubation, hypotension, pneumonia, or home bound life style
      3) After resuscitation: Coma, need for vasopressors, or arrest duration of greater than 15 minutes

6. Post Cardiac Arrest Care
   a. Acute MI: conventional treatment
   b. Chronic CHD
      1) Diagnostic testing: Cardiac catheterization, angiography, stress testing, or imaging
      2) Ischemic therapy: Medical or surgical management
      3) Electrophysiology evaluation: Surgery, devices, and/or medications
   c. Nonischemic heart disease
      1) Diagnostic testing: Cardiac catheterization, angiography, stress testing, imaging and electrophysiology evaluation (surgery, devices, and/or medications), if indicated
      2) Medical or surgical treatment
   d. Nonstructural arrhythmogenic factors
      1) Discontinue prodysrhythmic medications, correct electrolyte imbalance, and initiate treatment for hypoxemia

Acute Heart Failure and Pulmonary Edema

Acute Heart Failure (HF) and Pulmonary Edema is a complex syndrome that is characterized by an abnormality of cardiac function that results in the heart's inability to pump blood to the tissues at the required rate to meet metabolic needs. Decreased cardiac output, inadequate tissue perfusion, and acute pulmonary congestion characterize the syndrome. Pulmonary edema is caused by increased fluid in the interstitial compartment and alveoli due to elevated pulmonary capillary pressures.

1. Etiology
   a. Left ventricular systolic and diastolic dysfunction may lead to biventricular failure
   b. Aortic or mitral valve dysfunction
   c. Congenital arteriovenous fistulas
   d. Acute cardiac events associated with elevated left atrial and pulmonary capillary pressures
2. Risk factors
   a. Exacerbation of cardiac condition associated with acute HF
   b. Inadequate treatment, lack of compliance, uncontrolled hypertension (HTN), dysrhythmia, MI, and administration of cardiac depressant medications
3. Assessment
   a. History
      1) HTN, MI, aortic or mitral valvular dysfunction, rheumatic heart disease, dysrhythmia, cardiomyopathy, congenital arteriovenous fistula, and cardiotoxic drugs.
      2) Symptoms of left-sided HF: Dyspnea on exertion, paroxysmal nocturnal dyspnea, orthopnea, nocturia, activity intolerance, and fatigue
      3) Symptoms of right-sided HF: Weight gain, anorexia, nausea, early satiety, and abdominal pain
   b. Physical findings
      1) Left-sided HF: Rales, wheezes, S_3, S_4, and tachycardia
      2) Right-sided HF: Increased jugular venous pressure (JVP), increased central venous pressure (CVP), hepatojugular reflux, dependent edema, and hepatomegaly
   c. Diagnostic tests
      1) Chest roentgenogram (x-ray) to detect ventricular hypertrophy, pleural effusion, and pulmonary edema
      2) Electrocardiogram (ECG) to identify areas of infarction or ischemia, ventricular hypertrophy, and dysrhythmia
      3) Echocardiogram to evaluate ventricular function, ejection fraction (EF), valvular function, and wall motion abnormalities

4) Coronary angiography to evaluate ventricular filling pressures, EF, and coronary artery stenosis
5) Arterial blood gases (ABG) to determine acid-base imbalance and hypoxemia
6) Laboratory tests to detect electrolyte imbalance, renal insufficiency, and other causes of HF including anemia, and thyroid dysfunction

4. Management
   a. Invasive management
      1) Cardiac surgery to repair or replace impaired valves
      2) Intra-aortic balloon pump (IABP) or left ventricular assist device (VAD) to decrease workload of the left ventricle
      3) Continuous arteriovenous hemofiltration or continuous venovenous hemofiltration to decrease fluid overload
      4) Pacemaker or implanted cardioverter defibrillator for patients with symptomatic dysrhythmia or conduction defects
   b. Pharmacologic Management
      1) Morphine to decrease anxiety, decrease systemic vascular resistance (afterload), and increase venous capacitance (decrease preload)
      2) Vasodilators to decrease afterload
      3) Diuretics to remove excess fluid in the vascular compartment (decrease preload)
      4) Cardiac glycosides for cardiac rate control and to enhance contractility
      5) Inotropes to enhance myocardial contractility
      6) Antidysrhythmics for treatment of dysrhythmia; beta adrenergic blockers and calcium channel blockers may be contraindicated
      7) Vasopressor support to treat severe hypotension

Cardiogenic Shock

Cardiogenic Shock is the failure of the heart as pump to meet the metabolic demands of the body.

1. Etiology
   a. MI
   b. Congenital cardiac defects
   c. Valvular dysfunction
   d. Dysrhythmia
   e. Cardiomyopathy
   f. Cardiac trauma

2. Risk factors

   A major risk factor for cardiogenic shock is MI. Cardiogenic shock usually occurs as a result of damage to the left ventricle that impairs the pumping and ejection of blood.

3. Assessment
   a. History
      1) History of MI, congenital cardiac defects, valvular dysfunction, cardiomyopathy, or cardiac trauma
      2) Typical or atypical symptoms associated with MI and other conditions causing HF
      3) Symptoms of left-sided HF: Dyspnea on exertion, paroxysmal nocturnal dyspnea, orthopnea, nocturia, activity intolerance, and fatigue
      4) Symptoms of right-sided HF: Weight gain, anorexia, nausea, early satiety, and abdominal pain
   b. Physical findings
      1) Left-sided HF: Rales, wheezes, S_3, S_4, tachycardia, and hypotension
      2) Right-sided HF: Elevated JVP, increased CVP, hepatojugular reflux, dependent edema, and hepatomegaly
      3) Cardiac dysrhythmia
      4) Impaired tissue perfusion: Mottled or cyanotic extremities; cool, clammy skin; gastric hypomotility; oliguria; or change in level of consciousness
   c. Diagnostic tests
      1) ECG to identify MI, myocardial ischemia, or dysrhythmia
      2) Chest x-ray to detect cardiomegaly and pulmonary edema
      3) Echocardiogram to evaluate ventricular function, EF, and valvular function
      4) Laboratory tests to detect electrolyte imbalance, renal or liver impairment, anemia, and shock state (such as lactic acid level and ABG)

4. Management
   a. Invasive management
      1) Intubation and mechanical ventilation to improve oxygen supply to the myocardium
      2) Pulmonary artery catheter to monitor hemodynamic parameters (cardiac output, cardiac index, systemic vascular resistance, pulmonary artery and pulmonary capillary wedge pressure) at base line and effect of treatment. CVP is elevated in right and bi-ventricular failure.
      3) IABP or left VAD to decrease ventricular workload
      4) Cardiac surgery to repair the cause of cardiogenic shock

b. Pharmacologic management
   1) Inotropes to enhance myocardial contractility
   2) Vasodilators to decrease afterload
   3) Antidysrhythmics for treatment of dysrhythmia; beta adrenergic blockers and calcium channel blockers may be contraindicated
   4) Vasopressors to treat severe hypotension

Cardiac Tamponade

Cardiac tamponade is compression of the heart due to an accumulation of fluid in the pericardial space. Cardiac compression by pericardial fluid causes increased intracardiac pressures, decreased diastolic filling, and reduced cardiac output.

1. Etiology
   Pericarditis, cancer, uremia, MI, diagnostic cardiac procedures, cardiac trauma, bacterial infection, cardiomyopathy, and cardiac surgery
2. Risk factors
   a. Diseases or illnesses that cause the excessive accumulation of pericardial fluid
   b. Diagnostic procedures that result in the movement of fluid into the pericardial space
3. Assessment
   a History
      1) Acute or chronic pericarditis, cardiac disease, renal failure, infection, injury to the heart or systemic diseases
   b. Physical findings
      1) Hypotension
      2) Tachycardia
      3) Diminished heart sounds
      4) Pericardial friction rub
      5) Pulsus paradoxus
      6) Tachypnea
   c. Diagnostic tests
      1) Chest x-ray to identify enlarged cardiac silhouette
      2) ECG to detect electrical alternans of the QRS complex
      3) Echocardiogram to diagnose the presence of pericardial effusion
      4) Angiography
4. Management
   a. Invasive management
      1) Pericardiocentesis (percutaneously with a needle or catheter), pericardiotomy, or surgical pericardiectomy to remove pericardial fluid

Aortic Dissection

Aortic dissection usually starts with either a tear in the intima or medial hemorrhage that ruptures the integrity of the aortic wall. Blood penetrates into the aortic wall, separates the layers, and creates a false lumen.

1. Etiology
   a. Medial degeneration is the most common cause
   b. Trauma
2. Risk factors
   a. Hereditary connective tissue diseases such as Marfan and Ehlers-Danlos syndromes
   b. HTN
   c. Increasing age — peak incidence is the sixth and seventh decades
   d. Gender — affects men twice as frequently as women
3. Assessment
   a. History
      1) In acute dissection the pain often has a sudden onset. If the chest pain is located anteriorly, the site of dissection is often the ascending aorta. Other associated symptoms for this site may be neck, throat, or jaw pain. If the pain is located in the interscapular region, the area of involvement is usually the descending thoracic aorta. Pain in the back, abdomen, or lower extremities is frequently indicative of a dissection of the descending aorta.
   b. Physical findings
      1) HTN or hypotension
      2) Pulse deficits
      3) With proximal aortic dissection, decrescendo diastolic murmur of aortic regurgitation
      4) With involvement of the inominate or left common carotid arteries, changes in level of consciousness
      5) Paraparesis or paraplegia may occur as a result of changes in spinal cord perfusion.
   c. Diagnostic tests
      1) Aortography to identify the presence and extent of aortic dissection
      2) CT Scan or MRI study to detect extent of aortic dissection
      3) Transthoracic or transesophageal echocardiography to identify aortic dissection
4. Management
   a. Invasive management
      1) Aortic aneurysm repair is indicated for acute proximal dissection and those distal aortic dissections that are

complicated by continued pain, rupture, expansion, saccular aneurysm, Marfan's syndrome, and ischemia of organs and/or lower extremities.

b. Medical management

1) For those patients with uncomplicated distal aortic dissection, particularly the elderly, medical therapy is associated with similar outcomes as surgical repair.
2) Medical management is also recommended for those patients with stable arch dissection or uncomplicated distal dissection.
3) Patients experiencing acute aortic dissection should be admitted to the hospital for monitoring of their hemodynamic status and emergent surgical intervention.
   a) Acute reduction of arterial pressure may be accomplished with intravenous medications such as beta adrenergic blockers, calcium channel blockers, ACE inhibitors, or nitrates.
   b) Unstable patients or those requiring short acting intravenous medications should be admitted to an intensive care unit or operating suite.

Acute Arterial Occlusion

Acute Arterial Occlusion occurs when a thrombus or embolism obstructs an artery producing significant tissue ischemia. Prompt recognition and treatment are critical to avoid loss of limb or death.

1. Etiology
   a. Embolism from atrial fibrillation, recent MI, valvular heart disease, or ventricular aneurysm
   b. Thrombosis due to atherosclerosis, aneurysms, hypercoagulable diseases, and vascular grafts
   c. Iatrogenic emboli (eg, catheter tips, dislodged atherosclerotic debris)
2. Risk factors
   a. Presence of diseases or conditions that can cause either embolism or thrombosis
3. Assessment
   a. History
      1) History of prior peripheral vascular disease, aortic aneurysm, or other conditions associated with embolism or thrombosis
      2) Sudden onset of symptoms such as pain, coolness, and paresthesia distal to the arterial occlusion
   b. Physical findings
      1) Absence of peripheral pulses — may be acute loss of pulse distal to occlusion

   2) Pallor
   3) Poikilothermia (cold)
   4) Paralysis
  c. Diagnostic tests
   1) Arterial doppler studies
   2) Arteriography before embolectomy
   3) Echocardiogram may be indicated to evaluate cardiac source
4. Management
  a. Invasive management
   1) Balloon embolectomy
   2) Arterial bypass procedure
   3) Fasciotomy may be required after revascularization is achieved
  b. Pharmacologic management
   1) Fibrinolytic therapy
   2) Emergent heparinization to prevent propagation of the clot

Race, Ethnic, Gender, and Cultural Considerations

Race and Ethnicity

Heart disease is the leading and stroke the third highest cause of death for people in the US. Despite the gains achieved with the programs associated with Healthy People 2000, health disparities for specific racial and ethnic groups remain. There has been a decrease in the overall number of cardiovascular deaths but there are disparities related to race and ethnicity. African-Americans or Blacks have the highest rates of CHD deaths, HF hospitalizations, and stroke. They also have the highest rate of death from HTN of any racial or ethnic group. Statistics related to cardiac and vascular disease morbidity and mortality rates for specific racial and ethnic groups are:

1. American Indian or Alaska Native
   a. CHD deaths 134 per 100,000
   b. HF hospitalization data not statistically reliable
   c. Stroke 39 per 100,000
   d. HTN data not statistically reliable
   e. Total blood cholesterol level of 240 mg/dl or greater data not statistically reliable
2. Asian or Pacific Islander
   a. CHD deaths not collected
   b. HF hospitalizations data not statistically reliable
   c. Stroke 55 per 100,000

   d. HTN data not statistically reliable
   e. Total blood cholesterol level of 240 mg/dl or greater data not statistically reliable
3. Black or African-Americans
   a. Coronary heart disease deaths 257 per 100,000
   b. HF hospitalizations age 85 years or older 47.6 per 1,000
   c. Stroke 82 per 100,000
   d. HTN 40%
   e. Total blood cholesterol level of 240 mg/dl or greater 19%
4. Hispanic or Latino
   a. CHD deaths 151 per 100,000
   b. HF hospitalizations data not statistically reliable
   c. Stroke 40 per 100,000
   d. HTN not collected; Mexican Americans 29%
   e. Total blood cholesterol level of 240 mg/dl. or greater data not collected; Mexican American 18%
5. White or Caucasians
   a. CHD deaths 214 per 100,000
   b. HF hospitalizations age 85 years or older 42.1 per 1,000
   c. Stroke 60 per 100,000
   d. HTN 27%
   e. Total blood cholesterol level of 240 mg/dl or greater 21%

Gender

Women experience major cardiovascular events approximately ten years later than men. The difference between men and women decreases with advancing age. Because of the older age at onset of CHD and the presence of co-morbid conditions, women are more likely to die in the first few weeks after a MI than men. Black females and white males have the highest rate of CHD deaths of any racial or ethnic group. Statistics related to cardiac and vascular disease morbidity and mortality rates for men and women are:

1. Men
   a. CHD deaths 276 per 100,000
   b. HF hospitalization age 85 years or older — 59.3 per 1,000
   c. Stroke 64 per 100,000
   d. HTN 30%
2. Women
   a. CHD deaths 170 per 100,000
   b. HF hospitalization age 85 years or older — 50.6 per 1,000
   c. Stroke 60 per 100,000
   d. HTN 26%

Cultural Considerations

1. Cultural phenomena that vary among racial and ethnic groups may affect their receptivity to care delivered by health care providers. Some factors related to culture include:
   a. Environmental control is the ability of people to control nature. Cultural groups that believe they have mastery over nature or the environment may accept medications or invasive procedures. Cultural groups that believe they do not have control over nature or the environment may not accept medications and procedure and may seek alternative treatments such as folk medicine.
   b. Biologic variation is the genetic susceptibility of people to illness. Racial and ethnic variations in the incidence of cardiac and vascular diseases and the presence of risk factors (described previously) may have a genetic component.
   c. Social organization is the family unit and the role of family members. There are cultural differences in the composition (nuclear or extended) of families and the value placed on the respective roles. Some cultural groups have extended family units with multiple members involved in decision-making. Other cultural groups are matriarchal in their decision-making processes.
   d. Communication is the verbal and nonverbal behaviors that are used in personal interactions. Acceptable forms of expression for people are often culturally based. Some cultures are formal while others are informal in their conversations with health care providers.
   e. Space refers to the boundaries or acceptable distances between people that affects their personal comfort. Some cultural groups are comfortable with close contact with health care providers while others are not. Space or closeness is an important concern for nurses caring for cardiac and vascular patients because many procedures cross these boundaries and may result in personal discomfort.
   f. Time orientation has to do with culture's view of the past, present, and future. Some cultures are future oriented while others have strong beliefs in practices of their ancestors.
2. Cultural competency for health care providers. Nursing care that is culturally competent is knowledgeable and sensitive to patient's cultural needs. Care of people from different cultures should be based on the following principles:
   a. Care is designed for the specific patient.

b. Care is based on the patient's cultural norms and values.
c. Care incorporates interventions that facilitate patients' decisionmaking about their care.
d. Care is sensitive to the patient's cultural uniqueness.

Co-morbid or Concomitant Conditions

Cardiopulmonary Disease

Cardiopulmonary diseases and their related risk factors contribute to an increased incidence of cardiac and vascular health problems. Smoking is linked to CHD and chronic obstructive pulmonary diseases (COPD). Pulmonary health problems such as COPD may result in secondary pulmonary HTN and cardiac disorders such as cor pulmonale. The presence of cardiopulmonary diseases among patients experiencing cardiac or vascular health problems can complicate recovery and increase mortality.

Diabetes

Diabetes mellitus is a major risk factor for the development of cardiovascular diseases including CHD, stroke, and arterial occlusive diseases. The rate of newly diagnosed cases of non-insulin dependent diabetes mellitus in the US is 798,000 per year. Diabetes is a leading associated cause of mortality for men and women in this country. Approximately, two thirds of the people with diabetes will die of cardiovascular disease. People with diabetes who have intensive or tight control of their blood glucose have lower incidence of diabetic complications including retinopathy, microalbuminuria, and neuropathy as well as lower LDL-C and total cholesterol levels than people with less intensive control. Cardiovascular mortality is less when hemoglobin A1c levels are low. Diabetes mellitus complicates the recovery of people from cardiovascular events. Hyperglycemia increases risk of post-operative wound infections in people having surgical procedures such as coronary artery bypass surgery.

Renovascular Disease

Renovascular diseases contribute to an increased incidence of cardiac and vascular problems. The development of end stage renal disease has been linked to HTN. In 1998, there were 85,520 people newly diagnosed with this health problem. End stage renal disease (ESRD) and its sequel, chronic renal failure, has been associated with the development of HF, hypertrophic cardiomyopathy, and accelerated coronary atherosclerosis. In 1998, 65,153 people died from ESRD. The perioperative care of cardiac and vascular patients with renovascular disease presents many challenges because of complications associated with their disease including HTN, electrolyte imbalance, and fluid management issues.

Cerebrovascular Disease

Cerebrovascular diseases can be risk factors for the development of cardiac diseases and abnormalities of the heart can also cause acute cerebrovascular injury. Patients may have carotid artery occlusive disease and coexisting CHD because the risk factors are similar. Increased incidences of dysrhythmia, MI, and cardiopulmonary arrest have been associated with acute cerebrovascular injury. The presence of CHD adversely affects survival of patients with CVA. Stroke is the third leading cause of death and most CVAs are due to atherosclerosis. Patients undergoing cardiac or vascular surgical procedures may have an increased incidence of acute cerebral injury because of embolization from the aorta or carotid arteries, respectively.

Specific Nursing Interventions

General measures

1. Activity progression including bedrest, out of bed to the chair or commode, or ambulation is based on the patient's diagnosis and activity tolerance.
2. Vital signs are monitored to detect any changes in the patient's condition. The frequency of vital signs depends on the patient's acuity.
3. Neurovascular checks are used to assess the temperature, color, capillary refill, sensation, movement, and pulses of the upper and lower extremities. The frequency of neurovascular checks is determined by the presence of vascular disease or procedures that may cause changes in the peripheral circulation.
4. Intravenous access is indicated for acutely ill patients with cardiac and vascular diseases and those at risk for complications.
5. Oxygen is used for patients with ischemic symptoms or respiratory distress. Pulse oximetry or ABGs are used to monitor the effectiveness of oxygen therapy.
6. Intake and output are monitored to determine the patient's fluid status. The frequency of intake and output is based on the patient's diagnosis and acuity.
7. Daily weights are used to measure the patient's overall volume status and may used as an indicator for diuretic or fluid therapies.

Specific Interventions

1. A cardiac monitor may be used to continuously assess the electrical activity of the heart. It is used to identify cardiac dysrhythmia and ischemia in high-risk patients and those with acute health problems.
2. ECG is a graphic recording of the electrical impulses generated during the cardiac cycle. This procedure provides information on the electrical activity of specific segments of the heart. The ECG may be used to measure electrical impulses, identify cardiac dysrhythmia, and diagnose MI.
3. Unna boots are used in the management of venous ulcers. The plaster boot is a dressing composed of gauze moistened with specific medications.14 The boot is changed at specific time intervals (every 1 to 2 weeks) depending upon the amount of ulcer drainage. A boot should not be used and is discontinued if signs of infection are present.
4. Compression stockings promote venous return and are also used to decrease leg swelling and prevent ulceration. Patients are measured for these stockings to ensure proper fit. The pressure at the ankle should be at least 30–40 mm Hg and should decrease proximally.

CHAPTER 17

Psychosocial Aspects

Cardiovascular health problems affect not only the physiological status of patients but can also have a major impact on their coping and adaptation. The psychosocial aspects of illness can result in adaptive and maladaptive responses that can influence a person's interpersonal relationships, vocation, sexuality, and spirituality. Nurses can encourage patients to use positive coping mechanisms as they adapt to their cardiovascular health problems.

Coping and Adaptation

Coping is the continuously changing cognitive and behavioral actions used by an individual to manage the external and/or internal demands that are appraised as challenging or exceeding personal resources. Coping is a dynamic process between the individual and the environment.

Functions of Coping

1. Reduce tension and maintain equilibrium
2. Facilitate independence and freedom
3. Enhance personal decision-making
4. Manage reactions to stressors
5. Facilitate meeting social environmental demands
6. Avoid negative self-evaluation
7. Maintain a stable psychological, social, and physiological state

Coping Styles

1. An individual's way of coping may change according to specific situational variables.
2. A flexible coping style is more adaptive to different events and stressors than one that is rigid.
3. Coping styles involve a continuum of behaviors from approaching the situation to advoidance.

Adaptive Responses

1. Life-style modification: The individual changes certain aspects of their life-style to meet the demands of the illness. For the patient with newly diagnosed cardiac or vascular disease, life-style modification may mean starting an exercise routine, losing weight, and following a low fat diet. The patient learns to avoid those activities that may exacerbate their disease.
2. Enhancing knowledge and self-care strategies: The individual increases his or her understanding about the disease and its treatment. The individual copes by being aware of his or her symptoms and based on his or her assessment of the symptom either alters self-care activities or seeks help from health care providers.
3. Maintaining a positive self-concept: The individual integrates the illness and treatment into the sense of self to maintain feelings of normalcy. The individual engages in activities to enhance self-esteem and adapts to an altered body image.
4. Adjusting to changes in social relationships: The individual's illness and decreased energy alter his or her participation in social activities. Other individuals in social relationships may choose to limit contact with the individual either because of their discomfort with the situation or because of the need for respite. The ill individual must adapt to decreasing contacts and inquiries from other individuals and modifies his or her support systems.
5. Grieving over losses: The individual grieves over the losses associated with illness such as functional ability, energy, body image, roles, sexuality, and social relationships. The individual works to maintain self-concept by adapting to these losses.
6. Dealing with role changes: The individual adapts to changes in personal, social, and professional roles. Adaptation means either relinquishing or modifying previous roles and responsibilities. The individual assumes the new role of patient also.
7. Adjusting to physical discomfort: The individual attempts to cope with the discomfort associated with the illness and/or its treatment. The individual seeks ways to alleviate or decrease the discomfort through pharmacological and nonpharmacological interventions.
8. Maintaining a sense of control: The individual has multiple intrusions into his or her personal space and privacy because of the illness. The individual attempts to maintain privacy and preserve personal dignity. Maintaining control involves making decisions about treatments and the subsequent timing of this care.
9. Maintaining hope: The individual embraces a positive attitude that he or she will recover from the illness with the use of new

therapies. The person adjusts to deteriorating physical health and declining treatment options by having hope and attempts to avoid feelings of despair about the illness.

10. Confronting impending death: The individual realizes that his or her life will be short. The person has comfort in his or her personal accomplishments and relationships. Confronting death involves the anticipation and acceptance of the prognosis.

Maladaptive Responses

The individual who is unable to cope with his or her illness is at risk for developing maladaptive responses. Maladaptive responses include anxiety, anger, depression, denial, dependence, and noncompliance.

1. Anxiety is a response to an actual or perceived threat. It is characterized by feelings of apprehension, tension, and uneasiness. Anxiety may result from a fear of the illness and its associated diagnostic and therapeutic procedures. It can also occur because of fear of disfigurement and death. Mild anxiety has been associated with enhanced performance related to learning. Severe symptoms of acute anxiety, such as panic, include agitation and feeling out of control.
2. Anger is a reaction that is associated with feelings of extreme displeasure, hostility, or rage. The stimulus for this emotion may be an actual or perceived threat to the individual's self-concept. Anger occurs as a result of the person's perceived vulnerability because of the illness and the loss of independence and roles.
3. Depression is a state that is associated with the loss of roles, functional status, and changes in self-concept. Symptoms associated with depression include feeling sad, guilty, anxious, apathetic, or confused. The person may experience disturbances in sleep and appetite and may have somatic complaints also. Severe or major depression can impair the ability to function at work and in social situations. The person with major depression often has feelings of hopelessness, worthlessness, and fearfulness and may be at risk for committing suicide.
4. Denial is a defense mechanism that involves avoiding emotional conflict or anxiety by refusing to acknowledge thoughts, feelings, or facts that are intolerable. An individual may deny the presence of an illness or the need for prescribed therapy.
5. Dependence is a condition in which the person is overly dependent on others to meet his or her physical and emotional needs. This response may be precipitated also by a significant other's response to the illness.
6. Noncompliance is a reaction to the limitations imposed by the illness and its related treatment. The individual refuses to comply

with the management of the condition. The response may be a rebellion against the feelings of vulnerability, temporary respite from the prescribed therapies, or a depressive withdrawal from the stress.

7. Treatment of Maladaptive Responses
   a. Nonpharmacological interventions
      1) Cognitive behavioral therapy
      2) Psychotherapy
      3) Electroconvulsive therapy for selected depressive disorders
      4) Light therapy for seasonal affective disorder
   b. Pharmacological therapy
      1) Serotonin selective reuptake inhibitors (SSRIs) such as fluoxetine, sertraline, paroxetine, and fluoxamine are the first line of treatment for most anxiety disorders. They are also the medications of choice for depressive disorders.
      2) Tricylic antidepressants including imipramine, nortriptyline, desipramine, amitriptyline, and doxepin are useful in the treatment of generalized anxiety disorders and panic disorder. They are also used in the treatment of depressive disorders.
         a) Tricyclics are extremely dangerous when taken in overdose quantities.
         b) May cause cardiovascular adverse effects such as orthostatic hypotension, conduction defects, and dysrhythmia
      3) Benzodiazepines such as diazepam, lorazepam, and oxazepam are effective in the treatment of generalized anxiety. Alprazolam and clonazepam are usually used for panic disorder.
      4) Monoamine oxidase inhibitors (MAOIs) are used to treat atypical depression and treatment resistant patients. MAOIs include phenelzine, traylcypromine, L-deprenyl, and moclobemide.
      5) Atypical antidepressants include bupropion, mirtazapine, nefazodone and trazodone.

Nursing Diagnoses Related to Coping and Adaptation

1. Ineffective Coping is the inability to form a valid appraisal of the stressors, inadequate choices of practiced responses, and/or inability to use available resources.
2. Defensive Coping is the repeated projection of falsely positive self-evaluation based on a self-protective pattern that defends against underlying perceived threats to positive self-regard.

3. Compromised family coping occurs when the usually supportive primary person provides insufficient, ineffective, or compromised support, comfort, assistance or encouragement to manage adaptive tasks.
4. Ineffective denial is the conscious or unconscious attempt to disavow knowledge or meaning of an event to reduce anxiety, but leading to the detriment of health.

Nursing Interventions to Enhance Coping and Adaptation

1. Assess the patient's psychosocial responses to the illness and its treatment.
2. Identify whether these responses are adaptive or maladaptive.
3. Determine if there is a physiological cause of the maladaptive response.
4. Plan an individualized psychosocial nursing care plan with the patient and family.
5. Establish a therapeutic relationship with the patient and family.
6. Promote the use of adaptive coping mechanisms by the patient and family.
7. Provide educational materials to enhance knowledge about the disease and prescribed therapies.
8. Encourage patient and family participation in support groups composed of people with similar illnesses.
9. Consult with the patient's physician or advanced practice nurse about referral for psychiatric evaluation for maladaptive responses. Some patients may benefit from psychotherapy and/or psychopharmacology.
10. Evaluate the effectiveness of the psychosocial nursing care plan for the patient and family and revise as necessary.

Quality of Life

The World Health Organization defined quality of life as "a broad ranging concept affected in a complex way by the person's physical health, psychological state, level of independence, social relationships, and relationships to salient features of the environment." An individual's perception of his or her quality of life, either positive or negative, can have broad implications for the ability to cope with cardiovascular disease and treatment.

Influencing Factors

Factors influencing an individual's perception of his or her quality of life include health, functional status, symptoms, and life satisfaction. The acuity or chronic nature of the illness afflicting the person affects these factors.

1. Health is the "state of physical, mental, and social well-being and not merely the absence of disease or infirmity." Health exists on a continuum with health and illness being on opposite ends.
2. Functional status is the individual's ability to perform his or her roles and related activities. The activities that may be affected by cardiovascular disease include the individual's physical, psychological, and social interactions.
3. Symptoms are the individual's responses to his or her physical, emotional, or cognitive states. These responses may be manifested as adaptive and/or maladaptive coping mechanisms.
4. Life satisfaction is the fulfillment or contentment that an individual feels from different facets of life including family, health, sexuality, spirituality, friendships, job, education, housing, standard of living, and finances.

Support Systems

1. The spouse, family members, and significant others have an important role in the support of individuals with cardiovascular health problems. Individuals who have a high level of social integration or social links to family and friends have better outcomes after acute myocardial infarction. As a result of their positive support systems, these individuals often have a perceived higher quality of life. The care by the spouse or significant other may come at a physiological or psychological cost to the caregiver. For some caregivers, the burden of caring may result in physical exhaustion and negative emotional responses. These factors can have a negative effect on the perceived quality of life of the caregivers.
2. Community resources such as support groups, counseling services, and health care agencies can assist patients, their families, and significant others in their psychosocial adjustment to illness. Health care providers can help to improve the quality of life for patients and their family members. In some areas, respite care is also available to provide caregivers temporary relief from care giving responsibilities.

Work

Vocational issues are related to quality of life for people with cardiovascular diseases. For many people, self-concept is linked to the roles in their life including their occupation. Depending upon the type of work that the individual does, there may be changes in some or all of their responsibilities especially for those with physically demanding positions. Changes in work responsibilities and routines can cause stress and lowered self-esteem. These factors can have an effect on an individual's perceived quality of life and psychosocial responses to the illness. The time that an individual can return to work along with any work limitations should be discussed with their health care provider.

Sexuality

Sexuality is a concern for many cardiovascular patients. It is a subject that is not easily discussed in the therapeutic relationship. Some patients and their significant others may fear that sexual activity will result in angina or death. There are guidelines related to sexual activity after cardiovascular illnesses. For example, the American Heart Association recommends that patients having an uncomplicated myocardial infarction may resume sexual intercourse in seven to 10 days. Some medications used to treat individuals with cardiovascular conditions such as angiotensin converting enzyme inhibitors, beta adrenergic blockers, and calcium channel blockers may have a negative effect on libido. Sexual dysfunction can cause feelings of anxiety, anger, or depression for the patient and partner. Patients with sexual dysfunction should be referred to their health care provider for an evaluation.

Spirituality

Spirituality and religion give value to people's beliefs and behaviors. People may be spiritual but may not endorse a religion. Religious involvement has been associated with a lower incidence of cardiovascular disease and mortality. Additionally, individuals who have religious involvement and spirituality have a lower incidence of depression and anxiety related to physical illness. These factors have also been linked to higher levels of perceived quality of life for people with cardiovascular and other illnesses.

Stress Management

Stress management techniques are strategies that can be used to enhance an individual's ability to cope with stressors. Conditions that may activate the stress response may be physical, emotional, cognitive, social, economic, or spiritual. Stressors may be events that have actually occurred or may be perceived as threats that are not reality-based. The body's response to the actual or perceived threat results in physiologic and psychological responses.

General Adaptation Syndrome

The General Adaptation Syndrome, identified by Hans Selye, depicts the stages associated with the body's response to a stressor.

1. Alarm Stage is the initial response to the stressor. The central nervous system is stimulated and physiologic defense mechanisms are activated. This process is often called the fight or flight syndrome.
2. Stage of Resistance or Adaptation is the process whereby the individual continues the fight or flight response.
3. Stage of Exhaustion is the point in which the continued stress precipitates the disruption of the compensatory mechanisms leading to the onset of stress related dysfunction such as disease or illness.

Physiologic and Psychologic Responses

1. Physiologic responses to stress include the interaction between the sympathetic nervous system, anterior and posterior pituitary gland, and adrenal gland.
   a. Sympathetic stimulation causes the release of norepinephrine resulting in increased blood pressure, pupil dilation, skeletal muscle vasodilation, bronchodilation, and decreased gastric secretion.
   b. Adrenal medulla activation stimulates epinephrine secretion causing increased cardiac output, bronchodilation, increased glycogenolysis, increased gluconeogenesis, increased glucagon, increased free fatty acids, increased serum cholesterol, and decreased insulin.
   c. Anterior pituitary stimulation causes the release of ACTH, Growth Hormone, and Prolactin. ACTH acts on the adrenal cortex to secrete aldosterone and cortisol resulting in increased sodium and water retention, increased blood glucose from gluconeogenesis, increased amino acids from protein catabolism, increase polymorphonucleocytes, decreased monocytes/macrophages, decreased lymphocytes, and decreased eosinophils.
   d. Posterior pituitary activation causes the release of vasopressin or antidiuretic hormone thereby stimulating increased water retention.

2. Psychologic responses to stress such as cardiovascular illness may result in the use of adaptive and maladaptive coping mechanisms.

Identification of Personal Traits and Responses

1. Self-concept plays an important role in a individual's response to actual or perceived stressors. Those individuals with high self-esteem use more adaptive coping responses. Those individuals with lower self-esteem are more vulnerable to psychological stressors and may respond with feelings of anger, denial, or depression. Negative self-concept has been proposed to have a significant role in the eventual onset of disease in vulnerable individuals.
2. The "Type A Personality" was originally identified by Friedman and Rosenman. Personality traits of people with this syndrome include the need to accomplish tasks in the shortest amount of time, aggressive behavior that borders on hostility, highly motivated, very competitive, achievement oriented, labile temper, and involvement in multiple tasks at the same time. Individuals with this profile have been associated with a higher incidence of coronary heart disease. It has been proposed that these individuals have a heightened sympathetic responsiveness to stressors, which may be the key factor in pathological process leading to their increased cardiovascular risk.

Stress Management Techniques

1. Autogenics is a technique used to promote deep relaxation. It is centered around formulas that involve the repeating of repetitive verbal phases and concentrating on sensations and actions in certain parts of the body. The formulas are focused on exercises that involve muscular relaxation, vascular dilation, regulation of the heart, regulation of breathing, regulation of visceral organs, and regulation of the head.
2. Cognitive restructuring involves using the mind to alter the stress response. Negative feelings can trigger physiological aspects of the stress response. This technique requires the patient to identify maladaptive negative thoughts to stressors and to counter these feelings with adaptive positive thoughts.
3. Imagery is another method for stress reduction. The individual creates a place that is relaxing. Imagery is especially effective when combined with physical relaxation techniques such as diaphragmatic breathing exercises.
4. Progressive muscle relaxation reduces stress by interfering with the autonomic arousal of the sympathetic nervous system by decreasing muscle tension. This technique involves tension-relaxation

exercises of each of the major muscle groups of the body. It is used to decrease the impact of the physiological responses to stress and to enable the individual to learn adaptive responses to stimuli.

5. Meditation is a process that produces deep physiological relaxation. It involves limiting stimuli from conscious awareness, repeating verbal phrases or mantra, and concentrating on a focal point to relax the body.
6. Aerobic exercise reduces anxiety and stress along with having a positive effect on subjective mood states. The exercise prescription usually involves repetitive movement of large muscle groups. The goal of aerobic exercise is to elevate the heart rate to a specified level. There are often positive cardiovascular benefits from aerobic exercise.

Self-monitoring Techniques

Instructions for the individual learning self-monitoring techniques include:

1. Change your life-style by having a well balanced diet, regular exercise, adequate sleep, leisure activities, and using stress management techniques.
2. Modify stressful situations by managing time and finances, being assertive, engaging in problem-solving and possibly changing work situations or relationships.
3. Change thinking by being positive, seeing problems as new opportunities, decreasing negative thoughts, and having a sense of humor.
4. Modify reactions to stressors by being aware of your feelings. Learn to control these reactions with positive adaptive behaviours.

APPENDIX A
Selected Bibliography

Chapter 1

American Hospital Association (1990). *A patient's bill of rights.* Chicago, IL: Author.

American Nurses Association (2001). *Code of ethics for nurses with interpretive statements.* Washington, DC: American Nurses Publishing.

American Nurses Association (2003). *Nursing: Scope and Standards of Practice.* Washington, DC: American Nurses Publishing.

American Nurses Association (2003). *Nursing's social policy statemen, 2nd edition.* Washington,DC: American Nurses Publishing.

Beauchamp TL & Childress JF (2001). *Principles of biomedical ethics, 5th edition.* New York: Oxford University Press.

Daly BJ (1996). Ethics in critical care. In JM Clochesey, C Breu, S Cardin, AA Whittaker & EB Rudy. *Critical Care Nursing, 2nd edition.* Philadelphia: Saunders.

Trandel-Korenchuk DM & Trandel-Korenchuk KM (1997). *Nursing & the law, 5th edition.* Gaithersburg, MD: Aspen.

Chapter 2

Aguilera DC (1998). Crisis intervention: *Theory and methodology,* 8th edition. St. Louis: Mosby.

Bandura, A (1986). *Social foundations ofthought and action: A social cognitive theory.* Englewood Cliffs, NJ: Prentice-Hall.

Bowen M (1978). *Family therapy in clinical practice.* New York: Jason Aronson.

Bridges W (1991). *Managing transitions: Making the most of change.* Reading, MA: Addison-Wesley.

Burr WR, Leigh GK, Day RD & Constantine J(1979). Symbolic interaction and the family. In WR Burr, R Hill, FI Nye and IL Reiss (Eds.) *Contemporary theories about the family.* New York: Free Press.

Chinn PL & Jacobs MK (1987). *Theory and nursing: A systematic approach, 2nd edition.* St. Louis: Mosby.

Erickson EH (1955). Growth and crises of the healthy personality. In C Kluckhorn, HA Murray & DM Scheider (Eds.) *Personality in nature, society and culture.* New York: Knopf.

Fawcett J & Downs FS (1992). *The relationship of theory and research, 2nd edition.* Philadelphia:FA Davis.

Fishbein M & Azjen I (1975). *Belief, attitude,intention and behavior: An introduction to theory and research.* Reading, MA: Addison-Wesley.

Huber, D (1996). *Leadership and nursing caremanagement.* Philadelphia: WB Saunders.

King KM, Humen DP, Smith HL, Phan CL &Teo KK (2001). Psychosocial components of cardiac recovery and rehabilitation attendance. *Heart, 85*(3), 290–294.

Lewin K (1951). *Field theory in social science.* New York: Harper & Row.

Pender NJ (1996). *Health promotion in nursing practice, 3rd edition.* Norwalk, CN: Appleton & Lange.

Prochaska JO & DiClemente CC (1984). *The transtheoretical approach: Crossing traditional boundaries of change.* Homewood, IL: Dow-Jones-Irwin.

Rosenstock IM (1974). Historical origins of the Health Belief Model. In MH Becker (Ed.), *The Health Belief Model and personal health behavior.* Thorofare, NJ: Slack.

Roy C & Roberts SL (1981). *Theory construction in nursing: An adaptation model.* EnglewoodCliffs, NJ: Prentice-Hall.

Smith, J (1983). *The idea of health: Implications for the nursing profession.* New York: Teachers College.

Sullivan MD, LaCroix AZ, Russo J & Katon WJ (1998). Self-efficacy and self-reported functional status in coronary heart disease: a six-month study. *Psychosomatic Medicine, 60*(4),473–478.

Chapter 3

Bleich MR (1999). Managing and leading. In P Yoder-Wise. *Leading and managing in nursing.* St. Louis: Mosby.

Burns J (1978). *Leadership.* New York: Harper & Row.

Case Management Society of America (2001). *Definition of case management.* www.cmsa.org.

Coile RC (1999). Nursing case management in the new millennium: Two perspectives. *Nursing Case Management, 4*(6),244–251.

Idvall E, Rooke L & Hamrin E (1997). Quality indicators in clinical nursing: A review of theliterature. *Journal of Advanced Nursing, 25*(1), 6–17.

McCallin A (2001). Interdisciplinary practice—a matter of teamwork: An integrated literaturereview. *Journal of Clinical Nursing, 10*(4), 419–428.

Millward LJ & Jeffries N (2001). The team survey: A tool for health care team development. *Journal of Advanced Nursing, 35*(2), 276–287.

Spradley B & Allender J (2001). The community health nurse as leader, change agent, andcase manager. In J Allender & B Spradley *Community health nursing.* Philadelphia: Lippincott.

Swansburg RC & Swansburg RJ (1999). *Introductory management and leadership for nurses, 2nd edition.* Sudbury, MA: Jones & Barlett.

Urden LD (2001). Outcome evaluation: An essential component of CNS practice. *Clinical Nurse Specialist, 15*(6), 260–268.

Chapter 4

Abraham I, Bottrell MM, Fulmer T & Mezey MD, Editors (2003). *Geriatric nursing protocols for best practice, 2nd ed.* New York: Springer.

Burns N & Gove SK (1997). *The practice of nursing research: Conduct, critique & utilization, 3rd edition.* Philadelphia: Saunders.

Kirchoff (Eds.) *Using and conducting nursing research in the clinical setting, 2nd edition.* Philadelphia: Saunders.

Mateo MA & Newton C (1999). Progressing from an idea to a research question. In MA Mateo & K. Benner P (1984). *From novice to expert: Excellence and power in clinical nursing practice.* Menlo Park, CA: Addison Wesley.

Norman EM (1999). *We band of angels: The untold story of American Nurses trapped on Bataan by the Japanese.* New York: Random House.

Chapter 5

Bandura A (1986). *Social foundations of thought & action: A social cognitive theory.* Englewood Cliffs NJ: Prentice-Hall.

Knowles M. (1975). The modern practice of adult education. New York: Associated Press.

North American Nursing Diagnosis Association (2001). *Nursing diagnoses: Definitions & classification 2001–2002.* Philadelphia: Author.

Pender N (1987). *Health promotion in nursing practice, 2nd edition.* Los Altos, CA: Appleton & Lange.

Rankin SH & Stallings KD (2001). *Patient education: Principles & practice, 4th edition.* Philadelphia: Lippincott..

Redman BK (2001). *The practice of patient education, 9th edition.* St. Louis: Mosby.

Report of the US Preventive Services Task Force(1996). *Guide to clinical preventive services, 2nd edition.* Baltimore, MD: Williams & Wilkins

Rotter JB (1966). Generalized expectancies for internal versus external control of reinforcement. *Psychological Monographs, 80,* 1.

Chapter 6

Spardley B & Allender J (2001). Opportunities and challenges of community health nursing. In J Allender & B Spradley, *Community health nursing.* Philadelphia: Lippincott.

The Mended Hearts, Inc (2002). *The purpose of mended hearts.* www.mendedhearts.org.

Administration on Aging (2000). *Older Americans 2000.* www.aoa.gov.

US Census Bureau. (2001). *Population Projections.* www.census.gov.states.

Maddox PJ (2001). Bioterrorism: A renewed public health threat. *Dermatology Nursing 13*(6), 437–441.

US Department of Health and Human Services (2000). *Healthy People 2010 2nd edition. With Understanding and Improving Health and Objectives for Improving Health.* Washington, DC: US Government Printing Office. Available online at www.health.gov/healthypeople

American Heart Association (2001) *My heart watch.* www.americanheart.org

American Heart Association (2001). *Take Wellness to Heart.* www.women.americanheart.org.

American Heart Association (2001). *Operation Heartbeat.* www.americanheart.org

NHLBI (2001). *Act in Time to Heart Attack Signs.* www.nhlbi.nih.gov.

NHLBI (2001). *National High Blood Pressure Education Program.* www.nhlbi.nih.gov.

NHLBI (2001). *Detection, Evaluation, and Treatment of High Blood Cholesterol in Adults.* www.nhlbi.nih.gov.

NHLBI (2001). *Obesity Education Initiative.* www.nhlbi.nih.gov.

NHLBI (2001). *Developing a Women's Heart Health Education Action Plan.* www.nhlbi.nih.gov.

Department of HedLth and Human Services. (2001). *Healthy People in Healthy Communities.* www.health.gov/healthypeople.

Chapter 7

American Heart Association. *2001 Heart and Stroke Statistical Update.* Dallas, TX: Author.

D'Agostino, RB, Russell MW, Huse DM, Ellison RC, Silbershatz H, Wilson PWF & Hartz SC. (2000). Primary and Subsequent Coronary Risk Appraisal: New Results from the Framingham Study. *American Heart Journal, 139*(2), 272–281.

Elifaf M. (2001). The Treatment of Coronary Heart Disease: An Update: Part 1: An Overview of the Risk Factors for Cardiovascular Disease. *Current Medical Research and Opinion, 17*(1), 18–26.

Expert Panel on Detection, Evaluation, and Treatment of High Blood Cholesterol in Adults. (2001). Executive Summary of the Third Report of the National Cholesterol Education Program (NCEP). Expert Panel on Detection, Evaluation, and Treatment of High Blood Cholesterol in Adults (Adult Treatment Panel III). *Journal of the American Medical Association, 285,* 2486–97.

Goldstein LB, Adams R, Becker K, Furberg C, Gorelick PB, et al. (2001). Primary Prevention of Ischemic Stroke: A Statement for Healthcare Professionals From the Stroke Council of the American Heart Association. *Circulation, 103*(1),163–183.

McKenney J (2001). New Guidelines for Managing Hypercholesterolemia. *Journal of the American Pharmacy Association, 41*(4), 596–607.

Mohsenin V. (2001). Sleep-Related Breathing Disorders and Risk of Stroke. *Stroke, 32*(6), 1271–1278.

Sacco RL. (2001). Newer Risk Factors for Stroke. *Neurology, 57*(5 Suppl 2), 831–834.

Tierney S, Fennessey F & Hayes D. (2000). ABC's of arterial and vascular disease: Secondary prevention of peripheral vascular disease. *British Medical Journal, 320,* 1262–1265.

Wienbergen H, Schiele R, Gitt AK, Schneider S, Heer T, et al. (2001). Incidence, Risk Factors, and Clinical Outcome of Stroke after Acute Myocardial Infarction in Clinical Practice. *American Journal of Cardiology, 87*(6), 782–785.

Wolf PA, D'Agostino RB, Belanger, AJ & Kannel WB. (1991). Probability of Stroke: A Risk Profile From the Framingham Study. *Stroke, 22,* 312–318.

Chapter 8

Adams MH, Sherrod RA, Packs DR, Forte, LI, et al. (2001). Levels of prevention: restructuring a curriculum to meet future healthcare needs. *Nurse Educator, 26,* 6–8.

Ades PA (2001). Medical progress: Cardiac rehabilitation and secondary prevention of coronary heart disease. *New England Journal of Medicine, 345,* 892–902.

American Heart Association. (2001). *Heart and stroke A-Z guide.* [On-line]. www.americanheart.org

American Heart Association. (2001). Heart and stroke facts:1998 statistical supplement. [On-line]. www.americanheart.org

American Heart Association Scientific Statement (1998). Primary prevention of coronary heart disease: Guidance from Framingham. *American Heart Association* (Reprint No. 71–0139). Dallas, TX: AHA. (Reprinted from *Circulation, 97,* 1876–1887).

Balady G, Ades PA, Comoss P, et al. (2000). Core components of cardiac rehabilitation/ secondary prevention programs: A statement for healthcare professionals from the American Heart Association and the American Association of Cardiovascular and Pulmonary Rehabilitation Writing Group. *Circulation, 102,* 1069–1073.

Carlson JJ, Johnson JA, Franklin BA. & VanderLaan RL (2000). Program participation, exercise adherence, cardiovascular outcomes, and program cost of traditional versus modified cardiac rehabilitation. *American Journal of Cardiology. 86,* 17–23.

Expert Panel on Detection, Evaluation and Treatment of High Blood Cholesterol in Adults (2001). Executive summary of the third report of the National Cholesterol Education Program (NCEP). Expert Panel on Detection, Evaluation, and Treatment of High Blood Cholesterol in Adults (ATP-III). *JAMA, 285,* 2486–2497.

Grundy SM, D'Agostino RB, Mosca L, Burke GL, et al. (1999). *Summary of National Heart, Lung, and Blood Institute Workshop on cardiovascular risk assessment.*

Grundy SM, Balady GJ, Criqui MH, et al. (1997) Guide to prevention of cardiovascular diseases: A statement for health care professionals from the task force on risk reduction [AHA Science Advisory]. *Circulation, 95,* 2329–2331.

National Heart, Lung, and Blood Institute (2001). *Report of the task force on research in prevention of cardiovascular disease.* [On-line]. http://www.nhlbi.gov.

Pitt B & Rubenfire M (1999). Risk stratification for the detection of preclinical coronary artery disease [Editorial]. Circulation, 99, 2610–2612.

Report of the U.S. Preventive Services Task Force (1996). *Guide to clinical preventive services, 2nd edition.* Baltimore, MD: Williams & Wilkins.

Shepard R & Franklin B (2001). Changes in the quality of life: A major goal of cardiac rehabilitation. *Journal of Cardiopulmonary Rehabilitation, 21,* 189–200.

Smith SC, Blair SN, Bonow RO, Brass LM, et al. (2001). AHA/ACC guidelines for preventing heart attack and death in patients with atherosclerotic cardiovascular disease: 2001 update. A statement for healthcare professionals from the American Heart Association and the American College of Cardiology. *Circulation, 104,* 1577–1579.

Wright J, Rys W, & Wilkinson J R (1998). Health needs assessment: Development and importance of health needs assessment. *British Medical Journal, 316,* 1310–1313.

Chapter 9

American Heart Association (2000). *2001 Heart and stroke statistical update.* Dallas, TX: Author.

Appel LJ, Moore TJ, Obarzanek E, et al. (1997). A clinical trial of the effects of dietary patterns on blood pressure. *New England Journal Medicine, 336,* 1117–1124.

Cooper RS (1999). Geographic patterns of hypertension: A global perspective. In JL Izzo & HR Black (Eds.) *Hypertension primer, 2nd edition.* Baltimore, MD: Lippincott William & Wilkins.

Guidelines Sub-Committee (1999). 1999 World Health Organization-International Society of Hypertension Guidelines for the Management of Hypertension. *Journal Hypertension, 17,* 15–183.

Iowa Intervention Project (1996). *Nursing interventions classification (NIC), 2nd edition.* St. Louis: Mosby.

Iowa Intervention Project (1997). *Nursing outcomes classification (NOC).* St. Louis: Mosby.

Kannel WB & Wilson PWF (1999). Cardiovascular risk factors and hypertension. In JL Izzo & HR Black (Eds.) *Hypertension primer, 2nd edition.* Baltimore, MD: Lippincott William & Wilkins.

The Seventh Report of the Joint National Committee on Prevention, Detection, Evaluation, and Treatment of High Blood Pressure. Bethesda, MD: National Institutes of Health, National Heart, Lung and Blood Institute; August 2004. NIH Publication 04–5230.

Chapter 10

Ahmed SM, Clasen M E, & Donnelly J F (1998). Management of dyslipidemia in adults. *American Family Physician, 57,* 2192–2204.

Ballantyne CM, Olsson AG, Cook TJ, Mercuri MF, Pedersen TR, & Kjekshus J (2001). Influence of low high-density lipoprotein cholesterol and elevated triglyceride on coronary heart disease events and response to Simvastatin therapy in 4S. *Circulation, 104,* 3046–3051.

Expert Panel on Detection, Evaluation, and Treatment of High Blood Cholesterol in Adults. (2001). Executive summary of the third report of the National Cholesterol Education Program (NCEP) Expert Panel on Detection, Evaluation, and Treatment of High Blood Cholesterol in Adults (Adult Treatment Panel III). *JAMA, 285,* 2486–2497.

Ford ES, Giles W H & Dietz WH (2002). Prevalence of metabolic syndrome among US adults: Finding from the national health and nutrition examination survey. *JAMA, 287,* 356–359.

Maron DJ, Fazios S & Linton MF (2000). Current perspectives on statins. *Circulation, 101,* 207–213.

Papadakis JA, Ganotakis ES, Jagroop IA, Winder, AF & Mikhailidis DP (1999). Statin + fibrate combination therapy: Fluvastatin with bezafibrate or ciprofibrate in high-risk patients with vascular disease. *International Journal of Cardiology, 69,* 237–244.

Smilde TJ, van Wissen S, Wollersheim H, Trip MD, Kastelein JJP & Stalenhoef AFH (2001). Effect of aggressive versus conventional lipid lowering on atherosclerosis progression in familial hypercholesterolemia (ASAP): A prospective, randomized, double blind trial. *Lancet, 357,* 577–581

White CW, Gobel FL, Campeau L, Knatterud GL, Forman SA & Post-Coronary Artery Bypass Graft Trial Investigators (2001). Effect of an aggressive lipid-lowering strategy on progression of atherosclerosis in the left main coronary artery from patients in the post coronary artery bypass graft trial. *Circulation, 104,* 2660–2665.

Chapter 11

Bullock BA & Henze RL (2000). *Focus on pathophysiology.* Philadelphia: Lippincott.

Cotran RS, Kumar V & Collins T (1999). *Robbins: Pathologic basis of disease, 6th edition.* Philadelphia: WB Saunders.

McCance KL & Heuther SE (2002). *Pathophysiology: The biologic basis for disease in adults and children, 4th edition.* St. Louis: Mosby.

Woods SL, Sivarajan Froelicher ES & Underhill Motzer S (2000). *Cardiac nursing, 4th edition.* Philadelphia: Lippincott.

Chapter 12

Bickley LS & Hoekelman RA (2003). *Bates' Guide to physical examination and history taking, 8th edition.* Philadelphia: Lippincott.

Jarvis C (2000). *Physical examination and health assessment, 3rd edition.* Philadelphia: WB Saunders.

LeFever Kee J (2004). *Laboratory and diagnostic tests, 7th edition.* Upper Saddle River, NJ: Prentice Hall.

Levine BS & Motzer SU (2000). History taking and physical examination. In SL Woods, ESS Froelicher & SAU Motzer (Eds.), *Cardiac nursing, 4th edition.* Philadelphia: Lippincott.

National Cholesterol Education Program Expert Panel on Detection, Evaluation, and Treatment of High Blood Cholesterol in Adults (Adult Treatment Panel III) (2002). Available on the web at www.nhlbi.gov.

Seller RH (2000). *Differential diagnosis of common complaints, 4th edition.* Philadelphia: WB Saunders.

Chapter 13

Ades PA (2001). Medical Progress: Cardiac rehabilitation and secondary prevention of coronary heart disease. *New England Journal of Medicine, 345,* 892–902.

Al-Khatib SM, Wilkinson WE, Sanders LL, McCarthy EA & Pritchett EL (2000). Electrophysiology,observations on the transition from intermittent to permanent atrial fibrillation. *American Heart Journal, 140,* 142–145.

American Heart Association. (2000). Guideline 2000 for cardiopulmonary resuscitation and emergency cardiovascular care: International consensus on science. *Circulation (Suppl.), 102*(8).

American Heart Association (2001). *Heart and stroke statistical update.* Dallas, TX: Author.

American Heart Association. (2001). *Risk factors and coronary heart disease.*

Asorian B (2000). Cardiac Surgery. In Logan, P. *Principles of practice for the acute care nurse practitioner.* Stamford, CT: Appleton & Lange.

Braunwald E. (2001). *Heart disease: A textbook of cardiovascular medicine, 6th edition.* Philadelphia: Saunders.

Braunwald E, Antman EM, Beasley JW, Califf RM, Cheitlin MD, et al. (2000). ACC/AHA guidelines for the management of patients with unstable angina and non-ST-segment elevation myocardial infarction: Executive summary and recommendation: A report of the American College of Cardiology/American Heart Association Task Force on Practice Guidelines (Committee on Management of Patients with Unstable Angina). *Circulation, 102,* 1193–1209.

Callans DJ (2000). Arrhythmias. In Logan, P. *Principles of practice for the acute care nurse practitioner.* Stamford, CT: Appleton & Lange.

Cazeau S Leclercq C, Lavergne T, Walker S, Varma C, et al. (2001). Effects of multisite biventricular pacing in patients with heart failure and intraventricular conduction delay. *New England Journal of Medicine 344,* 873–880.

Chavey WE, Blaum CS, Bleske BE, Van Harrison B, Kesterson S & Nicklas JM (2001). Guideline for the management of heart failure caused by systolic dysfunction: Part I. Guideline development, etiology and diagnosis. *American Family Physician, 64,* 769–774.

Chavey WE, Blaum CS, Bleske BE, Van Harrison B, Kesterson S & Nicklas JM (2001). Guideline for the management of heart failure caused by systolic dysfunction: Parts II. Treatment. *American Family Physician, 64,* 1045–1054.

Diop D (2001). Definition, classification, and pathophysiology of acute coronary ischemic syndromes. *Emergency Medicine Clinics of North America, 19,* 259–267.

Futterman LG & Lemberg L (2001). Heart failure: Update on treatment and prognosis. *American Journal of Critical Care, 10,* 285–293.

Granger BB & Miller CM (2001). Acute coronary syndromes: Putting the new guidelines to work. *Nursing 2001 31,* 36–45.

Hunt SA, Baker DW, Chin MH, Cinquegrani MP, Feldman AM, et al. (2001). ACC/AHA guidelines for the evaluation and management of chronic heart failure in the adult: a report of the American College of Cardiology/American Heart Association Task Force on Practice Guidelines (Committee to revise the 1995 guidelines for the evaluation and management of heart failure). American College of Cardiology

Jacobson CJ (2004). Arrhythmias and conduction disturbances. In SL Woods, SSS Froelicher & SAU Motzer *Cardiac nursing. 5th edition.* Philadelphia: Lippincott.

Lakkis N (2000). New treatment methods for patients with hypertrophic obstructive cardiomyopathy. Current Opinion in Cardiology 15, 172–177.

Laurent-Bopp D. (2000). Heart failure. In SL Woods, SSS Froelicher & SAU Motzer *Cardiac nursing. 4th edition.* Philadelphia, Lippincott.

Maron BJ (2000). Role of alcohol septal ablation in treatment of obstructive hypertrophic cardiomyopathy. *Lancet, 355,* 425–426.

Packer M, Coats AJ, Fowler MB, Katus HA, Krum H, et al. (2001). Effect of carvedilol on the survival of patients with severe chronic heart failure. *New England Journal of Medicine, 344,* 1651–1658.

Peters RW, Gold MR (2000). Pacing for patients with congestive heart failure and dilated cardiomyopathy. *Cardiology Clinics, 18,* 55–66.

Schomig A, Kastrati A, Dirschinger J, Mehilli J, Schriche U, Pache J, Martinoff S, Neumann FJ & Schwaiger M. (2000). Coronary stenting plus platelet glycoprotein IIb/IIa blockade compared with tissue plasminogen activator in acute myocardial infarction. *New England Journal of Medicine, 343,* 385–391.

Smolens IA, Bolling SF (2000). Surgical approaches to dilated cardiomyopathy. *Current Cardiology Reports, 2,* 99–105.

Sorajja P, Elliott PM & McKenna WJ (2000). Pacing in hypertrophic cardiomyopathy. *Cardiology Clinics, 18,* 67–79.

Thompson PL (2001). Clinical relevance of statins: Instituting treatment early in acute coronary syndrome patients. *Atherosclerosis Supplements 2,* 15–19.

Wolfgang-MF, Muller OJ & Katus HA (2001). Cardiomyopathies: From genetics to the prospect of treatment. *Lancet 358,* 1627–1637

Chapter 14

Blum U, McCollum P, Hopkinson BR et al. (2000). Endovascular repair of abdominal aortic aneurysms. In JF Dyet, DF Ettles, AA Nicholson, et al (Eds). *Textbook of endovascular procedures.* New York: Churchill Livingstone.

Fogarty TJ, Biswas A, Newman CE (1999). Catheter thromboembolecctomy. In RA White, TJ Fogarty (Eds). *Peripheral endocvascular interventions. 2nd edition.* New York: Springer Verlag.

Hoffman R (2000). Coronary atherectomy devices. In S Apple, L Lindsay (Eds.) *Interventional cardiology.* Baltimore: Lippincott Williams & Wilkins.

Kornowski R, Kehoe K (2000). Percutaneous transluminal coronary angioplasty. In S Apple, L Lindsay (Eds.) *Interventional cardiology.* Baltimore, MD: Lippincott Williams & Wilkins.

Mathias K, Jager H, Beard JD (2000). Endoluminal treatment of carotid and vertebral artery stenosis. In Dyet JF, Ettles DF, Nicholson AA, et al (Eds.). *Textbook of endovascular procedures.* New York: Churchill Livingstone.

Moses HW, Miller BD, Moulton KP, Schneider JA (Eds.) (2000). *A Practical guide to cardiac pacing. 5th edition.* Philadelphia: Lippincott Williams & Wilkins.

Woods SL, Sivarajan Froelicher ES, Underhill Motzer SA (2004) (Eds). *Cardiac nursing, 5th edition.* Philadelphia: Lippincott Williams & Wilkins.

Chapter 15

Crawford MH (2001). Drug therapy in cardiovascular disease. *Cardiology Clinics. 19*(2), 195341.

The Expert Panel (2001). Detection, evaluation, and treatment of high blood cholesterol in adults (adult treatment panel III). *Third Report of the National Cholesterol Education Program (NCEP),* National Cholesterol Education Program, National Heart, Lung, and Blood Institute, NIH.

Frishman WH (2000). Recent advances in cardiovascular pharmacology. Current Problems in *Cardiology. 25*(4), 227–295.

Hardman JG & Limbird LE (2001). *Goodman and Gilman's the Pharmacological basis of therapeutics, 10th edition.* New York: McGraw-Hill.

Karch AM (2000). *Focus on nursing pharmacology.* Philadelphia, PA: Lippincott.

Katzung BG (2001). *Basic and clinical pharmacology, 8th edition.* New York: McGraw-Hill.

Sprague JE (2001). Teaching cardiac arrhythmias: a focus on pathophysiology and pharmacology. *American Journal Pharmacy Educuation, 65,* 169–77.

Chapter 16

American Heart Association (2001). *Heart and stroke statistical update.* Dallas, TX: Author.

Bedell SE (1983). Survival after cardiopulmonary resuscitation in the hospital. *New England Journal of Medicine, 309*(10), 569–576.

Braunwald E (2001). *Heart disease: A textbook of cardiovascular medicine, 6th edition.* Philadelphia: Saunders.

Department of Health and Human Services (2001). *Healthy people 2010.*

Fahey V (2003). *Vascular nursing, 4th edition.* Philadelphia: Saunders.

Jacob SR & Carnegie ME (2002). In B. Cherry & SR Jacob, *Contemporary nursing. 2nd edition.* St. Louis: Mosby.

Khaw KT, Wareham N, Luben R, et al. (2001). Glycated haemoglobin, diabetes, and mortality in men in Norfolk cohort of European Prospective Investigation of Cancer and Nutrition. *British Medical Journal, 322*(1), 15–18.

Myerburg RJ.& Kessler KM (1986). Management of patients who survive cardiac arrest. *Modern Concepts of Cardiovascular Diseases, 55*(1), 61–65.

National Institute of Diabetes, Digestive and Kidney Diseases (2001). *U.S. Renal data system report.*

Chapter 17

American College of Cardiology & American Heart Association (1999). *ACC/AHA guidelines for the management of patients with acute myocardial infarction.*

Anderson KL (1999). Conceptualization and measurement of quality of life as an outcome variable for health care intervention and research. *Journal of Advanced Nursing, 29*(2), 298–306.

Fricchione G & Marcantonio E (1998). Approach to the patient with chronic medical illness. In TA Stern, JB Herman & PL Slavin (Eds.) *The MGH Guide to psychiatry in primary care.* New York: McGraw-Hill.

Koenig HG, McCullough ME, & Larson DB (2001). *Handbook of religion and health.* New York: Oxford University.

Lazarus RS & Folkman S. (1984). *Stress, appraisal and coping.* New York: Springer.

Miller JF (2000). Analysis of coping with illness. In JF Miller, *Coping with chronic illness.* Philadelphia: FA Davis.

Pollack MH, Smoller JW, & Lee DK (1998). Approach to the anxious patient. In TA Stern, JB Herman & PL Slavin (Eds.) *The MGH Guide to psychiatry in primary care.* New York: McGraw-Hill.

Posen DB (1998). *Stress management for patient and physician.*

Rosenbaum JF & Fava M (1998). *Approach to the patient with depression. The MGH Guide to psychiatry in primary care.* New York: McGraw-Hill.

Selye H (1956). *The stress of life.* New York: McGraw-Hill.

World Health Organization. (1947). *Constitution of the World Health Organization: Chronicle of the World Health Organization.* Geneva: World Health Organization.

APPENDIX B

Review Questions

1. On her application for a nursing license, A nurse indicates on her application for a nursing license that she received a baccalaureate degree in nursing from a state university; however, she actually received an associate's degree from the university and has completed all but one course required for the baccalaureate. This nurse's actions are an example of:
   A. fraud.
   B. miscarriage of justice.
   C. intentional tort.
   D. invasion of privacy.

2. When a client begins to explore ways to quit smoking he is in which stage of the transtheoretical model of behavior change?
   A. Contemplation
   B. Preparation
   C. Action
   D. Termination

3. A case management model that focuses on employee health and wellness and return to work is:
   A. long-term health care.
   B. occupational health.
   C. managed care.
   D. private.

4. A researcher wants to know "What is the relationship between perceived self-efficacy and attendance at a cardiac rehabilitation program?" Which design helps to best answer this question?
   A. Descriptive
   B. Correlational
   C. Phenomenological
   D. Controlled clinical trial

5. The measurement scale in which data are rank ordered with equal distance between classes is:
   A. Nominal
   B. Ordinal
   C. Interval
   D. Ratio

6. Which strategy is most effective to use when teaching a patient to fill his weekly medication box (Mediset™)?
   A. Lecture with discussion
   B. Role playing with feedback
   C. Demonstration with return demonstration
   D. Instructional manual or booklet with illustrations

7. Which type of prevention is described as an intervention used to alter the susceptibility of individuals to illness?
   A. Primary
   B. Secondary
   C. Tertiary
   D. Quadra

8. What has been the major role of professional and national health care organizations in promoting the health of the country?
   A. Rely on federal initiatives such as *Healthy People 2010*.
   B. Assist local governments to develop regulations for their constituents.
   C. Develop community education programs focused on the public and health care providers.
   D. Work with academic institutions to research common health problems.

9. A desirable fasting lipid profile for a patient with CHD or CHD equivalent is:
   A. Total cholesterol 210, HDL 45, LDL 96, Triglycerides 126.
   B. Total cholesterol 223, HDL 38, LDL 116, Triglycerides 163.
   C. Total cholesterol 183, HDL 42, LDL 92, Triglycerides 135.
   D. Total cholesterol 146, HDL 44, LDL 110, Triglycerides 178.

10. While conducting a CVD risk assessment, the nurse discovers that a female patient has a waist circumference of 36 inches, a fasting glucose level of 124 mg/dL, and blood pressure of 140/90 mm Hg. From this information the nurse concludes that the patient has:
   A. obesity.
   B. hypertension.
   C. metabolic syndrome.
   D. hyperlipidemia.

11. The diagnosis of hypertension is based on:
   A. one (1) BP reading of 140/90 mmHg or greater.
   B. at least 3 BP readings with an average of 140/90 mmHg or greater.
   C. average BP reading of 140/90 mmHg or greater on 3 different occasions.
   D. positional decrease in BP of 10 mmHg or greater.

12. What is the first intervention for dyslipidemia in individuals with low to medium risk?
   A. Increase physical activity
   B. Decrease intake of dietary fat
   C. Control of blood glucose
   D. Increase soluble fiber

13. Water moves from an area of lesser sodium concentration to an area of greater sodium concentration by:
   A. filtration.
   B. diffusion.
   C. osmosis.
   D. facilitated diffusion.

14. The usual sequence of examination techniques is:
   A. inspection, palpation, percussion, and auscultation.
   B. palpation, auscultation, inspection and percussion.
   C. auscultation, inspection, percussion, and palpation.
   D. inspection, auscultation, palpation and percussion.

15. Which diagnostic imaging test provides the most information about soft tissue?
   A. X-ray
   B. Computed tomography (CT) scan
   C. MRI
   D. Contrast enhanced CT scan

16. Which risk factor is considered unmodifiable?
   A. Family history
   B. Hypertension
   C. Obesity
   D. Diabetes mellitus

17. On auscultation, the sound of mitral stenosis is a:
   A. pansystolic murmur.
   B. decrescendo, diastolic murmur.
   C. systolic ejection crescendo–decrescendo murmur.
   D. holodiastolic murmur.

18. The triad of treatment for systolic dysfunction includes:
   A. diuretics, anticoagulants, and inotropes.
   B. diuretics, vasodilators, and a permanent pacemaker.
   C. diuretics, vasodilators, and inotropes.
   D. vasodilators, inotropes, and mitral valve repair.

19. Which long-term therapy is considered for patients with heart failure when medical therapy fails and surgical revascularization is not appropriate?
   A. Coronary artery bypass graft (CABG) surgery
   B. Left ventricular assist device
   C. Cardiac transplantation
   D. Implantable cardiac defibrillator

20. Primary pulmonary hypertension is caused by:
   A. an unknown etiology.
   B. cardiac dysfunction.
   C. lung parenchymal disease.
   D. pulmonary vascular obstruction.

21. A 66-year-old man, is hospitalized with a diagnosis of acute myocardial infarction. Four hours after his admission, his left arm has a purplish rubor and has diminished pulses. His vital signs are: Temp: 97.2°F (36.2°C); HR: 166 bpm and irregular; Resp: 24 bpm; and BP: 82/50 mmHg. The most likely cause of this patient's left arm symptoms is:
   A. embolism from atrial fibrillation.
   B. thrombosis from venous catheters.
   C. intimal damage from chronic repetitive work.
   D. thromboembolism from trauma.

22. What does the cardiac/vascular nurse include in the teaching for a patient scheduled for a percutaneous transluminal coronary angioplasty (PTCA)?
   A. The procedure is done in the operating room under general anesthesia.
   B. After the procedure, angina will be completely gone.
   C. There are no complications associated with the procedure when it is done at this facility.
   D. A special catheter will be inserted through the femoral or brachial artery.

23. Which nursing intervention has highest priority when a home health care nurse visits a patient after discharge following surgical repair of an abdominal aneurysm?
   A. Assess understanding of the activity prescription
   B. Monitor and control blood pressure and circulation
   C. Assess wound healing and reapply a sterile dressing
   D. Instruct the patient and his spouse about a low fat, high carbohydrate diet.

24. Fosinopril (Monopril) is which type of medication?
   A. Calcium channel blocker
   B. Vasodilator
   C. Angiotensin II antagonist
   D. ACE inhibitor

25. A syndrome that results in the failure of the heart as a pump to meet the metabolic demands of the body is:
   A. myocardial infarction.
   B. cardiogenic shock.
   C. unstable angina pectoris.
   D. acute coronary syndrome.

26. Which intervention can be used in the treatment of draining venous stasis ulcers?
   A. Neurovascular monitoring
   B. Compression stockings
   C. Unna boots
   D. Elastic stockings

27. A 26-year-old woman has cardiomyopathy that was diagnosed two years ago after a viral illness. She has been informed that the only treatment option for her is a heart transplant. Lately, she has been feeling sad and has experienced symptoms of insomnia and anorexia. This patient's feelings are indicative of:
   A. depression.
   B. anxiety.
   C. anger.
   D. dependence.

28. Some individuals limit their contacts with someone who is ill because of their discomfort with the disease. An individual's adaptive response to changes in their support systems is:
   A. adjusting to changes in social relationships.
   B. grieving over losses.
   C. maintaining a positive self-concept.
   D. dealing with role changes.

29. The major factor associated with the increased survival of individuals experiencing cardiac arrest outside of the hospital is:
   A. initiation of cardiopulmonary bystander resuscitation.
   B. activation of resources for emergency care, e.g., 911, by family members.
   C. accurate assessment by health care personnel that the collapse is a cardiac arrest.
   D. initiation of ACLS protocols in the emergency room.

30. Which diuretic agent has been associated with hearing loss when administered intravenously?
   A. Spironolactone (Aldactone)
   B. Furosemide (Lasix)
   C. Chlorothiazide (Diuril)
   D. Mannitol (Osmitrol)

31. When caring for a patient with a temporary transvenous pacemaker, the cardiac/vascular nurse:
   A. keeps the patient in a semi-fowler position.
   B. encourage active range of motion at the insertion site to prevent frozen shoulder.
   C. maintain an electrically safe environment.
   D. obtain a physician's order for a broad-spectrum antibiotic.

32. Which statements best describes intermittent claudication?
    A. Muscle pain of the lower extremity that is aggravated by increased activity.
    B. Rest pain that is decreased by putting the lower extremity in a dependent position.
    C. Cramping pain of the lower extremity that is precipitated by activity and is relieved by rest.
    D. Activity pain of the lower extremity from diminished vascular flow that is not affected by position or rest.

33. Use of a transcutaneous pacemaker is indicated for which dysrhythmia?
    A. Atrial flutter
    B. Ventricular tachycardia,
    C. Second degree AVB type II
    D. First degree AVB

34. The most common cause of systolic heart failure is:
    A. coronary ischemia or infarction.
    B. hypertension.
    C. valvular dysfunction.
    D. anemia.

35. A 65-year-old man comes to the clinic with a chief complaint of retrosternal chest pain that radiates to his back. The pain decreases when he leans forward in a sitting position and increases when he lies down. The patient had coronary artery bypass graft (CABG) surgery four weeks ago. Based on his symptoms and past surgical history, the cardiac/vascular nurse suspects:
    A. rheumatic fever.
    B. endocarditis.
    C. pericarditis.
    D. angina pectoris.

36. Which is the appropriate medication to treat substernal chest pain that radiates to the left arm in a patient on a coronary telemetry unit?
    A. Maalox
    B. Ranitidine (Zantac)
    C. Nitroglycerin (Nitrostat)
    D. Metoprolol (Lopressor)

37. Which lipid profiles presents the lowest risk for cardiac and vascular disease?
   A. Total cholesterol, 190; LDL cholesterol, 100; HDL cholesterol 45
   B. Total cholesterol, 190; LDL cholesterol, 90; HDL cholesterol 45
   C. Total cholesterol, 200; LDL cholesterol, 90; HDL cholesterol 65
   D. Total cholesterol, 200; LDL cholesterol, 100; HDL cholesterol 65

38. Which is characterized by arterial spasm?
   A. Abdominal aortic aneurysm
   B. Takayasu disease
   C. Temporal arteritis
   D. Raynaud disease

39. When is lipid-lowering drug therapy started in individuals with dyslipidemia, but without other risk factors?
   A. When dyslipidemia is identified
   B. After 6 months if therapeutic lifestyle changes are not effective
   C. After 3 months if therapeutic lifestyle changes are not effective
   D. The decision to start drug treatment depends on the age of the patient.

40. The goal of treatment for hypertension is to reduce:
   A. symptoms.
   B. risk of cardiac and vascular disease.
   C. SBP to less than 120 mmHg.
   D. DBP to less than 70 mmHg.

41. Which statement about peripheral vascular disease(PVD) is true?
   A. PVD is an independent predictor for increased risk of cardiac death.
   B. If symptomatic, PVD carries a 30% risk of death within 10 years.
   C. PVD is more likely to develop in patients with hypertension than with diabetes.
   D. Symptomatic PVD carries a two-to five-fold increased risk of fatal or nonfatal CV events.

42. Diabetes mellitus is identified as a CHD equivalent because:
   A. individuals with diabetes have a poor prognosis after a myocardial infarction.
   B. age adjusted rates for CHD are 2-3 times higher in individuals with diabetes.
   C. diabetes is associated with an accelerated atheromatous process.
   D. by age 50, CHD is the leading cause of death in men with diabetes.

43. Which term describes a group of people seeking to solve a problem?
   A. Geographic community
   B. Common interest community
   C. Community of solution
   D. Population

44. Learning the signs and symptoms of peripheral vascular disease is an example of which domain of learning?
   A. Affective
   B. Cognitive
   C. Psychomotor
   D. Behavioral

45. A researcher concludes that there is no difference between two groups when, in fact, a real difference exists. This is an example of:
   A. measurement error.
   B. type I error.
   C. type II error.
   D. poor judgment.

46. The major population trend that will have the largest effect on the future of case management is:
   A. aging of the population.
   B. early discharges from hospitals.
   C. diversity of the population
   D. acuity of patients.

47. The nurse encourages a patient with intermittent claudication to begin walking a few blocks and gradually increase the distance. Which theorethical process supports this intervention?
   A. Negligence
   B. Vicarious learning
   C. Mastery
   D. Theory of reasoned action

48. A 74-year-old man with vascular dementia is admitted to the hospital from the nursing home with dehydration. He has difficulty swallowing liquids and has been restricted to thickened liquids. He does not have any advance directives and his wife believes a feeding tube is in his best interest. This situation poses an ethical dilemma based on which principles?
   A. Justice versus autonomy
   B. Beneficence versus autonomy
   C. Beneficence versus nonmaleficence
   D. This does not represent an ethical dilemma

49. What is the physiologic stimulus that promotes inflammation in atherosclerosis?
   A. High density cholesterol
   B. Foam cells
   C. Damage to the vascular endothelium
   D. Oxidized LDL cholesterol

50. Patients with valvular disorders scheduled for dental procedures need which type of medication?
   A. Anti-inflammatory to prevent gingival infections
   B. Aspirin to prevent clot formation
   C. Antibiotics for endocarditis prophylaxis
   D. Analgesics for pain management

APPENDIX C

Review Question Answers

1. **Correct Answer: A.** The provision of false or misleading information to a legal body is fraud. The BON has the right and duty to deny a license to persons who provide false information.
2. **Correct Answer: B.** In the preparation stage of behavior change the individual explores ways to quit smoking.
3. **Correct Answer: B.** The long-term care model targets people with extended care needs. The managed care model manages access to services and advocates cost-effective care for its subscribers. The private model coordinates services for individuals or other groups as a subcontractor.
4. **Correct Answer: B.** The research question asks about the relationship between two concepts. There is a relatively mature body of knowledge about both perceived self-efficacy and cardiac rehabilitation. Therefore, a correlational design is appropriate.
5. **Correct Answer: C.** Interval level data meet the following criteria: numbers are mutually exclusive and exhaustive, they are ordered, and there is an equal interval between data points. The interval level measurement scale does not include absolute zero.
6. **Correct Answer: C.** Demonstration with return demonstration is an effective strategy for teaching psychomotor skills. Information, discussion, cuing, and feedback may all be used with this strategy to enhance learning and build skill.
7. **Correct Answer: A.** Secondary prevention involves those strategies aimed at the early identification and treatment of disease. Tertiary prevention is focused on preserving or restoring function in people with health problems.
8. **Correct Answer: C.** Professional health care organizations have been involved with raising funds to support research on health problems. Their greatest contribution has been the development of community education programs to educate the public and health care providers about risk factors and health problems affecting individuals in this country. Many professional health care organizations are using the *Healthy People 2010* initiatives.
9. **Correct Answer: C.** ATP III treatment goals for patients with CHD or CHD equivalent are total cholesterol < 200, HDL > 40, LDL < 100, and triglycerides < 150.
10. **Correct Answer: C.** Metabolic syndrome is defined clinically as the presence of at least 3 of the following factors: abdominal obesity (waist circumference > 35 inches in women; > 40 inches in men), triglycerides ≥150

mg/dL, low HDL cholesterol (< 50 mg/dL in women; < 40 mg/dL in men), elevated blood pressure (≥130/≥85 mm Hg) and a fasting blood glucose ≥110 mg/dL. The other answers are incorrect because obesity is defined by body mass index (BMI >30), hypertension can not be diagnosed from a single reading, and there is no information provided about lipid levels.

11. **Correct Answer: C.** The diagnosis of hypertension is based on the average of two or more BP readings taken at each of 2 or more visits after an initial screening.

12. **Correct Answer: B.** The first intervention for most individuals with dyslipidemia is to reduce the intake of dietary fat.

13. **Correct Answer: C.** Water moves from an area of lesser sodium concentration to an area of greater sodium concentration by osmosis.

14. **Correct Answer: A.** The usual sequence of examination technique is inspection, palpation, percussion, and auscultation. This sequence is different for the abdominal examination where auscultation precedes palpation and percussion.

15. **Correct Answer: C.** Of these studies, the MRI provides the most detailed information about soft tissue structures.

16. **Correct Answer: A.** The effects of other risk factors such as hypertension, obesity, and diabetes mellitus may be modified with lifestyle changes such as diet, exercise, and weight reduction.

17. **Correct Answer: B.** Mitral regurgitation has a pansystolic murmur. The sound from aortic stenosis is a systolic ejection murmur while aortic regurgitation produces a holodiastolic murmur.

18. **Correct Answer: C.** Diuretics, vasodilators and inotropes are known as the triad for treatment of systolic dysfunction. Permanent pacemakers are used later in the disease process and not exclusively for systolic dysfunction. Mitral valve repair is only indicated if mitral valve disease is present.

19. **Correct Answer: C.** Cardiac transplantation is used when medical management is no longer effective and surgery is not considered an option. Coronary artery bypass graft surgery is contraindicated in this situation. Left ventricular assist devices are not approved for long-term management of heart failure. Implantable cardiac defibrillators are used for the management of problems such as ventricular fibrillation.

20. **Correct Answer: A.** There are several risk factors associated with the development of primary pulmonary hypertension but the actual cause has not been determined.

21. **Correct Answer: A.** This patient's symptoms are from arterial ischemia and the most likely cause based on his diagnosis of myocardial infarction and vital signs is atrial fibrillation.

22. **Correct Answer: D.** A special catheter will be inserted through a peripheral artery. PTCA is done in the cardiac catheterization laboratory under conscious sedation. Complications of the procedure include coronary

restenosis (reoccurrence of angina), abrupt closure of the coronary artery, myocardial infarction, bleeding or hematoma at the vascular access site, arterial embolization, pseudoaneurysm, retroperitoneal bleeding, and death.

23. **Correct Answer: B.** Hypertension is the major risk factor for aneurysm formation and must be controlled for life.

24. **Correct Answer: D.** Fosinopril is an angiotensin converting enzyme (ACE) inhibitor used in the treatment of heart failure and hypertension. All generic (chemical) names of ACE inhibitors end in "pril."

25. **Correct Answer: B.** The other health problems may result in the development of cardiogenic shock but are actually caused by inadequate blood flow to the myocardium.

26. **Correct Answer: C.** The Unna boot is a gauze dressing with specific medications that is used to treat this health problem.

27. **Correct Answer: A.** Anxiety is characterized by feelings of apprehension, tension, and uneasiness. Anger is associated with feelings of extreme displeasure and hostility. Dependence is a regressive reaction that causes the person who is ill to rely on others for their physical and emotional needs.

28. **Correct Answer: A.** The individual who is ill must adjust to changes in their social relationships. Other individuals impose some of the limitations. The individual who is ill may also limit their interactions because of discomfort and fatigues associated with the disease.

29. **Correct Answer: A.** The start of CPR immediately after cardiac arrest as part of prehospital care is associated with increased survival.

30. **Correct Answer: B.** The loop diuretics are associated with ototoxicity and hearing loss; therefore, furosemide is a diuretic associated with this adverse effect.

31. **Correct Answer: C.** A pacing wire goes directly from the skin (insertion site) to the heart; even small electrical currents can cause cardiac dysrhythmia or arrest.

32. **Correct Answer: C.** This pain results in an activity rest cycle. Intermittent claudication is a manifestation of lower arterial occlusive disease.

33. **Correct Answer: C.** Second degree AVB type II and complete heart block are considered high degrees of heart block. The rate that results from these blocks is often not fast enough to support adequate cardiac output. Medications such as atropine are ineffective. Transcutaneous pacemakers can be used effectively to increase the heart rate until the blood pressure stabilizes.

34. **Correct Answer: A.** CHD is the cause for approximately two-thirds of the people with systolic dysfunction.

35. **Correct Answer: C.** These are the classic symptoms of acute pericarditis. A risk factor for this health problem is invasive procedures such as cardiac surgery.

36. **Correct Answer: C.** The patient is probably experiencing angina pectoris

and needs to be treated with a vasodilator such as nitroglycerin.

37. **Correct Answer: C.** Although total cholesterol < 200 is desirable, in this case the total cholesterol is explained, in part, by the level of HDL (protective). LDL cholesterol is < 100, which is optimal.

38. **Correct Answer: D.**

39. **Correct Answer: C.** Therapeutic lifestyle change (diet, activity, and weight loss) is tried for 6 weeks. If target lipid levels are not reached, plant stanol/sterol is added. If target lipid levels are not reached at 12 weeks, pharmacotherapy is initiated.

40. **Correct Answer: B.** The goal of treatment for hypertension is to reduce the risk of cardiac and vascular disease. Hypertension is symptom-less unless target organ damage or very high levels of BP are present. The desired BP level for average risk individuals with hypertension is less than 140/90 mmHg.

41. **Correct Answer: A.** If symptomatic, PVD carries a 30% risk of death within 5 years, not 10. PVD is more likely to develop in patients with diabetes rather than hypertension due to the tendency of diabetes toward smaller distal vessels. If asymptomatic, patients have a two- to five-fold increased risk of CV events.

42. **Correct Answer: C.** It is the accelerated pathology of atherosclerosis that places diabetes in the category of a CHD equivalent. After an MI, individuals with diabetes have a higher mortality rate than those without diabetes. Age adjusted rates for CHD in individuals with diabetes are 2-3 x for men and 3-7 times for women. By age 40 the leading cause of death is CHD in both men and women with diabetes.

43. **Correct Answer: C.** A geographic community is defined by the boundaries of towns, cities, or neighborhoods while a common interest community is composed of people with similar interests.

44. **Correct Answer: B.** Cognitive learning deals with the intellectual or knowledge area and involves acquiring facts, reaching conclusions, or making decisions.

45. **Correct Answer: C.** Type II error occurs when a study does not have sufficient power to detect a real difference between groups. Type I error occurs when the researcher erroneously rejects the null hypothesis concluding that a difference exists when it does not.

46. **Correct Answer: A.** Even though all of these factors will have an effect on case management and the delivery of health care services, the aging of the population will have the greatest impact because of the increasing numbers of older adults requiring care.

47. **Correct Answer: C.** Mastery is a source of efficacy information. It provides the patient with positive reinforcement through achievement.

48. **Correct Answer: D.** An ethical dilemma requires a choice between courses of action that involve fundamental concepts of right and wrong. Because

there is no advance directive, the surrogate decision maker (the wife) is legally and ethically bound to make the decision she believes to be in the best interest of the patient.

49. **Correct Answer: C.** Damage to the vascular endothelium initiates the inflammatory process in atherosclerosis. Endothelial damage may be caused by wear and tear, microorganisms, e.g., *chlamydia pneumoniae,* or other cardio-vascular risk factors.

50. **Correct Answer: C.** Patients with valvular disorders are at risk for endo-carditis and need to receive antibiotic prophylaxis.

Index

B

C

D

E

F

M

N

O

P

R

S

T